American Medical Association

Physicians dedicated to the health of America

cpt

1993

Physicians' Current Procedural Terminology

Celeste G. Kirschner, MHSA
Robin C. Burkett, BA
Judy A. Coy, RN, MGS
Nancy K. Edwards, MA
Gina Leoni, RRA
Mary R. McNamara O'Heron, RRA
Karen E. Neary, BS
Ann Pollack, MBA
Karen R. Scholten
Maurine G. Spillman, MPH
Dianne M. Willard, RRA, MBA

Library of Congress Catalog Card Number: 78-13816

ISBN: 0-89970-510-3
ISSN: 0276-8283

1st Edition printed 1966
2nd Edition printed 1970
3rd Edition printed 1973
4th Edition printed 1977
revised: 1978, 1979, 1980, 1981
reprinted: 1980, 1982
CPT-1984 — First printing, November 1983
Second printing, January 1984
Third printing, June 1984
Fourth printing, September 1984
CPT-1985 — First printing, November 1984
Second printing, January 1985
CPT-1986 — First printing, November 1985
Second printing, February 1986
Third printing, August 1986
CPT-1987 — First printing, November 1986
Second printing, April 1987
Third printing, July 1987
CPT-1988 — First printing, November 1987
Second printing, January 1988
Third printing, March 1988
Fourth printing, April 1988
CPT-1989 — First printing, November 1988
Second printing, February 1989
Third printing, April 1989
CPT-1990 — First printing, November 1989
CPT-1991 — First printing, November 1990
CPT-1992 — First printing, October 1991
CPT-1993 — First printing, October 1992

For other correspondence address inquiries to:
Department of Coding & Nomenclature
American Medical Association
515 North State Street
Chicago, Illinois 60610

Additional books may be purchased from:
Order Department: OP054193
American Medical Association
P.O. Box 109050
Chicago, Illinois 60610

AC22:92-382:400MM:11/92

Foreword

Physicians' *Current Procedural Terminology,* Fourth Edition (CPT) is a listing of descriptive terms and identifying codes for reporting medical services and procedures performed by physicians. The purpose of the terminology is to provide a uniform language that will accurately describe medical, surgical, and diagnostic services, and will thereby provide an effective means for reliable nationwide communication among physicians, patients, and third parties. CPT 1993 is the most recent revision of a work that first appeared in 1966.

CPT descriptive terms and identifying codes currently serve a wide variety of important functions in the field of medical nomenclature. This system of terminology is the most widely accepted nomenclature for the reporting of physician procedures and services under government and private health insurance programs. CPT is also useful for administrative management purposes such as claims processing and for the development of guidelines for medical care review. The uniform language is likewise applicable to medical education and research by providing a useful basis for local, regional, and national utilization comparisons.

The changes that appear in this revision have been prepared by the CPT Editorial Panel with the assistance of physicians representing all specialties of medicine, and with important contributions from many third party payors and governmental agencies.

With the introduction of new codes for evaluation and management services in CPT 1992, important changes were made in the way that physicans report many of their services. These revisions were responsive to changes in the medical practice environment. Further experience with the use of these new codes provides strong evidence that this new system will provide greater uniformity, will be easier for physicians to use, and will be flexible enough to accommodate additional medical practice changes for many years.

As we continue to gain experience with the new system, we continue to expect that there will be a period of adjustment and continued refinement. This period will require efforts by both physicians and by third party payors to learn and adapt to the concepts inherent in the new system.

The American Medical Association trusts that this revision will continue the usefulness of its predecessors in identifying, describing, and coding medical, surgical, and diagnostic services performed by practicing physicians.

James S. Todd, M.D.
Executive Vice President

November 1, 1992

AMA CPT Editorial Panel

AMA CPT Advisory Committee

Curtis W. Hawkins, M.D.	Society for Investigative Dermatology
Terry C. Hicks, M.D.	American Society of Colon & Rectal Surgeons
Timmothy Holt, M.D.	American Geriatric Society
Raymond V. Janevicius, M.D.	American Society of Plastic & Reconstructive Surgeons, Inc.
Christine L. Kasser, M.D.	American Society of Addiction Medicine
Richard T. Katz, M.D.	American Association of Electromyography & Electrodiagnosis
Robert Katz, M.D.	American College of Occupational Medicine
Gerald R. Kerby, M.D.	American Thoracic Society
Kenneth L. Kidd, M.D.	American Roentgen Ray Society
Eileen B. King, M.D.	American Society of Cytology
George F. Kwass, M.D.	College of American Pathologists
Sidney Levitsky, M.D.	Society of Thoracic Surgeons
Victor L. Lewis, M.D.	American Association of Plastic Surgeons
Philipp M. Lippe, M.D.	American Academy of Pain Medicine
Glenn Littenberg, M.D.	American Society of Internal Medicine
James Maberry, M.D.	American Academy of Dermatology
Robert H. Maisel, M.D.	American Laryngological, Rhinological & Otological Society, Inc.
David R. Musher, M.D.	American College of Gastroenterology
Stanley J. Myers, M.D.	American Academy of Physical Medicine & Rehabilitation
Loren D. Nelson, M.D.	Society of Critical Care Medicine
Fred T. Nobrega, M.D.	American College of Preventive Medicine
Walter J. Pedowitz, M.D.	American Orthopaedic Foot and Ankle Society
Robert L. Peters, Jr., DO	American Osteopathic Association
Byron C. Pevehouse, M.D.	American Association of Neurological Surgeons
Merton A. Quaife, M.D.	American College of Nuclear Physicians
Merton A. Quaife, M.D.	The Society of Nuclear Medicine
Michael X. Repka, M.D.	American Academy of Ophthalmology, Inc.
Nigel K. Roberts, M.D.	Association of Life Insurance Medical Directors of America
June K. Robinson, M.D.	American Society for Dermatologic Surgery, Inc.
Demostene Romanucci, M.D.	American Society of Abdominal Surgeons
Arnold M. Rosen, M.D.	American Society for Gastrointestinal Endoscopy
Herbert E. Rosenbaum, M.D.	American Academy of Neurology
Jacob M. Rowe, M.D.	American Society of Hematology
Andrew C. Ruoff III, M.D.	The Society of Medical Consultants to the Armed Forces
Maurice Sandler, M.D.	American Urological Association, Inc.
Chester W. Schmidt, Jr., M.D.	American Psychiatric Association
Jon D. Shanser, M.D.	American College of Radiology
Karl W. Stevenson, M.D.	American Academy of Child & Adolescent Psychiatry
Willis W. Stogsdill, M.D.	American Society of Anesthesiologists, Inc.

Dennis Stone, M.D.	American Medical Directors Association
Douglas L. Stringer, M.D.	Congress of Neurological Surgeons
Roger F. Suchyta, M.D.	American Academy of Pediatrics
Donald G. Vidt, M.D.	American Society for Clinical Pharmacology & Therapeutics
F. Stephen Vogel, M.D.	United States & Canadian Academy of Pathology
Theodore A. Watson, M.D.	American Academy of Otolaryngic Allergy
Milton Weinberg, Jr., M.D.	American Association for Thoracic Surgery
Edward Weisberger, M.D.	American Academy of Otolaryngology, Head & Neck Surgery, Inc.
Jonathan B. Weisbuch, M.D.	American Association of Public Health Physicians
Douglas L. Wood, M.D.	American College of Cardiology

Acknowledgements

The publication of CPT 1993 represents a product of the combined efforts of many individuals and organizations. The editors accordingly express their gratitude to the many national medical specialty societies, state medical associations, health insurance organizations and agencies, and to the many individual physicians who devoted their energies and expertise to the preparation of this revision. Thanks are due to Jean A. Harris, Health Care Financing Administration, Bonnie Balkin and David Tennenbaum, Blue Cross and Blue Shield Association, Thomas Musco, Health Insurance Association of America, Donna Ganzer and Donna Pickett, American Hospital Association, and to Toula Nicholas, American Health Information Management Association, for their invaluable assistance in enhancing CPT. Finally, the editors are grateful to Barry S. Eisenberg, Director, Division of Payment Policy and Programs, for his helpful invaluable assistance.

body areas

head, face
neck
chest, breast, axilla
abdomen
genitalia, groin & buttocks
back
extremities

Dedication

This publication is dedicated to William R. Felts, M.D., former chairman of the CPT Editorial Panel, and Charles B. Clayman, M.D., for their immeasurable contribution to CPT.

body systems - CPT Definition

- Eyes
- Ears, Nose, & throat
- Cardiovasular
- Respiratory
- Gastro intestinal
- Genitourinary
- Musculoskeletal
- Skin
- Neurologic
- Psychiatric
- Hematologic / Lymphatic / Immunologic

Contents

Introduction

Physicians' *Current Procedural Terminology*, Fourth Edition (CPT) is a systematic listing and coding of procedures and services performed by physicians. Each procedure or service is identified with a five digit code. The use of CPT codes simplifies the reporting of services. With this coding and recording system, the procedure or service rendered by the physician is accurately identified.

Inclusion of a descriptor and its associated specific five-digit identifying code number in CPT is generally based upon the procedure being consistent with contemporary medical practice and being performed by many physicians in clinical practice (not on an investigational basis) in multiple locations. Inclusion in CPT does not represent endorsement by the American Medical Association of any particular diagnostic or therapeutic procedure. Inclusion or exclusion of a procedure does not imply any health insurance coverage or reimbursement policy.

The main body of the material is listed in six sections. Within each section are subsections with anatomic, procedural, condition, or descriptor subheadings. The procedures and services with their identifying codes are presented in numeric order with one exception—the entire **EVALUATION AND MANAGEMENT** section (99201-99499) has been placed at the beginning of the listed procedures. These items are used by most physicians in reporting a significant portion of their services. The **MEDICINE** (procedures) section now follows **PATHOLOGY**.

The section numbers and their sequence are as follows:

EVALUATION AND MANAGEMENT	99201 to 99499
ANESTHESIOLOGY	00100 to 01999, 99100 to 99140
SURGERY	10040 to 69999
RADIOLOGY (INCLUDING NUCLEAR MEDICINE AND DIAGNOSTIC ULTRASOUND)	70010 to 79999
PATHOLOGY AND LABORATORY	80002 to 89999
MEDICINE (except Anesthesiology)	90701 to 99199

The first and last code numbers and the subsection name of the items appear at the top of each page (eg, "20000—20206 Musculoskeletal System"). The continuous pagination of CPT is found on the lower, outer margin of each page along with the section name.

Instructions for Use of CPT

A physician using CPT terminology and coding selects the name of the procedure or service that most accurately identifies the service performed. In surgery, it may be an operation; in medicine, a diagnostic or therapeutic procedure; in radiology, a radiograph. The physician then may list other additional procedures performed or pertinent special services. When necessary, he lists any modifying or extenuating circumstance. **Any service or procedure should be adequately documented in the medical record.**

It is important to recognize that the listing of a service or procedure and its code number in a specific section of this book does not restrict its use to a specific specialty group. Any procedure or service in any section of this book may be used to designate the services rendered by any qualified physician.

Format of the Terminology

CPT procedure terminology has been developed as stand-alone descriptions of medical procedures. However, some of the procedures in CPT are not printed in their entirety but refer back to a common portion of the procedure listed in a preceding entry. This is evident when an entry is followed by one or more indentations. This is done in an effort to conserve space.

For example:

25100 Arthrotomy, wrist joint; for biopsy
25105   for synovectomy

Note that the common part of code 25100 (that part before the semicolon) should be considered part of code 25105. Therefore the full procedure represented by code 25105 should read:

25105 Arthrotomy, wrist joint; for synovectomy

Requests to Update CPT

The effectiveness of Physicians' *Current Procedural Terminology* is dependent upon constant updating to reflect changes in medical practice. This can only be accomplished through the interest and timely suggestions of practicing physicians, medical specialty societies, state medical associations, and other organizations and agencies. Accordingly, the American Medical Association welcomes correspondence, inquiries, and suggestions concerning old and new procedures, as well as other matters such as codes and indices.

For suggestions concerning the introduction of new procedures, or the coding, deleting, or revising of procedures contained in CPT 1993, correspondence should be directed to:

Department of Coding and Nomenclature
American Medical Association
515 North State Street
Chicago, Illinois 60610

All proposed additions to, or modifications of, CPT 1993 will be by decision of the CPT Editorial Panel after consultation with appropriate medical specialty societies.

Guidelines

Specific "Guidelines" are presented at the beginning of each of the six sections. These Guidelines define items that are necessary to appropriately interpret and report the procedures and services contained in that section. For example, in the **MEDICINE** section, specific instructions are provided for handling unlisted services or procedures, special reports, and supplies and materials provided by the physician. Guidelines also provide explanations regarding terms that apply only to a particular section. For instance, **SURGERY** guidelines provide an explanation of the use of the star, while in **RADIOLOGY,** the unique term, "radiological supervision and interpretation" is defined.

Starred Procedures

The star "⋆" is used to identify certain surgical procedures. A description of this reporting mechanism will be found in the SURGERY "Guidelines."

Modifiers

A modifier provides the means by which the reporting physician can indicate that a service or procedure that has been performed has been altered by some specific circumstance but not changed in its definition or code. The judicious application of modifiers obviates the necessity for separate procedure listings that may describe the modifying circumstance. Modifiers may be used to indicate to the recipient of a report that:

- A service or procedure has both a professional and technical component.
- A service or procedure was performed by more than one physician and/or in more than one location.
- A service or procedure has been increased or reduced.
- Only part of a service was performed.
- An adjunctive service was performed.
- A bilateral procedure was performed.
- A service or procedure was provided more than once.
- Unusual events occurred.

For example:

A physician providing diagnostic or therapeutic radiology services, ultrasound or nuclear medicine services in a hospital would use either modifier -26 or 09926 to report the professional component.

For example:

73090-26 = Professional component only for an x-ray of the forearm

OR

73090 AND 09926 = Professional component only for an x-ray of the forearm

Two surgeons, usually with different skills, may be required to manage a specific surgical problem. The modifier-62 or the alternative modifier five digit code 09962 would be applicable. Modifier -62 would be appropriate only when both surgeons are reporting the same code number and descriptor. For instance, a neurological surgeon and an otolaryngologist are working as co-surgeons in performing transsphenoidal excision of a pituitary neoplasm.

For example:

61546-62 = Craniotomy for hypophysectomy or excision of pituitary tumor, intracranial approach + two surgeons modifier

OR

61546 AND 09962 = Craniotomy for hypophysectomy or excision of pituitary tumor, intracranial approach + two surgeons modifier

AND the second surgeon would report:

61546-62 = Craniotomy for hypophysectomy or excision of pituitary tumor, intracranial approach + two surgeons modifier

OR

61546 AND 09962 = Craniotomy for hypophysectomy or excision of pituitary tumor, intracranial approach + two surgeons modifier

A listing of modifiers pertinent to **EVALUATION AND MANAGEMENT, ANESTHESIA, SURGERY, RADIOLOGY, PATHOLOGY,** and **MEDICINE** are located in the Guidelines of each section. A complete listing of modifiers is found in Appendix A.

Unlisted Procedure or Service

It is recognized that there may be services or procedures performed by physicians that are not found in CPT. Therefore, a number of specific code numbers have been designated for reporting unlisted procedures. When an unlisted procedure number is used, the service or procedure should be described. Each of these unlisted procedural code numbers (with the appropriate accompanying topical entry) relates to a specific section of the book and is presented in the Guidelines of that section.

Special Report

A service that is rarely provided, unusual, variable, or new may require a special report in determining medical appropriateness of the service. Pertinent information should include an adequate definition or description of the nature, extent, and need for the procedure; and the time, effort, and equipment necessary to provide the service. Additional items which may be included are:

> Complexity of symptoms, final diagnosis, pertinent physical findings, diagnostic and therapeutic procedures, concurrent problems, and follow-up care.

Code Changes

A summary listing of additions, deletions and revisions applicable to CPT 1993 is found in Appendix B. New procedure numbers added to CPT are identified throughout the text with the symbol "●" placed before the code number. In instances where a code revision has resulted in a substantially altered procedure descriptor, the symbol "▲" is placed before the code number.

Short Procedure Tape Revision

Appendix C has been included for those users who have purchased a CPT 1992 short procedure description tape or floppy disk or have a tape/disk current through CPT 1992. The listing includes changes and/or corrections necessary to update the CPT 1993 data file. For additional information regarding the availability of CPT magnetic computer tapes and floppy disks, see page xvii of the **INTRODUCTION.**

Alphabetical Reference Index

A complete alphabetical index is found in the back of the book. It includes listings by procedure and anatomic site. Procedures and services commonly known by their eponyms or other designations are also included.

Magnetic Computer Tapes and Floppy Disk

CPT 1993 procedure codes and descriptors are also available on magnetic computer tapes in the three formats listed below.

CPT Full Procedure Tape contains the complete procedural text of the CPT manual. The procedures in this tape are constructed of 80-byte line records. In cases where the procedural narrative exceeds the 80-byte line limit, the header record is followed by several trailing line records. The start of each procedure is indicated by a change in "procedure number" or the presence of 01, 02 etc. in the sequence fields.

CPT Short Description Tape also contains the complete listing of procedural codes found in the CPT manual; however, each has an abbreviated narrative written in non-technical or layman's terms. Each code and description is limited to 28 characters or less on a single line.

Both CPT computer tapes are identical technically, each having the following line specifications:

record format	fixed
logical record length	80 bytes
block size	80 bytes
label	no label
tracks	9
tape density	1600 or 6250 BPI
content	EBCDIC or ASCII

CPT Floppy Disk is identical in content to the short description tape. That is, each code and description is limited to 28 characters or less on a single line.

Technical Description of Disk

- Standard PC format with a maximum length of 36 characters per record
- Content: ASCII
- PC requirements: IBM PC, XT, AT or compatible
- 3½″ double side/double density (720K) disk OR 5¼″ double side/double density (360K) disk

Using Compatible Software

Please bear in mind that the disks and tapes contain *only* a CPT data file. They are *not* programs or other operations software. We have deliberately not included programs with this data file, as each user has different needs.

Order information for the CPT magnetic computer tapes/disk may be found at the back of this book. Questions or suggestions concerning the CPT magnetic computer tapes/disk may be directed to:

Department of Coding and Nomenclature
CPT Magnetic Computer Tapes
American Medical Association
515 N. State Street
Chicago, Illinois 60610

Evaluation and Management (E/M) Services

Guidelines

In addition to the information presented in the **INTRODUCTION,** several other items unique to this section are defined or identified here:

1. **CLASSIFICATION OF EVALUATION AND MANAGEMENT (E/M) SERVICES:** The E/M section is divided into broad categories such as office visits, hospital visits and consultations. Most of the categories are further divided into two or more subcategories of E/M services. For example, there are two subcategories of office visits (new patient and established patient) and there are two subcategories of hospital visits (initial and subsequent). The subcategories of E/M services are further classified into levels of E/M services that are identified by specific codes. This classification is important because the nature of physician work varies by type of service, place of service, and the patient's status.

   The basic format of the levels of E/M services is the same for most categories. First, a unique code number is listed. Second, the place and/or type of service is specified, eg, office consultation. Third, the content of the service is defined, eg, comprehensive history and comprehensive examination. (See levels of E/M services following for details on the content of E/M services.) Fourth, the nature of the presenting problem(s) usually associated with a given level is described. Fifth, the time typically required to provide the service is specified. (A detailed discussion of time is provided on pages 5-7.)

2. **DEFINITIONS OF COMMONLY USED TERMS:** Certain key words and phrases are used throughout the E/M section. The following definitions are intended to reduce the potential for differing interpretations and to increase the consistency of reporting by physicians in differing specialties.

NEW AND ESTABLISHED PATIENT: A new patient is one who has not received any professional services from the physician or another physician of the same specialty who belongs to the same group practice, within the past three years.

An established patient is one who has received professional services from the physician or another physician of the same specialty who belongs to the same group practice, within the past three years.

In the instance where a physician is on call for or covering for another physician, the patient's encounter will be classified as it would have been by the physician who is not available.

No distinction is made between new and established patients in the emergency department. E/M services in the emergency department category may be reported for any new or established patient who presents for treatment in the emergency department.

CONCURRENT CARE is the provision of similar services, eg, hospital visits, to the same patient by more than one physician on the same day. When concurrent care is provided, no special reporting is required. Modifier -75 has been deleted.

COUNSELING is a discussion with a patient and/or family concerning one or more of the following areas:

- diagnostic results, impressions, and/or recommended diagnostic studies;
- prognosis;
- risks and benefits of management (treatment) options;
- instructions for management (treatment) and/or follow-up;
- importance of compliance with chosen management (treatment) options;
- risk factor reduction; and
- patient and family education.

(For psychotherapy, see 90841-90857)

LEVELS OF E/M SERVICES: Within each category or subcategory of E/M service, there are three to five levels of E/M services available for reporting purposes. Levels of E/M services are **not** interchangeable among the different categories or subcategories of service. For example, the first level of E/M services in the subcategory of office visit, new patient, does not have the same definition as the first level of E/M services in the subcategory of office visit, established patient.

The levels of E/M services include examinations, evaluations, treatments, conferences with or concerning patients, preventive pediatric and adult health supervision, and similar medical services. The levels of E/M services encompass the wide variations in skill, effort, time, responsibility and medical knowledge required for the prevention or diagnosis and treatment of illness or injury and the promotion of optimal health. Each level of E/M services may be used by all physicians.

The descriptors for the levels of E/M services recognize seven components, six of which are used in defining the levels of E/M services. These components are:

- history;
- examination;
- medical decision making;
- counseling;
- coordination of care;
- nature of presenting problem; and
- time.

The first three of these components (history, examination and medical decision making) are considered the **key** components in selecting a level of E/M services. (See 7. c., pages 10-11.)

The next three components (counseling, coordination of care, and the nature of the presenting problem) are considered **contributory** factors in the majority of encounters. Although the first two of these contributory factors are important E/M services, it is not required that these services be provided at every patient encounter.

Coordination of care with other providers or agencies without a patient encounter on that day is reported using the case management codes.

The final component, time, is discussed in detail following (see pages 5-7).

The actual performance of diagnostic tests/studies for which specific CPT codes are available is **not** included in the levels of E/M services. Physician performance of diagnostic tests/studies for which specific CPT codes are available should be reported separately, *in addition* to the appropriate E/M code.

NATURE OF PRESENTING PROBLEM: A presenting problem is a disease, condition, illness, injury, symptom, sign, finding, complaint, or other reason for encounter, with or without a diagnosis being established at the time of the encounter. The E/M codes recognize five types of presenting problems that are defined as follows:

- Minimal—A problem that may not require the presence of the physician, but service is provided under the physician's supervision.
- Self-limited or Minor—A problem that runs a definite and prescribed course, is transient in nature and is not likely to permanently alter health status OR has a good prognosis with management/compliance.
- Low severity—A problem where the risk of morbidity without treatment is low; there is little to no risk of mortality without treatment; full recovery without functional impairment is expected.
- Moderate severity—A problem where the risk of morbidity without treatment is moderate; there is moderate risk of mortality without treatment; uncertain prognosis OR increased probability of prolonged functional impairment.
- High severity—A problem where the risk of morbidity without treatment is high to extreme; there is a moderate to high risk of mortality without treatment OR high probability of severe, prolonged functional impairment.

TIME: The inclusion of time in the definitions of levels of E/M services has been implicit in prior editions of CPT. The inclusion of time as an explicit factor beginning in CPT 1992 is done to assist physicians in selecting the most appropriate level of E/M services. It should be recognized that the specific times expressed in the visit code descriptors are averages, and therefore represent a range of times which may be higher or lower depending on actual clinical circumstances.

Time is **not** a descriptive component for the emergency department levels of E/M services because emergency department services are typically provided on a variable intensity basis, often involving multiple encounters with several patients over an extended period of time. Therefore, it is often difficult for physicians to provide accurate estimates of the time spent face-to-face with the patient.

Studies to establish levels of E/M services employed surveys of practicing physicians to obtain data on the amount of time and work associated with typical E/M services. Since "work" is not easily quantifiable, the codes must rely on other objective, verifiable measures that correlate with physicians' estimates of their "work". It has been demonstrated that physicians' estimations of **intra-service time** (as explained below), both within and across specialties, is a variable that is predictive of the "work" of E/M services. This same research has shown there is a strong relationship between intra-service time and total time for E/M services. Intra-service time, rather than total time, was chosen for inclusion with the codes because of its relative ease of measurement and because of its direct correlation with measurements of the total amount of time and work associated with typical E/M services.

Intra-service times are defined as **face-to-face** time for office and other outpatient visits and as **unit/floor** time for hospital and other inpatient visits. This distinction is necessary because most of the work of typical office visits takes place during the face-to-face time with the patient, while most of the work of typical hospital visits takes place during the time spent on the patient's floor or unit.

a. **Face-to-face time (office and other outpatient visits and office consultations):** For coding purposes, face-to-face time for these services is defined as only that time that the physician spends face-to-face with the patient and/or family. This includes the time in which the physician performs such tasks as obtaining a history, performing an examination, and counseling the patient.

Physicians also spend time doing work before or after the face-to-face time with the patient, performing such tasks as reviewing records and tests, arranging for further services, and communicating further with other professionals and the patient through written reports and telephone contact.

This *non* face-to-face time for office services—also called pre- and post-encounter time—is not included in the time component described in the E/M codes. However, the pre and post face-to-face work associated with an encounter was included in calculating the total work of typical services in physician surveys.

Thus, the face-to-face time associated with the services described by any E/M code is a valid proxy for the total work done before, during, and after the visit.

b. **Unit/floor time (hospital observation services, inpatient hospital care, initial and follow-up hospital consultations, nursing facility):** For reporting purposes, intra-service time for these services is defined as unit/floor time, which includes the time that the physician is present on the patient's hospital unit and at the bedside rendering services for that patient. This includes the time in which the physician establishes and/or reviews the patient's chart, examines the patient, writes notes and communicates with other professionals and the patient's family.

In the hospital, pre- and post-time includes time spent off the patient's floor performing such tasks as reviewing pathology and radiology findings in another part of the hospital.

This pre- and post-visit time is not included in the time component described in these codes. However, the pre- and post-work performed during the time spent off the floor or unit was included in calculating the total work of typical services in physician surveys.

Thus, the unit/floor time associated with the services described by any code is a valid proxy for the total work done before, during, and after the visit.

3. **UNLISTED SERVICE:** An E/M service may be provided that is not listed in this section of CPT. When reporting such a service, the appropriate "Unlisted" code may be used to indicate the service, identifying it by "Special Report" as discussed in item 4. The "Unlisted Services" and accompanying codes for the E/M section are as follows:

   99429 Unlisted preventive medicine service
   99499 Unlisted evaluation and management service

4. **SPECIAL REPORT:** An unlisted service or one that is unusual, variable, or new may require a special report demonstrating the medical appropriateness of the service. Pertinent information should include an adequate definition or description of the nature, extent, and need for the procedure; and the time, effort and equipment necessary to provide the service. Additional items which may be included are complexity of symptoms, final diagnosis, pertinent physical findings, diagnostic and therapeutic procedures, concurrent problems, and follow-up care.

5. **CLINICAL EXAMPLES:** of the codes for E/M services are provided to assist physicians in understanding the meaning of the descriptors and selecting the correct code. Each example was developed by physicians in the specialties shown.

   The same problem, when seen by physicians in different specialties, may involve different amounts of work. Therefore, the appropriate level of encounter should be reported using the descriptors rather than the examples.

   The examples have been tested for validity and approved by the CPT Editorial Panel. Physicians were given the examples and asked to assign a code or assess the amount of time and work involved. Only those examples that were rated consistently have been included.

6. **MODIFIERS:** Listed services may be modified under certain circumstances. When applicable, the modifying circumstance against general guidelines should be identified by the addition of the appropriate modifier code, which may be reported in either of two ways. The modifier may be reported by a two digit number placed after the usual procedure number from which it is separated by a hyphen. Or, the modifier may be reported by a separate five digit code that is used in addition to the procedure code. Modifiers available in E/M are as follows:

   -21 Prolonged Evaluation and Management Services: When the service(s) provided is prolonged or otherwise greater than that usually required for the highest level of E/M service within a given category, it may be identified by adding modifier '-21' to the E/M code number or by use of the separate five digit modifier code 09921. A report may also be appropriate.

   -24 Unrelated Evaluation and Management Service by the Same Physician During a Postoperative Period: The physician may need to indicate that an evaluation and management service was performed during a postoperative period for a reason(s) unrelated to the original procedure. This circumstance may be reported by adding the modifier '-24' to the appropriate level of E/M service, or the separate five digit modifier 09924 may be used.

   -25 Significant, Separately Identifiable Evaluation and Management Service by the Same Physician on the Day of a Procedure: The physician may need to indicate that on the day a procedure or service identified by a CPT code was performed, the patient's condition required a significant, separately identifiable E/M service above and beyond the usual preoperative and postoperative care associated with the procedure that was performed. This circumstance may be reported by adding the modifier '-25' to the appropriate level of E/M service, or the separate five digit modifier 09925 may be used.

-32 Mandated Services: Services related to *mandated* consultation and/or related services (eg, PRO, 3rd party payor) may be identified by adding the modifier '-32' to the basic procedure or the service may be reported by use of the five digit modifier 09932.

-52 Reduced Services: Under certain circumstances a service or procedure is partially reduced or eliminated at the physician's election. Under these circumstances the service provided can be identified by its usual procedure number and the addition of the modifier '-52,' signifying that the service is reduced. This provides a means of reporting reduced services without disturbing the identification of the basic service. Modifier code 09952 may be used as an alternative to modifier '-52.'

7. INSTRUCTIONS FOR SELECTING A LEVEL OF E/M SERVICE:

a. **Identify the category and subcategory of service:** The categories and subcategories of codes available for reporting E/M services are as follows:

Category/Subcategory	Code Numbers
Office or Other Outpatient Services	
New Patient	99201-99205
Established Patient	99211-99215
Hospital Observation Services	99218-99220
Hospital Inpatient Services	
Initial Hospital Care	99221-99223
Subsequent Hospital Care	99231-99233
Hospital Discharge Services	99238
Consultations	
Office Consultations	99241-99245
Initial Inpatient Consultations	99251-99255
Follow-up Inpatient Consultations	99261-99263
Confirmatory Consultations	99271-99275
Emergency Department Services	99281-99288
Critical Care Services	99291-99292
Neonatal Intensive Care	99295-99297

Category/Subcategory	Code Numbers
Nursing Facility Services	
Comprehensive Nursing Facility Assessments	99301-99303
Subsequent Nursing Facility Care	99311-99313
Domiciliary, Rest Home or Custodial Care Services	
New Patient	99321-99323
Established Patient	99331-99333
Home Services	
New Patient	99341-99343
Established Patient	99351-99353
Case Management Services	
Team Conferences	99361-99362
Telephone Calls	99371-99373
Preventive Medicine Services	
New Patient	99381-99387
Established Patient	99391-99397
Individual Counseling	99401-99404
Group Counseling	99411-99412
Other	99420-99429
Newborn Care	99431-99440
Other E/M Services	99499

b. **Review the reporting instructions for the selected category or subcategory**: Most of the categories and many of the subcategories of service have special guidelines or instructions unique to that category or subcategory. Where these are indicated, eg, "Inpatient Hospital Care", special instructions will be presented preceding the levels of E/M services.

c. **Review the level of E/M service descriptors and examples in the selected category or subcategory:** The descriptors for the levels of E/M services recognize seven components, six of which are used in defining the levels of E/M services. These components are:

- history;
- examination;
- medical decision making;

- counseling;
- coordination of care;
- nature of presenting problem; and
- time.

The first three of these components (ie, history, examination and medical decision making) should be considered the **key components** in selecting the level of E/M services. An exception to this rule is in the case of visits which consist predominantly of counseling or coordination of care (See g. 3, page 13.)

The nature of the presenting problem and time are provided in some levels to assist the physician in determining the appropriate level of E/M service.

d. **Determine the extent of HISTORY obtained:** The levels of E/M services recognize four types of history that are defined as follows:

- Problem Focused—chief complaint; brief history of present illness or problem.
- Expanded Problem Focused—chief complaint; brief history of present illness; problem pertinent system review.
- Detailed—chief complaint; extended history of present illness; extended system review; **pertinent** past, family and/or social history.
- Comprehensive—chief complaint; extended history of present illness; complete system review; **complete** past, family and social history.

e. **Determine the extent of EXAMINATION performed:** The levels of E/M services recognize four types of examination that are defined as follows:

- Problem Focused—an examination that is limited to the affected body area or organ system.
- Expanded Problem Focused—an examination of the affected body area or organ system and other symptomatic or related organ systems.

- Detailed—an extended examination of the affected body area(s) and other symptomatic or related organ system(s).

- Comprehensive—a complete single system specialty examination or a complete multi-system examination.

f. **Determine the complexity of MEDICAL DECISION MAKING:** Medical decision making refers to the complexity of establishing a diagnosis and/or selecting a management option as measured by:

- the number of possible diagnoses and/or the number of management options that must be considered;

- the amount and/or complexity of medical records, diagnostic tests, and/or other information that must be obtained, reviewed and analyzed; and

- the risk of significant complications, morbidity and/or mortality, as well as comorbidities, associated with the patient's presenting problems(s), the diagnostic procedure(s) and/or the possible management options.

Four types of medical decision making are recognized: straightforward; low complexity; moderate complexity; and, high complexity. To qualify for a given type of decision making, two of the three elements in the table following must be met or exceeded:

Number of diagnoses or management options	Amount and/or complexity of data to be reviewed	Risk of complications and/or morbidity or mortality	Type of decision making
minimal	minimal or none	minimal	**straight-forward**
limited	limited	low	**low complexity**
multiple	moderate	moderate	**moderate complexity**
extensive	extensive	high	**high complexity**

Comorbidities/underlying diseases, in and of themselves, are not considered in selecting a level of E/M services *unless* their presence significantly increases the complexity of the medical decision making.

g. **Select the appropriate level of E/M services based on the following:**

1. For the following categories/subcategories, **ALL OF THE KEY COMPONENTS** ie, history, examination, and medical decision making, must meet or exceed the stated requirements to qualify for a particular level of E/M service: office, new patient; hospital observation services; initial hospital care; office consultations; initial inpatient consultations; confirmatory consultations; emergency department services; comprehensive nursing facility assessments; domiciliary care, new patient; and home, new patient.

2. For the following categories/subcategories, **TWO OF THE THREE KEY COMPONENTS** (ie, history, examination, and medical decision making) must meet or exceed the stated requirements to qualify for a particular level of E/M services: office, established patient; subsequent hospital care; follow-up inpatient consultations; subsequent nursing facility care; domiciliary care, established patient; and home, established patient.

3. In the case where counseling and/or coordination of care dominates (more than 50%) of the physician/patient and/or family encounter (face-to-face time in the office or other outpatient setting or floor/unit time in the hospital or nursing facility), then **time** is considered the key or controlling factor to qualify for a particular level of E/M services. The extent of counseling and/or coordination of care must be documented in the medical record.

EVALUATION AND MANAGEMENT

Office or Other Outpatient Services

The following codes are used to report evaluation and management services provided in the physician's office or in an outpatient or other ambulatory facility. A patient is considered an outpatient until inpatient admission to a health care facility occurs.

To report services provided to a patient who is admitted to a hospital or nursing facility in the course of an encounter in the office or other ambulatory facility, see the notes for initial hospital inpatient care (page 25) or comprehensive nursing facility assessments (pages 54-55).

For services provided by physicians in the Emergency Department, see 99281-99285.

For observation care, see 99218-99220.

For definitions of key components, see Evaluation and Management Services Guidelines.

NEW PATIENT

99201 Office or other outpatient visit for the evaluation and management of a new patient, which requires these three key components:

- **a problem focused history;**
- **a problem focused examination; and**
- **straightforward medical decision making.**

Counseling and/or coordination of care with other providers or agencies are provided consistent with the nature of the problem(s) and the patient's and/or family's needs.

Usually, the presenting problems are self limited or minor. Physicians typically spend 10 minutes face-to-face with the patient and/or family.

Examples

Initial office visit with 65-year-old male for reassurance about an isolated seborrheic keratosis on the upper back. (Dermatology/Plastic Surgery)

Initial office visit with 9-month-old female with diaper rash. (Pediatrics)

Initial office visit to advise for or against the removal of wisdom teeth, 18-year-old male referred by an orthodontist. (Oral & Maxillofacial Surgery)

Initial office visit for a 22-year-old male with a small area of sunburn requiring first aid. (Dermatology/Family Medicine/Internal Medicine)

Initial office visit with an out-of-town visitor who needs a prescription refilled because she forgot her hay fever medication. (Allergy & Immunology/Internal Medicine)

Initial office visit with 10-year-old male with severe rash and itching for the past 24 hours, positive history for contact with poison oak 48 hours prior to the visit. (Family Medicine)

Initial office visit with 5-year-old female to remove sutures from simple wound, placed by another physician. (Plastic Surgery)

Initial office visit for the evaluation and management of a contusion of a finger. (Orthopaedic Surgery)

99202 Office or other outpatient visit for the evaluation and management of a new patient, which requires these three key components:

- **an expanded problem focused history;**
- **an expanded problem focused examination; and**
- **straightforward medical decision making.**

Counseling and/or coordination of care with other providers or agencies are provided consistent with the nature of the problem(s) and the patient's and/or family's needs.

Usually, the presenting problem(s) are of low to moderate severity. Physicians typically spend 20 minutes face-to-face with the patient and/or family.

Examples

Initial office visit, 16-year-old male with severe cystic acne, new patient. (Dermatology)

Initial office evaluation for gradual hearing loss, 58-year-old male, history and physical examination, with interpretation of complete audiogram, air bone, etc. (Otolaryngology)

Initial office visit for evaluation and management of recurrent urinary infection in female. (Internal Medicine)

Initial office visit for a 10-year-old female with acute maxillary sinusitis. (Family Medicine)

Initial office visit for a 25-year-old patient with single season allergic rhinitis. (Allergy & Immunology)

Initial office visit with 10-year-old girl with history of chronic otitis media and a draining ear. (Pediatrics)

Initial office visit for a patient with recurring episodes of herpes simplex who has developed a clustering of vesicles on the upper lip. (Internal Medicine)

Initial office visit to plan transient dialysis for a 56-year-old stable dialysis patient who has accompanying records. (Nephrology)

99203 Office or other outpatient visit for the evaluation and management of a new patient, which requires these three key components:

- **a detailed history;**
- **a detailed examination; and**
- **medical decision making of low complexity.**

Counseling and/or coordination of care with other providers or agencies are provided consistent with the nature of the problem(s) and the patient's and/or family's needs.

Usually, the presenting problem(s) are of moderate severity. Physicians typically spend 30 minutes face-to-face with the patient and/or family.

Examples

Initial office visit for evaluation of a 48-year-old man with recurrent low back pain radiating to the leg. (General Surgery)

Initial office visit with couple for counseling concerning voluntary vasectomy for sterility. Spent 30 minutes discussing procedure, risks and benefits, and answering questions. (Urology)

Initial office visit for evaluation of 13-year-old female with progressive scoliosis. (Physical Medicine & Rehabilitation)

Initial office evaluation for diagnosis and management of painless gross hematuria in new patient, without cystoscopy. (Internal Medicine)

Initial office evaluation of 49-year-old male with nasal obstruction. Detailed exam with topical anesthesia. (Plastic Surgery)

Initial office visit for 21-year-old female desiring counseling and evaluation of initiation of contraception. (Family Medicine/ Internal Medicine/Obstetrics & Gynecology)

Initial office visit for 49-year-old male presenting with painless blood per rectum associated with bowel movement.
(Colon & Rectal Surgery)

Initial office visit for 19-year-old football player with 3 day old acute knee injury; now with swelling and pain. (Orthopaedic Surgery)

99204 Office or other outpatient visit for the evaluation and management of a new patient, which requires these three key components:

- **a comprehensive history;**
- **a comprehensive examination; and**
- **medical decision making of moderate complexity.**

Counseling and/or coordination of care with other providers or agencies are provided consistent with the nature of the problem(s) and the patient's and/or family's needs.

Usually, the presenting problem(s) are of moderate to high severity. Physicians typically spend 45 minutes face-to-face with the patient and/or family.

Examples

Initial office visit for evaluation of a 63-year-old male with chest pain on exertion.
(Cardiology/Internal Medicine)

Initial office visit for 7-year-old female with juvenile diabetes mellitus, new to area, past history of hospitalization times three.
(Pediatrics)

Initial office visit of a 50-year-old female with progressive solid food dysphagia. (Gastroenterology)

Initial office evaluation of 70-year-old female with polyarthralgia.
(Rheumatology)

Initial office evaluation of a 70-year-old patient with recent onset of episodic confusion.
(Internal Medicine)

Initial office visit for 34-year-old patient with primary infertility, including counseling.
(Obstetrics & Gynecology)

Initial office visit for a patient with papulosquamous eruption involving 60% of the cutaneous surface with joint pain. Combinations of topical and systemic treatments discussed.
(Dermatology)

99205 Office or other outpatient visit for the evaluation and management of a new patient, which requires these three key components:

- **a comprehensive history;**
- **a comprehensive examination; and**
- **medical decision making of high complexity.**

Counseling and/or coordination of care with other providers or agencies are provided consistent with the nature of the problem(s) and the patient's and/or family's needs.

Usually, the presenting problem(s) are of moderate to high severity. Physicians typically spend 60 minutes face-to-face with the patient and/or family.

Examples

Initial office evaluation of a 65-year-old female with exertional chest pain, intermittent claudication, syncope and a murmur of aortic stenosis. (Cardiology)

Initial office evaluation, patient with systemic lupus erythematosus, fever, seizures and profound thrombocytopenia.
(Allergy & Immunology/Internal Medicine/Rheumatology)

Initial office visit for a 24-year-old homosexual male who has a fever, a cough, and shortness of breath.
(Infectious Disease)

Initial office visit for a 17-year-old female, who is having school problems and has told a friend she is considering suicide. The patient and her family are consulted in regards to treatment options.
(Psychiatry)

Initial office visit for a female with severe hirsutism, amenorrhea, weight loss and a desire to have children.
(Endocrinology/Obstetrics & Gynecology)

Initial office visit for a 73-year-old male with an unexplained 20-pound weight loss. (Hematology/Oncology)

Initial office evaluation and management of patient with systemic vasculitis and compromised circulation to the limbs. (Rheumatology)

Initial outpatient evaluation of a 69-year-old male with severe chronic obstructive pulmonary disease, congestive heart failure, and hypertension. (Family Medicine)

Initial office visit for a 42-year-old male on hypertensive medication, newly arrived to the area, with diastolic blood pressure of 110, history of recurrent renal calculi, episodic headaches, intermittent chest pain and orthopnea.
(Internal Medicine)

ESTABLISHED PATIENT

The following codes are used to report the evaluation and management services provided to established patients who present for follow-up and/or periodic reevaluation of problems or for the evaluation and management of new problem(s) in established patients.

99211 Office or other outpatient visit for the evaluation and management of an established patient, that may not require the presence of a physician.

Usually, the presenting problem(s) are minimal.

Typically, 5 minutes are spent performing or supervising these services.

Examples

Outpatient visit with 19-year-old male, established patient, for supervised drug screen. (Addiction Medicine)

Office visit with 31-year-old female, established patient, for return to work certificate. (Anesthesiology)

Office visit for 14-year-old established patient to re-dress an abrasion. (Orthopaedic Surgery)

Office visit for a 23-year-old established patient for instruction in use of peak flow meter. (Allergy & Immunology)

Office visit with 12-year-old male, established patient, for cursory check of hematoma one day after venipuncture. (Internal Medicine)

Office visit for a 42-year-old established patient to read tuberculin test results. (Allergy & Immunology)

Office visit for a 45-year-old female, established patient, for a blood pressure check. (Obstetrics & Gynecology)

Office visit for prescription refill for a 35-year-old female, established patient, with schizophrenia who is stable but has run out of neuroleptic and is scheduled to be seen in a week. (Psychiatry)

99212 Office or other outpatient visit for the evaluation and management of an established patient, which requires at least two of these three key components:

- **a problem focused history;**
- **a problem focused examination;**
- **straightforward medical decision making.**

Counseling and/or coordination of care with other providers or agencies are provided consistent with the nature of the problem(s) and the patient's and/or family's needs.

Usually, the presenting problem(s) are self limited or minor. Physicians typically spend 10 minutes face-to-face with the patient and/or family.

Examples

Office visit, established patient, 6-year-old child with sore throat and headache.
(Family Medicine/Pediatrics)

Office visit with 65-year-old female, established patient, returns for 3 week follow-up for resolving severe ankle sprain. (Orthopaedic Surgery)

Office visit with 33-year-old female, established patient, recently started on treatment for hemorrhoidal complaints, for re-evaluation.
(Colon & Rectal Surgery)

Office visit for 27-year-old female, established patient, with complaints of vaginal itching.
(Obstetrics & Gynecology)

Office evaluation for possible purulent bacterial conjunctivitis with 1-2 day history of redness and discharge, 16-year-old female, established patient. (Pediatrics/ Internal Medicine/Family Medicine)

Office visit, sore throat, fever and fatigue in 19-year-old college student, established patient.
(Internal Medicine)

Office visit with 36-year-old male, established patient, for follow-up on effectiveness of medicine management of oral candidiasis.
(Oral & Maxillofacial Surgery)

Office visit for a 65-year-old male, established patient, with eruptions on both arms from poison oak exposure. (Allergy & Immunology/ Internal Medicine)

99213 Office or other outpatient visit for the evaluation and management of an established patient, which requires at least two of these three key components:

- **an expanded problem focused history;**
- **an expanded problem focused examination;**
- **medical decision making of low complexity.**

Counseling and coordination of care with other providers or agencies are provided consistent with the nature of the problem(s) and the patient's and/or family's needs.

Usually, the presenting problem(s) are of low to moderate severity. Physicians typically spend 15 minutes face-to-face with the patient and/or family.

Examples

Office visit with 55-year-old male, established patient, for management of hypertension, mild fatigue, on beta blocker/thiazide regimen.
(Family Medicine/Internal Medicine)

Outpatient visit with 37-year-old male, established patient, who is 3 years post total colectomy for chronic ulcerative colitis, presents for increased irritation at his stoma.
(General Surgery)

Office visit for a 70-year-old diabetic hypertensive established patient with recent change in insulin requirement.
(Internal Medicine/Nephrology)

Office visit for an established patient with stable cirrhosis of the liver.
(Gastroenterology)

Quarterly follow-up office visit for a 45-year-old male, with stable chronic asthma, on steroid and bronchodilator therapy.
(Pulmonary Medicine)

Office visit with 80-year-old female established patient, for follow-up osteoporosis, status-post compression fractures.
(Rheumatology)

Routine, follow-up office evaluation at a three-month interval for a 77-year-old female with nodular small cleaved-cell lymphoma.
(Hematology/Oncology)

Office visit for a 50-year-old female, established patient, with insulin-dependent diabetes mellitus and stable coronary artery disease, for monitoring.
(Family Medicine/Internal Medicine)

99214 Office or other outpatient visit for the evaluation and management of an established patient, which requires at least two of these three key components:

- **a detailed history;**
- **a detailed examination;**
- **medical decision making of moderate complexity.**

Counseling and/or coordination of care with other providers or agencies are provided consistent with the nature of the problem(s) and the patient's and/or family's needs.

Usually, the presenting problem(s) are of moderate to high severity. Physicians typically spend 25 minutes face-to-face with the patient and/or family.

Examples

Office visit for a 68-year-old male, established patient, with stable angina, two months post myocardial infarction, who is not tolerating one of his medications. (Cardiology)

Follow-up office visit for a 60-year-old male, established patient, whose post-traumatic seizures have disappeared on medication, and who now raises the question of stopping the medication
(Neurology)

Weekly office visit for 5FU therapy for an ambulatory established patient with metastatic colon cancer and increasing shortness of breath.
(Hematology/Oncology)

Office evaluation on new onset RLQ pain in a 32-year-old woman, established patient.
(Urology/General Surgery/Internal Medicine/Family Medicine)

Office evaluation of 28-year-old established patient with regional enteritis, diarrhea and low grade fever. (Family Medicine/Internal Medicine)

Follow-up office visit for a 45-year-old established patient with rheumatoid arthritis on gold, methotrexate, or immunosuppressive therapy. (Rheumatology)

Office visit for 60-year-old male, established patient, 2 years post-removal of intracranial meningioma, now with new headaches and visual disturbance. (Neurosurgery)

Office visit with 50-year-old female, established patient, diabetic, blood sugar controlled by diet. She now complains of frequency of urination and weight loss, blood sugar of 320 and negative ketones on dipstick. (Internal Medicine)

Office visit with 63-year-old female, established patient, with familial polyposis, after a previous colectomy and sphincter sparing procedure, now with tenesmus, mucus, and increased stool frequency. (Colon & Rectal Surgery)

Office visit for a 68-year-old female, established patient, for routine review and follow-up of non-insulin dependent diabetes, obesity, hypertension and congestive heart failure. Complains of vision difficulties and admits dietary noncompliance. Patient is counseled concerning diet and current medications adjusted. (Family Medicine)

99215 Office or other outpatient visit for the evaluation and management of an established patient, which requires at least two of these three key components:

- **a comprehensive history;**
- **a comprehensive examination;**
- **medical decision making of high complexity.**

Counseling and/or coordination of care with other providers or agencies are provided consistent with the nature of the problem(s) and the patient's and/or family's needs.

Usually, the presenting problem(s) are of moderate to high severity. Physicians typically spend 40 minutes face-to-face with the patient and/or family.

Examples

Office visit with 30-year-old male, established patient for 3 month history of fatigue, weight loss, intermittent fever, and presenting with diffuse adenopathy and splenomegaly. (Family Medicine)

Office visit for restaging of an established patient with new lymphadenopathy one year post-therapy for lymphoma. (Hematology/Oncology)

Office visit for evaluation of recent onset syncopal attacks in a 70-year-old woman, established patient. (Internal Medicine)

Office evaluation and discussion of treatment options for a 68-year-old male, established patient, with a biopsy-proven rectal carcinoma. (General Surgery)

Office visit for a 75-year-old patient with ALS (amyotrophic lateral sclerosis), who is no longer able to swallow. (Neurology)

Office visit, 40-year-old mother of 3, established patient, with acute rheumatoid arthritis, anatomical Stage 3, ARA function Class 3 rheumatoid arthritis, and deteriorating function. (Rheumatology)

Office visit for a 65-year-old male, established patient, with a fever of recent onset while on outpatient antibiotic therapy for endocarditis. (Infectious Disease)

Office visit for a 70-year-old female, established patient, with diabetes mellitus and hypertension, presenting with a 2 month history of increasing confusion, agitation and short-term memory loss. (Family Medicine/Internal Medicine)

Hospital Observation Services

The following codes are used to report evaluation and management services provided to patients designated/admitted as "observation status" in a hospital. It is not necessary that the patient be located in an observation area designated by the hospital. If such an area does exist in a hospital (as a separate unit in the hospital, in the emergency department, etc.), these codes are to be utilized if the patient is placed in such an area.

For definitions of key components and commonly used terms, please see Evaluation and Management Services Guidelines.

Typical times have not yet been established for this category of services.

INITIAL OBSERVATION CARE

NEW OR ESTABLISHED PATIENT

The following codes are used to report the first encounter with the patient when designated as "observation status." For initial observation encounters by physicians other than the admitting physician, see office or other outpatient consultation codes (99241-99245).

To report services provided to a patient who is admitted to the hospital after receiving hospital observation care services on the same date, see the notes for initial hospital inpatient care (page 25). For a patient admitted to the hospital on a date subsequent to the date of observation status, the hospital admission would be reported with the appropriate initial hospital care codes (99221-99223). Do not report observation discharge in conjunction with the hospital admission.

When the patient is admitted to "observation status" in the course of an encounter in another site of service (eg, hospital emergency department, physician's office, nursing facility) all evaluation and management services provided by that physician in conjunction with admission to "observation status" are considered part of the initial observation care when performed on the same date as admission to "observation status." The observation care level of service reported by the admitting physician should include the services related to admission to "observation status" he/she provided in the other sites of service as well as in the observation setting. Evaluation and management services on the same date provided in sites other than the hospital that are related to admission to "observation status" should NOT be reported separately.

These codes may not be utilized for post-operative recovery if the procedure is considered a global surgical procedure. These codes apply to all physician services that are provided on the same date of patient admission to "observation status."

● **99218** Initial observation care, per day, for the evaluation and management of a patient which requires these three key components:

- **a detailed or comprehensive history;**
- **a detailed or comprehensive examination; and**
- **medical decision making that is straightforward or of low complexity.**

Counseling and/or coordination of care with other providers or agencies are provided consistent with the nature of the problem(s) and the patient's and/or family's needs.

Usually, the problem(s) requiring admission to "observation status" are of low severity.

● **99219** Initial observation care, per day, for the evaluation and management of a patient, which requires these three key components:

- **a comprehensive history;**
- **a comprehensive examination; and**
- **medical decision making of moderate complexity.**

Counseling and/or coordination of care with other providers or agencies are provided consistent with the nature of the problem(s) and the patient's and/or family's needs.

Usually, the problem(s) requiring admission to "observation status" are of moderate severity.

● **99220** Initial observation care, per day, for the evaluation and management of a patient, which requires these three key components:

- **a comprehensive history;**
- **a comprehensive examination; and**
- **medical decision making of high complexity.**

Counseling and/or coordination of care with other providers or agencies are provided consistent with the nature of the problem(s) and the patient's and/or family's needs.

Usually, the problem(s) requiring admission to "observation status" are of high severity.

Hospital Inpatient Services

The following codes are used to report evaluation and management services provided to hospital inpatients. Hospital inpatient services include those services provided to patients in a 'partial hospital' setting. These codes are to be used to report these partial hospitalization services. See also psychiatry notes in the full text of CPT.

For definitions of key components and commonly used terms, please see Evaluation and Management Services Guidelines. For hospital observation services, see 99218-99220.

INITIAL HOSPITAL CARE

NEW OR ESTABLISHED PATIENT

The following codes are used to report the first hospital inpatient encounter with the patient by the admitting physician. For initial inpatient encounters by physicians other than the admitting physician, see initial inpatient consultation codes (99251-99255) or subsequent hospital care codes (99231-99233) as appropriate.

When the patient is admitted to the hospital as an inpatient in the course of an encounter in another site of service (eg, hospital emergency department, observation status in a hospital, physician's office, nursing facility) all evaluation and management services provided by that physician in conjunction with that admission are considered part of the initial hospital care when performed on the same date as the admission. The inpatient care level of service reported by the admitting physician should include the services related to the admission he/she provided in the other sites of service as well as in the inpatient setting.

Evaluation and management services on the same date provided in sites other than the hospital that are related to the admission should NOT be reported separately.

▲99221 Initial hospital care, per day, for the evaluation and management of a patient which requires these three key components:

- **a detailed or comprehensive history;**
- **a detailed or comprehensive examination; and**
- **medical decision making that is straightforward or of low complexity.**

Counseling and/or coordination of care with other providers or agencies are provided consistent with the nature of the problem(s) and the patient's and/or family's needs.

Usually, the problem(s) requiring admission are of low severity. Physicians typically spend 30 minutes at the bedside and on the patient's hospital floor or unit.

Examples

Hospital admission, examination, and initiation of treatment program for a 67-year-old male with uncomplicated pneumonia who requires IV antibiotic therapy. (Internal Medicine)

Initial hospital visit for a 12-year-old with a laceration of the upper eyelid involving the lid margin and superior canaliculus, admitted prior to surgery for IV antibiotic therapy. (Ophthalmology)

Initial hospital visit for a patient with several large venous stasis ulcers not responding to outpatient therapy. (Dermatology)

Initial hospital visit for a 73-year-old female with acute pyelonephritis who is otherwise generally healthy. (Geriatrics)

Hospital admission for an 18-month-old child with 10 percent dehydration. (Pediatrics)

Hospital admission for a 32-year-old female with severe flank pain, hematuria and presumed diagnosis of ureteral calculus as determined by Emergency Department physician. (Urology)

Initial hospital visit for 21-year-old pregnant patient (9 weeks gestation) with hyperemesis gravidarum. (Obstetrics & Gynecology)

Initial hospital visit for 62-year-old patient with cellulitis of the foot requiring bedrest and intravenous antibiotics. (Orthopaedic Surgery)

99222 Initial hospital care, per day, for the evaluation and management of a patient, which requires these three key components:

- **a comprehensive history;**
- **a comprehensive examination; and**
- **medical decision making of moderate complexity.**

Counseling and/or coordination of care with other providers or agencies are provided consistent with the nature of the problem(s) and the patient's and/or family's needs.

Usually, the problem(s) requiring admission are of moderate severity. Physicians typically spend 50 minutes at the bedside and on the patient's hospital floor or unit.

Examples

Hospital admission, young adult patient, failed previous therapy and now presents in acute asthmatic attack.
(Family Medicine/Allergy & Immunology)

Hospital admission, examination, and initiation of a treatment program for a 65-year-old female with new onset of right-sided paralysis and aphasia. (Neurology)

Hospital admission, examination, and initiation of treatment program for a 66-year-old chronic hemodialysis patient with fever and a new pulmonary infiltrate.
(Nephrology)

Initial hospital visit for an 8-year-old febrile patient with chronic sinusitis and severe headache, unresponsive to oral antibiotics.
(Allergy & Immunology)

Hospital admission of a 62-year-old smoker, established patient, with bronchitis in acute respiratory distress. (Internal Medicine/ Pulmonary Medicine)

Hospital admission for a 50-year-old with left lower quadrant abdominal pain and increased temperature, but without septic picture.
(General Surgery)

Hospital admission for a 3-year-old with high temperature, limp and painful hip motion of 18 hours duration. (Orthopaedic Surgery)

Initial hospital visit for a 40-year-old male with submaxillary cellulitis and trismus from infected lower molar.
(Oral & Maxillofacial Surgery)

99223 Initial hospital care, per day, for the evaluation and management of a patient, which requires these three key components:

- **a comprehensive history;**
- **a comprehensive examination; and**
- **medical decision making of high complexity.**

Counseling and/or coordination of care with other providers or agencies are provided consistent with the nature of the problem(s) and the patient's and/or family's needs.

Usually, the problem(s) requiring admission are of high severity. Physicians typically spend 70 minutes at the bedside and on the patient's hospital floor or unit.

Examples

Hospital admission, examination, and initiation of treatment program for a previously unknown 58-year-old male who presents with acute chest pain. (Cardiology)

Hospital admission following a motor vehicle accident of a 24-year-old male with fracture dislocation of C5-6; neurologically intact. (Neurosurgery)

Hospital admission, examination, and initiation of treatment program for a 65-year-old immunosuppressed male with confusion, fever, and a headache. (Infectious Disease)

Initial hospital visit for a 65-year-old male who presents with acute myocardial infarction, oliguria, hypotension, and altered state of consciousness. (Cardiology)

Initial hospital visit for 89-year-old female with fulminant hepatic failure and encephalopathy. (Gastroenterology)

Hospital admission, examination, and initiation of induction chemotherapy for a 42-year-old patient with newly diagnosed acute myelogenous leukemia. (Hematology/Oncology)

Hospital admission for a 78-year-old female with left lower lobe pneumonia and a history of coronary artery disease, congestive heart failure, osteoarthritis and gout. (Family Medicine)

Hospital admission for a 9-year-old with vomiting, dehydration, fever, tachypnea and an admitting diagnosis of diabetic ketoacidosis. (Pediatrics)

Initial hospital visit for a hostile/ resistant adolescent patient who is severely depressed and involved in poly-substance abuse. Patient is experiencing significant conflict in his chaotic family situation and was suspended from school following an attack on a teacher with a baseball bat. (Psychiatry)

Initial hospital visit for a 42-year-old female with rapidly progressing scleroderma, malignant hypertension, digital infarcts, and oligourea. (Rheumatology)

SUBSEQUENT HOSPITAL CARE

All levels of subsequent hospital care include reviewing the medical record and reviewing the results of diagnostic studies and changes in the patient's status, (ie, changes in history, physical condition and response to management) since the last assessment by the physician.

99231 Subsequent hospital care, per day, for the evaluation and management of a patient, which requires at least two of these three key components:

- **a problem focused interval history;**
- **a problem focused examination;**
- **medical decision making that is straightforward or of low complexity.**

Counseling and/or coordination of care with other providers or agencies are provided consistent with the nature of the problem(s) and the patient's and/or family's needs.

Usually, the patient is stable, recovering or improving. Physicians typically spend 15 minutes at the bedside and on the patient's hospital floor or unit.

Examples

Subsequent hospital visit for a 50-year-old male with uncomplicated myocardial infarction who is clinically stable and without chest pain. (Family Medicine/Cardiology/Internal Medicine)

Subsequent hospital visit, two days post admission for a 65-year-old male with a CVA (cerebral vascular accident) and left hemiparesis, who is clinically stable. (Neurology/Physical Medicine & Rehabilitation)

Subsequent visit on third day of hospitalization for a 60-year-old female recovering from an uncomplicated pneumonia. (Infectious Disease/Internal Medicine/Pulmonary Medicine)

Subsequent hospital visit for a 4-year-old female, admitted for acute gastroenteritis and dehydration, requiring IV hydration; now stable. (Family Medicine/Internal Medicine)

Subsequent hospital visit for a stable 72-year-old lung cancer patient undergoing a five day course of infusion chemotherapy. (Hematology/Oncology)

Subsequent hospital visit for now stable, 33-year-old male, status post lower gastrointestinal bleeding. (General Surgery)

Subsequent hospital visit for a 3-year-old patient in traction for a congenital dislocation of the hip. (Orthopaedic Surgery)

Subsequent hospital visit for 50-year-old female with resolving uncomplicated acute pancreatitis. (Gastroenterology)

99232 Subsequent hospital care, per day, for the evaluation and management of a patient, which requires at least two of these three key components:

- **an expanded problem focused interval history;**
- **an expanded problem focused examination;**
- **medical decision making of moderate complexity.**

Counseling and/or coordination of care with other providers or agencies are provided consistent with the nature of the problem(s) and the patient's and/or family's needs.

Usually, the patient is responding inadequately to therapy or has developed a minor complication. Physicians typically spend 25 minutes at the bedside and on the patient's hospital floor or unit.

Examples

Subsequent hospital visit for a 54-year-old patient, post MI (myocardial infarction), who is out of the CCU (coronary care unit) but is now having frequent premature ventricular contractions on telemetry. (Cardiology/Internal Medicine)

Subsequent hospital visit for a 50-year-old male admitted two days ago for sub-acute renal allograft rejection. (Nephrology)

Subsequent hospital visit of a 81-year-old male with abdominal distention, nausea, and vomiting. (General Surgery)

Subsequent hospital visit for a 73-year-old female with recently diagnosed lung cancer, who complains of unsteady gait. (Pulmonary Medicine)

Subsequent hospital visit for 13-year-old male admitted with left lower quadrant abdominal pain and fever, not responding to therapy. (General Surgery)

Subsequent hospital visit for a patient with neutropenia, a fever responding to antibiotics, and continued slow gastrointestinal bleeding on platelet support. (Hematology/Oncology)

Subsequent hospital visit for a 35-year-old drug addict, not responding to initial antibiotic therapy for pyelonephritis. (Urology)

Subsequent hospital care for a 62-year-old female with congestive heart failure, who remains dyspneic and febrile. (Internal Medicine)

Subsequent hospital visit for a 20-month-old male with bacterial meningitis treated 1 week with antibiotic therapy; has now developed a temperature of 101.0°. (Pediatrics)

Subsequent hospital visit for a 65-year-old male with hemiplegia and painful paretic shoulder. (Physical Medicine & Rehabilitation)

99233 Subsequent hospital care, per day, for the evaluation and management of a patient, which requires at least two of these three key components:

- **a detailed interval history;**
- **a detailed examination;**
- **medical decision making of high complexity.**

Counseling and/or coordination of care with other providers or agencies are provided consistent with the nature of the problem(s) and the patient's and/or family's needs.

Usually, the patient is unstable or has developed a significant complication or a significant new problem. Physicians typically spend 35 minutes at the bedside and on the patient's hospital floor or unit.

Examples

Subsequent hospital visit for a 60-year-old female, 4 days post uncomplicated inferior myocardial infarction who has developed severe chest pain, dyspnea, diaphoresis and nausea. (Family Medicine)

Subsequent hospital visit for a 38-year-old quadriplegic male with acute autonomic hyperreflexia, who is not responsive to initial care. (Physical Medicine & Rehabilitation)

Subsequent hospital visit for a 60-year-old female with persistent leukocytosis and a fever seven days after a sigmoid colon resection for carcinoma. (Infectious Disease)

Subsequent hospital visit for a 65-year-old male with acute myocardial infarction who now demonstrates complete heart block and congestive heart failure. (Cardiology)

Subsequent hospital visit for a 55-year-old male with severe chronic obstructive pulmonary disease and bronchospasm; initially admitted for acute respiratory distress requiring ventilatory support in the ICU. The patient was stabilized, extubated and transferred to the floor, but has now developed acute fever, dyspnea, left lower lobe rhonchi and laboratory evidence of carbon dioxide retention and hypoxemia. (Family Medicine/Internal Medicine)

Subsequent hospital visit for a patient with AML (acute myelogenous leukemia), fever, elevated white count and uric acid undergoing induction chemotherapy. (Hematology/Oncology)

Subsequent hospital visit for a 65-year-old female post-op resection of abdominal aortic aneurysm, with suspected ischemic bowel. (General Surgery)

Subsequent hospital visit for a chronic renal failure patient on dialysis, who develops chest pain, shortness of breath and new onset of pericardial friction rub. (Nephrology)

Subsequent hospital visit for a 25-year-old female with hypertension and systemic lupus erythmatosus, admitted for fever and respiratory distress. On the third hospital day, the patient presented with purpuric skin lesions and acute renal failure. (Rheumatology)

Subsequent hospital visit for 46-year-old female, known liver cirrhosis patient, with recent upper gastrointestinal hemorrhage from varices; now with worsening ascites and encephalopathy. (Gastroenterology)

Subsequent hospital visit for 62-year-old female admitted with acute subarachnoid hemorrhage, negative cerebral arteriogram, increased lethargy and hemiparesis with fever. (Neurosurgery)

HOSPITAL DISCHARGE SERVICES

Final hospital discharge or observation care discharge of a patient from "observation status" includes final examination of the patient, discussion of the hospital stay, instructions for continuing care, and preparation of discharge records.

99238 Hospital discharge day management

(This code is to be utilized by the physician to report all services provided to a patient on the date of discharge if other than the initial date of inpatient or observation status. To report services to a patient who is admitted as an inpatient, or designated observation status, and discharged on the same date use only the codes for Initial Hospital Inpatient Services, 99221-99223, or Initial Observation Services, 99218-99220, as appropriate.)

Consultations

A consultation is a type of service provided by a physician whose opinion or advice regarding evaluation and/or management of a specific problem is requested by another physician or other appropriate source.

A physician consultant may initiate diagnostic and/or therapeutic services.

The request for a consultation from the attending physician or other appropriate source and the need for consultation must be documented in the patient's medical record. The consultant's opinion and any services that were ordered or performed must also be documented in the patient's medical record and communicated to the requesting physician or other appropriate source.

A "consultation" initiated by a patient and/or family, and not requested by a physician, is not reported using the initial consultation codes but may be reported using the codes for confirmatory consultation or office visits, as appropriate. If a confirmatory consultation is required, eg, by a third party payor, the modifier -32 or 09932, mandated services, should also be reported.

Any specifically identifiable procedure (ie, identified with a specific CPT code) performed on or subsequent to the date of the initial consultation should be reported separately.

If subsequent to the completion of a consultation, the consultant assumes responsibility for management of a portion or all of the patient's condition(s), the follow-up consultation codes should not be used. In the hospital setting, the physician receiving the patient for partial or complete transfer of care should use the appropriate inpatient hospital consultation code for the initial encounter and then subsequent hospital care codes (not follow-up consultation codes). In the office setting, the appropriate established patient code should be used.

There are four subcategories of consultations: office, initial inpatient, follow-up inpatient, and confirmatory. See each subcategory for specific reporting instructions.

For definitions of key components and commonly used terms, please see Evaluation and Management Services Guidelines.

OFFICE OR OTHER OUTPATIENT CONSULTATIONS

NEW OR ESTABLISHED PATIENT

The following codes are used to report consultations provided in the physician's office or in an outpatient or other ambulatory facility, including hospital observation services, home services, domiciliary, rest home, custodial care, or emergency department (See consultation definition, page 32).

Follow-up visits in the consultant's office or other outpatient facility that are initiated by the physician consultant are reported using office visit codes for established patients (99211-99215). If an additional request for an opinion or advice regarding the same or a new problem is received from the attending physician and documented in the medical record, the office consultation codes may be used again.

99241 Office consultation for a new or established patient, which requires these three key components:

- **a problem focused history;**
- **a problem focused examination; and**
- **straightforward medical decision making.**

Counseling and/or coordination of care with other providers or agencies are provided consistent with the nature of the problem(s) and the patient's and/or family's needs.

Usually, the presenting problem(s) are self limited or minor. Physicians typically spend 15 minutes face-to-face with the patient and/or family.

Examples

Initial office consultation with 25-year-old postpartum female with severe symptomatic hemorrhoids. (Colon & Rectal Surgery)

Initial office consultation for 30-year-old female tennis player with sprain or contusion of the forearm. (Orthopaedic Surgery)

Office consultation with 58-year-old male, referred for follow-up of creatinine level and evaluation of obstructive uropathy, relieved two months ago. (Nephrology)

Initial office consultation for a 45-year-old male, requested by his internist, with asymptomatic torus palatinus requiring no further treatment.
(Oral & Maxillofacial Surgery)

99242 Office consultation for a new or established patient, which requires these three key components:

- **an expanded problem focused history;**
- **an expanded problem focused examination; and**
- **straightforward medical decision making.**

Counseling and/or coordination of care with other providers or agencies are provided consistent with the nature of the problem(s) and the patient(s) and/or family's needs.

Usually, the presenting problem(s) are of low severity. Physicians typically spend 30 minutes face-to-face with the patient and/or family.

Examples

Office consultation for management of systolic hypertension in a 70-year-old male scheduled for elective prostate resection.
(Geriatrics)

Office consultation with 66-year-old female with wrist and hand pain, and finger numbness, secondary to suspected carpal tunnel syndrome.
(Orthopaedic Surgery)

Initial office consultation for a patient with papulosquamous eruption of elbow with pitting of nails and itchy scalp. (Dermatology)

Office consultation with 27-year-old female, with old amputation, for evaluation of existing above-knee prosthesis.
(Physical Medicine & Rehabilitation)

Initial office consultation for 61-year-old female, recently on antibiotic therapy, now with diarrhea and leukocytosis.
(Abdominal Surgery)

Initial office consultation for a 30-year-old female with single season allergic rhinitis.
(Allergy & Immunology)

99243 Office consultation for a new or established patient, which requires these three key components:

- **a detailed history;**
- **a detailed examination; and**
- **medical decision making of low complexity.**

Counseling and/or coordination of care with other providers or agencies are provided consistent with the nature of the problem(s) and the patient's and/or family's needs.

Usually, the presenting problem(s) are of moderate severity. Physicians typically spend 40 minutes face-to-face with the patient and/or family.

Examples

Office consultation for a 65-year-old female with persistent bronchitis. (Infectious Disease)

Office consultation for 23-year-old female with Crohn's disease not responding to therapy. (Abdominal Surgery/Colon & Rectal Surgery)

Office consultation for a 67-year-old patient with osteoporosis and mandibular atrophy with regard to reconstructive alternatives. (Oral & Maxillofacial Surgery)

Office consultation for a 65-year-old man with chronic low-back pain radiating to the leg. (Neurosurgery)

Office consultation for 25-year-old patient with symptomatic knee pain and swelling, with torn anterior cruciate ligament and/or torn meniscus. (Orthopaedic Surgery)

Office consultation for 39-year-old patient referred at a perimenopausal age for irregular menses and menopausal symptoms. (Obstetrics & Gynecology)

99244 Office consultation for a new or established patient, which requires these three key components:

- **a comprehensive history;**
- **a comprehensive examination; and**
- **medical decision making of moderate complexity.**

Counseling and/or coordination of care with other providers or agencies are provided consistent with the nature of the problem(s) and the patient's and/or family's needs.

Usually, the presenting problem(s) are of moderate to high severity. Physicians typically spend 60 minutes face-to-face with the patient and/or family.

Examples

Office consultation with 38-year-old female, with inflammatory bowel disease, who now presents with right lower quadrant pain and suspected intra-abdominal abscess.
(General Surgery/Colon & Rectal Surgery)

Office consultation for discussion of treatment options for a 40-year-old female with a two-centimeter adenocarcinoma of the breast.
(Radiation Oncology)

Office consultation for 66-year-old female, history of colon resection for adenocarcinoma 6 years earlier, now with severe mid-back pain; x-rays showing osteoporosis and multiple vertebral compression fractures.
(Neurosurgery)

Office consultation with 72-year-old male with esophageal carcinoma, symptoms of dysphagia and reflux.
(Thoracic Surgery)

Office consultation for young patient referred by pediatrician because of patient's short attention span, easy distractibility and hyperactivity.
(Psychiatry)

Office consultation for a patient with chronic pelvic inflammatory disease who now has left lower quadrant pain with a palpable pelvic mass.
(Obstetrics & Gynecology)

Office consultation for a patient with long-standing psoriasis with acute onset of erythroderma, pustular lesions, chills and fever. Combinations of topical and systemic treatments discussed and instituted. (Dermatology)

99245 Office consultation for a new or established patient, which requires these three key components:

- **a comprehensive history;**
- **a comprehensive examination; and**
- **medical decision making of high complexity.**

Counseling and/or coordination of care with other providers or agencies are provided consistent with the nature of the problem(s) and the patient's and/or family's needs.

Usually, the presenting problem(s) are of moderate to high severity. Physicians typically spend 80 minutes face-to-face with the patient and/or family.

Examples

Consultation in the emergency room for a 25-year-old male with severe, acute, closed head injury.
(Neurosurgery)

Office consultation for a 23-year-old female with Stage II A Hodgkins disease with positive supraclavicular and mediastinal nodes.
(Radiation Oncology)

Office consultation for a 27-year-old juvenile diabetic patient with severe diabetic retinopathy, gastric atony, nephrotic syndrome and progressive renal failure, now with a serum creatinine of 2.7, and a blood pressure of 170/114. (Nephrology)

Outpatient consultation for a 67-year-old male with a negative past ophthalmic history is referred with a 3-day history of a red, painful eye with blurred vision due to acute angle closure glaucoma. The patient is dehydrated from nausea and vomiting. (Ophthalmology)

Office consultation for a 6-year-old male for evaluation of severe muscle and joint pain and a diffuse rash. Well until 4-6 weeks earlier when he developed arthralgia, myalgias, and a fever of 102° for 1 week. (Rheumatology)

Office consultation for independent medical evaluation of a patient with a history of complicated low back and neck problems with previous multiple failed back surgeries. (Orthopaedic Surgery)

Office consultation for adolescent referred by pediatrician for recent onset of violent and self-injurious behavior. (Psychiatry)

INITIAL INPATIENT CONSULTATIONS

NEW OR ESTABLISHED PATIENT

The following codes are used to report physician consultations provided to hospital inpatients, residents of nursing facilities, or patients in a partial hospital setting. Only one initial consultation should be reported by a consultant per admission.

99251 Initial inpatient consultation for a new or established patient, which requires these three key components:

- **a problem focused history;**
- **a problem focused examination; and**
- **straightforward medical decision making.**

Counseling and/or coordination of care with other providers or agencies are provided consistent with the nature of the problem(s) and the patient's and/or family's needs.

Usually, the presenting problem(s) are self limited or minor. Physicians typically spend 20 minutes at the bedside and on the patient's hospital floor or unit.

Examples

Initial inpatient consultation for a 30-year-old female complaining of vaginal itching, post orthopaedic surgery. (Obstetrics & Gynecology)

Initial inpatient consultation for a 36-year-old male on orthopaedic service with complaint of localized dental pain.
(Oral & Maxillofacial Surgery)

99252 Initial inpatient consultation for a new or established patient, which requires these three key components:

- **an expanded problem focused history;**
- **an expanded problem focused examination; and**
- **straightforward medical decision making.**

Counseling and/or coordination of care with other providers or agencies are provided consistent with the nature of the problem(s) and the patient's and/or family's needs.

Usually, the presenting problem(s) are of low severity. Physicians typically spend 40 minutes at the bedside and on the patient's hospital floor or unit.

Examples

Initial inpatient consultation for recommendation of antibiotic prophylaxis for a patient with a synthetic heart valve who will undergo urologic surgery.
(Internal Medicine)

Initial inpatient consultation for evaluation of hypertension in a 60-year-old male who will undergo a cholecystectomy. Patient had a normal annual check-up in your office four months ago.
(Internal Medicine)

Initial inpatient consultation for a 66-year-old male smoker referred for pain management immediately status post-biliary tract surgery done via sub-costal incision.
(Anesthesiology/Pain Medicine)

Initial inpatient consultation for possible drug eruption in 50-year-old male. (Dermatology)

Initial inpatient consultation for 66-year-old patient with wrist and hand pain and finger numbness, secondary to carpal tunnel syndrome. (Orthopaedic Surgery/Plastic Surgery)

Initial inpatient consultation for a 45-year-old male previously abstinent alcoholic, who relapsed and was admitted for management of gastritis. The patient readily accepts the need for further treatment. (Addiction Medicine)

99253 Initial inpatient consultation for a new or established patient, which requires these three key components:

- **a detailed history;**
- **a detailed examination; and**
- **medical decision making of low complexity.**

Counseling and/or coordination of care with other providers or agencies are provided consistent with the nature of the problem(s) and the patient's and/or family's needs.

Usually, the presenting problem(s) are of moderate severity. Physicians typically spend 55 minutes at the bedside and on the patient's hospital floor or unit.

Examples

Initial inpatient consultation for a 57-year-old male, post lower endoscopy, for evaluation of abdominal pain and fever. (General Surgery)

Initial inpatient consultation for diagnosis/management of fever following abdominal surgery. (Internal Medicine)

Initial inpatient consultation for a 42-year-old non-diabetic patient, post-op cholecystectomy, now with an acute urinary tract infection. (Nephrology)

Initial inpatient consultation for 45-year-old patient with chronic neck pain with radicular pain of the left arm. (Orthopaedic Surgery)

Initial inpatient consultation for rehabilitation of a 73-year-old female one week after surgical management of a hip fracture. (Physical Medicine & Rehabilitation)

Initial inpatient consultation for a 35-year-old female with a fever and pulmonary infiltrate following caesarean section. (Pulmonary Medicine)

Initial inpatient consultation for 53-year-old female with moderate uncomplicated pancreatitis. (Gastroenterology)

Initial inpatient consultation for 8-year-old patient with new onset of seizures who has a normal examination and previous history. (Neurology)

99254 Initial inpatient consultation for a new or established patient, which requires three key components:

- **a comprehensive history;**
- **a comprehensive examination; and**
- **medical decision making of moderate complexity.**

Counseling and/or coordination of care with other providers or agencies are provided consistent with the nature of the problem(s) and the patient's and/or family's needs.

Usually, the presenting problem(s) are of moderate to high severity. Physicians typically spend 80 minutes at the bedside and on the patient's hospital floor or unit.

Examples

Initial inpatient consultation of a 63-year-old in the ICU with diabetes and chronic renal failure who develops acute respiratory distress syndrome 36 hours after a mitral valve replacement. (Anesthesiology)

Initial inpatient consultation for a 43-year-old female for evaluation of sudden painful visual loss, optic neuritis and episodic paresthesia. (Ophthalmology)

Initial hospital consultation for a 72-year-old male with emergency admission for possible bowel obstruction. (Internal Medicine/General Surgery)

Initial inpatient consultation for a 66-year-old female with enlarged supraclavicular lymph nodes, found on biopsy to be malignant. (Hematology/Oncology)

Initial inpatient consultation for evaluation of a 71-year-old male with hyponatremia (serum sodium 114) who was admitted to the hospital with pneumonia. (Nephrology)

Initial inpatient consultation for a 35-year-old female with fever, swollen joints, and rash of 1 week duration. (Rheumatology)

99255 Initial inpatient consultation for a new or established patient, which requires these three key components:

- **a comprehensive history;**
- **a comprehensive examination; and**
- **medical decision making of high complexity.**

Counseling and/or coordination of care with other providers or agencies are provided consistent with the nature of the problem(s) and the patient's and/or family's needs.

Usually, the presenting problem(s) are of moderate to high severity. Physicians typically spend 110 minutes at the bedside and on the patient's hospital floor or unit.

Examples

Initial inpatient consultation in the ICU for a 70-year-old male who experienced a cardiac arrest during surgery and was resuscitated. (Cardiology)

Initial inpatient consultation for a patient with severe pancreatitis complicated by respiratory insufficiency, acute renal failure and abscess formation. (Gastroenterology)

Initial inpatient consultation for a 70-year-old cirrhotic male admitted with ascites, jaundice, encephalopathy, and massive hematemesis. (Gastroenterology)

Initial evaluation and formulation of plan for management of multiple trauma patient with complex pelvic fracture, 35-year-old male. (General Surgery/Orthopaedics)

Initial inpatient consultation for 45-year-old male with recent, acute subarachnoid hemorrhage, hesitant speech, mildly confused, drowsy. High risk group for HIV+ status. (Neurosurgery)

Initial inpatient consultation in the ICU for a 51-year-old patient who is on a ventilator and has a fever two weeks after a renal transplantation. (Infectious Disease)

Initial inpatient consultation for a 50-year-old male with a history of previous myocardial infarction, now with acute pulmonary edema and hypotension. (Cardiology)

Initial inpatient consultation for 36-year-old female referred by her internist to evaluate a patient being followed for abdominal pain and fever. The patient has developed diffuse abdominal pain, guarding, rigidity and increased fever. (Obstetrics & Gynecology)

FOLLOW-UP INPATIENT CONSULTATIONS

ESTABLISHED PATIENT

Follow-up consultations are visits to complete the initial consultation OR subsequent consultative visits requested by the attending physician. A follow-up consultation includes monitoring progress, recommending management modifications or advising on a new plan of care in response to changes in the patient's status.

If the physician consultant has initiated treatment at the initial consultation, and participates thereafter in the patient's management, the codes for subsequent hospital care should be used (99231-99233).

The following codes are used to report follow-up consultations provided to hospital inpatients or nursing facility residents only. For consultative services provided in other settings, the codes for office or other outpatient consultations should be reported (99241-99245).

99261 Follow-up inpatient consultation for an established patient, which requires at least two of these three key components:

- **a problem focused interval history;**
- **a problem focused examination;**
- **medical decision making that is straightforward or of low complexity.**

Counseling and/or coordination of care with other providers or agencies are provided consistent with nature of the problem(s) and the patient's and/or family's needs.

Usually, the patient is stable, recovering or improving. Physicians typically spend 10 minutes at the bedside and on the patient's hospital floor or unit.

Examples

Follow-up inpatient consultation with 35-year-old female with pulmonary embolism post-op cesarean section, now stable, for assessment of response to anticoagulation and recommended adjustment of heparin dose. (Pulmonary Medicine)

Follow-up inpatient consultation with 67-year-old female, established patient for review of diagnostic studies ordered at time of first contact. (Internal Medicine)

Follow-up inpatient consultation for a 36-year-old female 2 days after spontaneous passage of 3mm stone. (Urology)

Follow-up inpatient consultation for a 50-year-old male, asymptomatic with borderline ECG abnormality, needs preoperative opinion after a thallium exercise perfusion scan. (Cardiology)

Follow-up inpatient consultation for a 74-year-old male whose postoperative facial paralysis after a cholecystectomy is now resolving. (Neurology)

Follow-up inpatient consultation for 78-year-old female nursing home resident for evaluation of medical management of pruritis ani. (General Surgery/Colon & Rectal Surgery)

Follow-up inpatient consultation for a 94-year-old male nursing home resident for re-evaluation of hemorrhoids following conservative therapy. (Colon & Rectal Surgery/General Surgery/Geriatrics)

99262 Follow-up inpatient consultation for an established patient which requires at least two of these three key components:

- **an expanded problem focused interval history;**
- **an expanded problem focused examination;**
- **medical decision making of moderate complexity.**

Counseling and/or coordination of care with other providers or agencies are provided consistent with the nature of the problem(s) and the patient's and/or family's needs.

Usually, the patient is responding inadequately to therapy or has developed a minor complication. Physicians typically spend 20 minutes at the bedside and on the patient's hospital floor or unit.

Examples

Follow-up inpatient consultation with 72-year-old female, established patient with bullous pemphigoid on combined oral therapy steroids and immunosuppressive to evaluate progress of cutaneous care orders and adjustment of oral/parenteral therapy dosages. (Dermatology)

Follow-up inpatient consultation with 68-year-old, incapacitated male, with spinal stenosis and failure to respond to bedrest, analgesics, and PT. (Neurosurgery)

Follow-up inpatient consultation for reevaluation of a stroke patient, and development of plan for initial rehabilitation services. (Neurology)

Follow-up inpatient consultation for an asymptomatic 35-year-old Type I diabetic patient with hyperkalemic, hyperchloremia acidosis, to review lab results. (Nephrology)

Follow-up inpatient consultation for a 71-year-old male who has developed a maculopapular skin rash while on antibiotics that you recommended for an uncomplicated pneumonia. (Infectious Disease)

Follow-up inpatient consultation with 51-year-old male, for evaluation and determination of the etiology of postoperative hyponatremia following TURP. (Family Medicine)

Follow-up inpatient consultation with 45-year-old male, established patient for discussion of CT scan which demonstrates a cavernous hemangioma. (Ophthalmology)

Follow-up inpatient consultation for an elderly male with a perioperative myocardial infarction requiring adjustment of vasoactive medications. (Anesthesiology)

99263 Follow-up inpatient consultation for an established patient which requires at least two of these three key components:

- **a detailed interval history;**
- **a detailed examination;**
- **medical decision making of high complexity.**

Counseling and/or coordination of care with other providers or agencies are provided consistent with the nature of the problem(s) and the patient's and/or family's needs.

Usually, the patient is unstable or has developed a significant complication or a significant new problem. Physicians typically spend 30 minutes at the bedside and on the patient's hospital floor or unit.

Examples

Follow-up inpatient consultation with 72-year-old male established patient admitted for management of alcohol withdrawl, now confused and febrile. (Addiction Medicine)

Follow-up inpatient hospital consultation for an HIV-positive patient with an increasing fever following ten days of antibiotic therapy for pneumocystis carinii pneumonia. (Infectious Disease)

Follow-up inpatient consultation with 58-year-old diabetic female, with bacterial endocarditis, continued fever after 2 weeks of intravenous antibiotic therapy, and new onset ventricular ectopia. (Cardiology)

Follow-up inpatient consultation for a 62-year-old male, status post-op acute small bowel obstruction; now with acute renal failure. (Family Medicine)

Follow-up inpatient consultation for 42-year-old male with persistent gastrointestinal bleeding, etiology undetermined, not responding to conservative therapy of transfusions. (General Surgery/Colon & Rectal Surgery)

Follow-up inpatient consultation for a 90-year-old female with urinary incontinence who has a complicated medical history requiring reassessment of multiple medical problems, recommendations for placement, further recommendation for management of incontinence and reevaluation of cognitive status because of competency issues. (Geriatrics/Psychiatry)

Follow-up inpatient consultation for a 62-year-old female with steroid-dependent asthma, diabetes mellitus, thyrotoxicosis, abdominal pain and possible vasculitis. (Rhematology)

CONFIRMATORY CONSULTATIONS

NEW OR ESTABLISHED PATIENT

The following codes are used to report the evaluation and management services provided to patients when the consulting physician is aware of the confirmatory nature of the opinion sought (eg, when a second/third opinion is requested or required on the necessity or appropriateness of a previously recommended medical treatment or surgical procedure). Confirmatory consultations may be provided in any setting.

A physician consultant providing a confirmatory consultation is expected to provide an opinion and/or advice only. Any services subsequent to the opinion are coded at the appropriate level of office visit, established patient, or subsequent hospital care. If a confirmatory consultation is required, eg, by a third party payor, the modifier -32 or 09932, mandated services, should also be reported. (See also Consultation Notes, page 32).

Typical times have not yet been established for this subcategory of services.

99271 Confirmatory consultation for a new or established patient, which requires these three key components:

- **a problem focused history;**
- **a problem focused examination; and**
- **straightforward medical decision making.**

Counseling and/or coordination of care with other providers or agencies are provided consistent with the nature of the problem(s) and the patient's and/or family's needs.

Usually, the presenting problem(s) are self limited or minor.

99272 Confirmatory consultation for a new or established patient, which requires these three key components:

- **an expanded problem focused history;**
- **an expanded problem focused examination; and**
- **straightforward medical decision making.**

Counseling and/or coordination of care with other providers or agencies are provided consistent with the nature of the problem(s) and the patient's and/or family's needs.

Usually, the presenting problem(s) are of low severity.

99273 Confirmatory consultation for a new or established patient, which requires these three key components:

- **a detailed history;**
- **a detailed examination; and**
- **medical decision making of low complexity.**

Counseling and/or coordination of care with other providers or agencies are provided consistent with the nature of the problem(s) and the patient's and/or family's needs.

Usually, the presenting problem(s) are of moderate severity.

99274 Confirmatory consultation for a patient, which requires these three key components:

- **a comprehensive history;**
- **a comprehensive examination; and**
- **medical decision making of moderate complexity.**

Counseling and/or coordination of care with other providers or agencies are provided consistent with the nature of the problem(s) and the patient's and/or family's needs.

Usually, the presenting problem(s) are of moderate to high severity.

99275 Confirmatory consultation for a patient, which requires these three key components:

- **a comprehensive history;**
- **a comprehensive examination; and**
- **medical decision making of high complexity.**

Counseling and/or coordination of care with other providers or agencies are provided consistent with the nature of the problem(s) and the patient's and/or family's needs.

Usually, the presenting problem(s) are of moderate to high severity.

Emergency Department Services

NEW OR ESTABLISHED PATIENT

The following codes are used to report evaluation and management services provided in the emergency department. No distinction is made between new and established patients in the emergency department.

An emergency department is defined as an organized hospital-based facility for the provision of unscheduled episodic services to patients who present for immediate medical attention. The facility must be available 24 hours a day.

For critical care services provided in the Emergency Department, see Critical Care notes and 99291, 99292.

For evaluation and management services provided to a patient in an observation area of a hospital, see 99218-99220.

For definitions of key components and commonly used terms, see Evaluation and Management Services Guidelines.

99281 Emergency department visit for the evaluation and management of a patient, which requires these three key components:

- **a problem focused history;**
- **a problem focused examination; and**
- **straightforward medical decision making.**

Counseling and/or coordination of care with other providers or agencies are provided consistent with the nature of the problem(s) and the patient's and/or family's needs.

Usually, the presenting problem(s) are self limited or minor.

Examples

Emergency department visit for a patient for removal of sutures from a well-healed, uncomplicated laceration. (Emergency Medicine)

Emergency department visit for a patient for tetanus toxoid immunization. (Emergency Medicine)

Emergency department visit for a patient with several uncomplicated insect bites. (Emergency Medicine)

99282 Emergency department visit for the evaluation and management of a patient, which requires these three key components:

- **an expanded problem focused history;**
- **an expanded problem focused examination; and**
- **medical decision making of low complexity.**

Counseling and/or coordination of care with other providers or agencies are provided consistent with the nature of the problem(s) and the patient's and/or family's needs.

Usually, the presenting problem(s) are of low to moderate severity.

Examples

Emergency department visit for a 20-year-old student who presents with a painful sunburn with blister formation on the back. (Emergency Medicine)

Emergency department visit for a patient with a minor traumatic injury of an extremity with localized pain, swelling, and bruising. (Emergency Medicine)

Emergency department visit for a child presenting with impetigo localized to the face. (Emergency Medicine)

Emergency department visit for an otherwise healthy patient whose chief complaint is a red, swollen cystic lesion on his/her back. (Emergency Medicine)

Emergency department visit for a young adult patient with infected sclera and purulent discharge from both eyes without pain, visual disturbance or history of foreign body in either eye. (Emergency Medicine)

Emergency department visit for a patient presenting with a rash on both legs after exposure to poison ivy. (Emergency Medicine)

▲99283 Emergency department visit for the evaluation and management of a patient, which requires these three key components:

- **an expanded problem focused history;**
- **an expanded problem focused examination; and**
- **medical decision making of moderate complexity.**

Counseling and/or coordination of care with other providers or agencies are provided consistent with the nature of the problem(s) and the patient's and/or family's needs.

Usually, the presenting problem(s) are of moderate severity.

Examples

Emergency department visit for a sexually active female complaining of vaginal discharge who is afebrile and denies experiencing abdominal or back pain. (Emergency Medicine)

Emergency department visit for a patient with an inversion ankle injury, who is unable to bear weight on the injured foot and ankle. (Emergency Medicine)

Emergency department visit for a healthy, young adult patient who sustained a blunt head injury with local swelling and bruising **without** subsequent confusion, loss of consciousness or memory deficit. (Emergency Medicine)

Emergency department visit for a well-appearing 8-year-old child who has a fever, diarrhea and abdominal cramps, is tolerating oral fluids and is not vomiting. (Emergency Medicine)

Emergency department visit for a patient who has a complaint of acute pain associated with a suspected foreign body in the painful eye. (Emergency Medicine)

99284 Emergency department visit for the evaluation and management of a patient, which requires these three key components:

- **a detailed history;**
- **a detailed examination; and**
- **medical decision making of moderate complexity.**

Counseling and/or coordination of care with other providers or agencies are provided consistent with the nature of the problem(s) and the patient's and/or family's needs.

Usually, the presenting problem(s) are of high severity, and require urgent evaluation by the physician but do not pose an immediate significant threat to life or physiologic function.

Examples

Emergency department visit for a 4-year-old child who fell off a bike sustaining a head injury with brief loss of consciousness. (Emergency Medicine)

Emergency department visit for a patient with flank pain and hematuria. (Emergency Medicine)

Emergency department visit for an elderly female who has fallen and is now complaining of pain in her right hip and is unable to walk. (Emergency Medicine)

Emergency department visit for a female presenting with lower abdominal pain and a vaginal discharge. (Emergency Medicine)

99285 Emergency department visit for the evaluation and management of a patient, which requires these three key components within the constraints imposed by the urgency of the patient's clinical condition and mental status:

- **a comprehensive history;**
- **a comprehensive examination; and**
- **medical decision making of high complexity.**

Counseling and/or coordination of care with other providers or agencies are provided consistent with the nature of the problem(s) and the patient's and/or family's needs.

Usually, the presenting problem(s) are of high severity and pose an immediate significant threat to life or physiologic function.

Examples

Emergency department visit for a patient with a complicated overdose requiring aggressive management to prevent side effects from the ingested materials. (Emergency Medicine)

Emergency department visit for a patient exhibiting active, upper gastrointestinal bleeding. (Emergency Medicine)

Emergency department visit for a patient with an acute onset of chest pain compatible with symptoms of cardiac ischemia and/or pulmonary embolus. (Emergency Medicine)

Emergency department visit for a patient with a new onset of a cerebral vascular accident. (Emergency Medicine)

Emergency department visit for a patient with a new onset of rapid heart rate requiring IV drugs. (Emergency Medicine)

Emergency department visit for a previously healthy young adult patient who is injured in an automobile accident and is brought to the emergency department immobilized and has symptoms compatible with intra-abdominal injuries or multiple extremity injuries. (Emergency Medicine)

Emergency department visit for a patient who presents with a sudden onset of "the worst headache of her life," and complains of a stiff neck, nausea, and inability to concentrate. (Emergency Medicine)

Emergency department visit for acute febrile illness in an adult, associated with shortness of breath and an altered level of alertness. (Emergency Medicine)

MISCELLANEOUS

In physician directed emergency care, advanced life support, the physician is located in a hospital emergency or critical care department, and is in two-way voice communication with ambulance or rescue personnel outside the hospital. The physician directs the performance of necessary medical procedures, including but not limited to: telemetry of cardiac rhythm; cardiac and/or pulmonary resuscitation; endotracheal or esophageal obturator airway intubation; administration of intravenous fluids and/or administration of intramuscular, intratracheal or subcutaneous drugs; and/or electrical conversion of arrhythmia.

99288 Physician direction of emergency medical systems (EMS) emergency care, advanced life support

Critical Care Services

Critical care includes the care of critically ill patients in a variety of medical emergencies that requires the constant attendance of the physician (eg, cardiac arrest, shock, bleeding, respiratory failure, postoperative complications). Critical care is usually, but not always, given in a critical care area, such as the coronary care unit, intensive care unit, respiratory care unit, or the emergency care facility.

Services for a patient who is not critically ill but happens to be in a critical care unit are reported using subsequent hospital care codes. (See 99231-99233)

The following services are included in reporting critical care when performed during the critical period by the physician providing critical care: the interpretation of cardiac output measurements (93561, 93562), chest x-rays (71010, 71020), blood gases, and information data stored in computers (eg, ECGs, blood pressures, hematologic data (99090)); gastric intubation (91105); temporary transcutaneous pacing (92953); ventilator management (94656, 94657); and, vascular access procedures (36000, 36410, 36415, 36600). Any services performed which are not listed above should be reported separately.

The critical care codes are used to report the total duration of time spent by a physician providing constant attention to a critically ill patient. Code 99291 is used to report the first hour of critical care on a given day. It should be used only once per day even if the time spent by the physician is not continuous on that day. Code 99292 is used to report each additional 30 minutes beyond the first hour. For example, if 1 hour of critical care is provided at 10AM and 2 hours provided from 3PM to 5PM, then report code 99291 once and 99292 four times to report the total of three hours on a single day.

▲**99291** Critical care, evaluation and management of the critically ill or critically injured patient, requiring the constant attendance of the physician; first hour

99292 each additional 30 minutes

Neonatal Intensive Care

The following codes (99295-99297) are used to report services provided by physicians directing the care of a neonate or infant in a neonatal intensive care unit (NICU). They represent care starting with the date of admission to the NICU and may be reported only once per day, per patient. Once the neonate is no longer considered to be critically ill, the codes for Subsequent Hospital Care (99231-99233) should be utilized.

These NICU codes are to be used in addition to codes 99150, 99151 and 99440 when the physician is present for the delivery and newborn resuscitation is required.

Care rendered includes management; monitoring and treatment of the patient including nutritional, metabolic and hematologic maintenance; parent counseling; and personal direct supervision of the health care team in the performance of cognitive and procedural activities.

The following procedures are also included as part of the global descriptors: umbilical, central or peripheral vessel catheterization, endotracheal intubation, lumbar puncture and suprapubic bladder aspiration. In addition, specific services are included in the parenthetic note following each NICU code. Any services performed which are not listed above or not listed with each NICU code should be reported separately.

(For additional instructions, see parenthetical descriptions listed for 99295-99297)

• **99295** Initial NICU care, per day, for the evaluation and management of a critically ill neonate or infant.

This care is provided on the date of admission of a neonate who requires cardiopulmonary monitoring and support.

Such care includes the following, as necessary: initiation of mechanical ventilation or continuous positive airway pressure (CPAP); surfactant administration; pharmacologic control of the circulatory system; intravascular fluid administration; transfusion of blood components; vascular punctures; and blood gas interpretation.

● **99296** Subsequent NICU care, per day, for the evaluation and management of a critically ill and unstable neonate or infant

A critically ill and unstable neonate represents a neonate whose cardiopulmonary and metabolic status is unstable; whose neurologic status may be unstable; who requires frequent ventilator changes, inotropic and chronotropic support; who requires frequent IV changes and whose condition is changing almost minute to minute. Such an infant requires almost constant attention by a neonatologist.

This description represents care provided on dates subsequent to the admission date.

Such care includes the following, as necessary: mechanical ventilation or CPAP; surfactant administration; pharmacologic control of the circulatory system; total parenteral nutrition; seizure management; invasive or non-invasive electronic monitoring of vital signs, and/or monitoring of blood gases or oxygen saturation.

● **99297** Subsequent NICU care, per day, for the evaluation and management of a critically ill and stable neonate or infant

A critically ill and stable neonate may represent an infant who is still intubated and requires invasive cardiopulmonary monitoring but whose vital signs are stable; who is not seizing; whose metabolic status is stable but who is still NPO and receiving parenteral nutrition and IV medications; and who is not yet over the acute phase of the initial problem.

This description represents care provided on dates subsequent to the admission date.

Such care includes the following, as necessary: ventilatory support and treatment; total parenteral nutrition; invasive or non-invasive electronic monitoring of vital signs; apnea management and/or monitoring of blood gases or oxygen saturation.

Nursing Facility Services

The following codes are used to report evaluation and management services to patients in Nursing Facilities (formerly called Skilled Nursing Facilities (SNFs), Intermediate Care Facilities (ICFs) or Long Term Care Facilities (LTCFs)).

These codes should also be used to report evaluation and management services provided to a patient in a psychiatric residential treatment center (a facility or a distinct part of a facility for psychiatric care, which provides a 24 hour therapeutically planned and professionally staffed group living and learning environment). If procedures such as medical psychotherapy are provided in addition to evaluation and management services, these should be reported in addition to the evaluation and management services provided.

Nursing facilities that provide convalescent, rehabilitative, or long term care are required to conduct comprehensive, accurate, standardized, and reproducible assessments of each resident's functional capacity using a Resident Assessment Instrument (RAI). All RAIs include the Minimum Data Set (MDS), Resident Assessment Protocols (RAPs) and utilization guidelines. The MDS is the primary screening and assessment tool; the RAPs trigger the identification of potential problems and provide guidelines for follow-up assessments.

Physicians have a central role in assuring that all residents receive thorough assessments and that medical plans of care are instituted or revised to enhance or maintain the residents' physical and psychosocial functioning.

Two subcategories of nursing facility services are recognized: Comprehensive Nursing Facility Assessments and Subsequent Nursing Facility Care. Both subcategories apply to new or established patients. Comprehensive Assessments may be performed at one or more sites in the assessment process: the hospital, office, nursing facility, domiciliary/non-nursing facility or patient's home.

For definitions of key components and commonly used terms, please see Evaluation and Management Services Guidelines.

COMPREHENSIVE NURSING FACILITY ASSESSMENTS

NEW OR ESTABLISHED PATIENT

When the patient is admitted to the nursing facility in the course of an encounter in another site of service (eg, hospital emergency department, physician's office), all evaluation and management services provided by that physician in conjunction with that admission are considered part of the initial nursing facility care when performed as part of the admission.

The nursing facility care level of service reported by the admitting physician should include the services related to the admission he/she provided in the other sites of service as well as in the nursing facility setting. With the exception of hospital discharge services, evaluation and management services on the same date provided in sites other than the nursing facility that are related to the admission should NOT be reported separately. Hospital discharge services may be reported separately.

More than one comprehensive assessment may be necessary during an inpatient confinement.

99301 Evaluation and management of a new or established patient involving an annual nursing facility assessment which requires these three key components:

- **a detailed interval history;**
- **a comprehensive examination; and**
- **medical decision making that is straightforward or of low complexity.**

Counseling and/or coordination of care with other providers or agencies are provided consistent with the nature of the problem(s) and the patient's and/or family's needs.

Usually, the patient is stable, recovering or improving. The review and affirmation of the medical plan of care is required. Physicians typically spend 30 minutes at the bedside and on the patient's facility floor or unit.

99302 Evaluation and management of a new or established patient involving a nursing facility assessment which requires these three key components:

- **a detailed interval history;**
- **a comprehensive examination; and**
- **medical decision making of moderate to high complexity.**

Counseling and/or coordination of care with other providers or agencies are provided consistent with the nature of the problem(s) and the patient's and/or family's needs.

Usually, the patient has developed a significant complication or a significant new problem and has had a major permanent change in status. The creation of a new medical plan of care is required. Physicians typically spend 40 minutes at the bedside and on the patient's facility floor or unit.

▲**99303** Evaluation and management of a new or established patient involving a nursing facility assessment at the time of initial admission or readmission to the facility, which requires these three key components:

- **a comprehensive history;**
- **a comprehensive examination; and**
- **medical decision making of moderate to high complexity.**

Counseling and/or coordination of care with other providers or agencies are provided consistent with the nature of the problem(s) and the patient's and/or family's needs. The creation of a medical plan of care is required. Physicians typically spend 50 minutes at the bedside and on the patient's facility floor or unit.

SUBSEQUENT NURSING FACILITY CARE

NEW OR ESTABLISHED PATIENT

The following codes are used to report the services provided to residents of nursing facilities who do not require a comprehensive assessment, and/or who have not had a major, permanent change of status.

All levels include reviewing the medical record, noting changes in the resident's status since the last visit, and reviewing and signing orders.

99311 Subsequent nursing facility care, per day, for the evaluation and management of a new or established patient, which requires at least two of these three key components:

- **a problem focused interval history;**
- **a problem focused examination;**
- **medical decision making that is straightforward or of low complexity.**

Counseling and/or coordination of care with other providers or agencies are provided consistent with the nature of the problem(s) and the patient's and/or family's needs.

Usually, the patient is stable, recovering or improving. Physicians typically spend 15 minutes at the bedside and on the patient's facility floor or unit.

99312 Subsequent nursing facility care, per day, for the evaluation and management of a new or established patient, which requires at least two of these three key components:

- **an expanded problem focused interval history;**
- **an expanded problem focused examination;**
- **medical decision making of moderate complexity.**

Counseling and/or coordination of care with other providers or agencies are provided consistent with the nature of the problem(s) and the patient's and/or family's needs.

Usually, the patient is responding inadequately to therapy or has developed a minor complication. Physicians typically spend 25 minutes at the bedside and on the patient's facility floor or unit.

99313 Subsequent nursing facility care, per day, for the evaluation and management of a new or established patient, which requires at least two of these three key components:

- **a detailed interval history;**
- **a detailed examination;**
- **medical decision making of moderate to high complexity.**

Counseling and/or coordination of care with other providers or agencies are provided consistent with the nature of the problem(s) and the patient's and/or family's needs.

Usually, the patient has developed a significant complication or a significant new problem. Physicians typically spend 35 minutes at the bedside and on the patient's facility floor or unit.

Domiciliary, Rest Home (eg, Boarding Home), or Custodial Care Services

The following codes are used to report evaluation and management services in a facility which provides room, board and other personal assistance services, generally on a long-term basis. The facility's services do not include a medical component.

For definitions of key components and commonly used terms, please see Evaluation and Management Services Guidelines.

Typical times have not yet been established for this category of services.

NEW PATIENT

99321 Domiciliary or rest home visit for the evaluation and management of a new patient which requires these three key components:

- **a problem focused history;**
- **a problem focused examination; and**
- **medical decision making that is straightforward or of low complexity.**

Counseling and/or coordination of care with other providers or agencies are provided consistent with the nature of the problem(s) and the patient's and/or family's needs.

Usually, the presenting problem(s) are of low severity.

99322 Domiciliary or rest home visit for the evaluation and management of a new patient, which requires these three key components:

- **an expanded problem focused history;**
- **an expanded problem focused examination; and**
- **medical decision making of moderate complexity.**

Counseling and/or coordination of care with other providers or agencies are provided consistent with the nature of the problem(s) and the patient's and/or family's needs.

Usually, the presenting problem(s) are of moderate severity.

99323 Domiciliary or rest home visit for the evaluation and management of a new patient, which requires these three key components:

- **a detailed history;**
- **a detailed examination; and**
- **medical decision making of high complexity.**

Counseling and/or coordination of care with other providers or agencies are provided consistent with the nature of the problem(s) and the patient's and/or family's needs.

Usually, the presenting problem(s) are of high complexity.

ESTABLISHED PATIENT

99331 Domiciliary or rest home visit for the evaluation and management of an established patient, which requires at least two of these three key components:

- **a problem focused interval history;**
- **a problem focused examination;**
- **medical decision making that is straightforward or of low complexity.**

Counseling and/or coordination of care with other providers or agencies are provided consistent with the nature of the problem(s) and the patient's and/or family's needs.

Usually, the patient is stable, recovering or improving.

99332 Domiciliary or rest home visit for the evaluation and management of an established patient, which requires at least two of these three key components:

- **an expanded problem focused interval history;**
- **an expanded problem focused examination;**
- **medical decision making of moderate complexity.**

Counseling and/or coordination of care with other providers or agencies are provided consistent with the nature of the problem(s) and the patient's and/or family's needs.

Usually, the patient is responding inadequately to therapy or has developed a minor complication.

99333 Domiciliary or rest home visit for the evaluation and management of an established patient, which requires at least two of these three key components:

- **a detailed interval history;**
- **a detailed examination;**
- **medical decision making of high complexity.**

Counseling and/or coordination of care with other providers or agencies are provided consistent with the nature of the problem(s) and the patient's and/or family's needs.

Usually, the patient is unstable or has developed a significant complication or a significant new problem.

Home Services

The following codes are used to report evaluation and management services provided in a private residence.

For definitions of key components and commonly used terms, please see Evaluation and Management Services Guidelines. Typical times have not yet been established for this category of services.

NEW PATIENT

99341 Home visit for the evaluation and management of a new patient, which requires these three key components:

- **a problem focused history;**
- **a problem focused examination; and**
- **medical decision making that is straightforward or of low complexity.**

Counseling and/or coordination of care with other providers or agencies are provided consistent with the nature of the problem(s) and the patient's and/or family's needs.

Usually, the presenting problem(s) are of low severity.

99342 Home visit for the evaluation and management of a new patient, which requires these three key components:

- **an expanded problem focused history;**
- **an expanded problem focused examination; and**
- **medical decision making of moderate complexity.**

Counseling and/or coordination of care with other providers or agencies are provided consistent with the nature of the problem(s) and the patient's and/or family's needs.

Usually, the presenting problem(s) are of moderate severity.

99343 Home visit for the evaluation and management of a new patient, which requires these three key components:

- **a detailed history;**
- **a detailed examination; and**
- **medical decision making of high complexity.**

Counseling and/or coordination of care with other providers or agencies are provided consistent with the nature of the problem(s) and the patient's and/or family's needs.

Usually, the presenting problem(s) are of high severity.

ESTABLISHED PATIENT

99351 Home visit for the evaluation and management of an established patient, which requires at least two of these three key components:

- **a problem focused interval history;**
- **a problem focused examination;**
- **medical decision making that is straightforward or of low complexity.**

Counseling and/or coordination of care with other providers or agencies are provided consistent with the nature of the problem(s) and the patient's and/or family's needs.

Usually, the patient is stable, recovering or improving.

99352 Home visit for the evaluation and management of an established patient, which requires at least two of these three key components:

- **an expanded problem focused interval history;**
- **an expanded problem focused examination;**
- **medical decision making of moderate complexity.**

Counseling and/or coordination of care with other providers or agencies are provided consistent with the nature of the problem(s) and the patient's and/or family's needs.

Usually, the patient is responding inadequately to therapy or has developed a minor complication.

99353 Home visit for the evaluation and management of an established patient, which requires at least two of these three key components:

- **a detailed interval history;**
- **a detailed examination;**
- **medical decision making of high complexity.**

Counseling and/or coordination of care with other providers or agencies are provided consistent with the nature of the problem(s) and the patient's and/or family's needs.

Usually, the patient is unstable or has developed a significant complication or a significant new problem.

Case Management Services

Physician case management is a process in which a physician is responsible for direct care of a patient, and for coordinating and controlling access to or initiating and/or supervising other health care services needed by the patient.

TEAM CONFERENCES

99361 Medical conference by a physician with interdisciplinary team of health professionals or representatives of community agencies to coordinate activities of patient care (patient not present); approximately 30 minutes

99362 approximately 60 minutes

TELEPHONE CALLS

99371 Telephone call by a physician to patient or for consultation or medical management or for coordinating medical management with other health care professionals (eg, nurses, therapists, social workers, nutritionists, physicians, pharmacists); simple or brief (eg, to report on tests and/or laboratory results, to clarify or alter previous instructions, to integrate new information from other health professionals into the medical treatment plan, or to adjust therapy)

99372 intermediate (eg, to provide advice to an established patient on a new problem, to initiate therapy that can be handled by telephone, to discuss test results in detail, to coordinate medical management of a new problem in an established patient, to discuss and evaluate new information and details, or to initiate new plan of care)

99373 complex or lengthy (eg, lengthly counseling session with anxious or distraught patient, detailed or prolonged discussion with family members regarding seriously ill patient, lengthy communication necessary to coordinate complex services of several different health professionals working on different aspects of the total patient care plan)

Preventive Medicine Services

The following codes are used to report the routine evaluation and management of adults and children when these services are performed in the absence of patient complaints. The extent and focus of the services will largely depend on the age of the patient, the circumstances of the examination, and the abnormalities encountered.

Codes 99381-99397 do not include counseling, risk factor reduction interventions or immunizations. If risk management services are provided at the same session as a preventive medicine visit, both codes should be reported. For counseling and/or risk factor reduction interventions, see 99401-99412. For immunizations, see 90701-90749.

Ancillary studies involving laboratory, radiology, or other procedures are reported separately.

NEW PATIENT

99381 Initial evaluation and management of a healthy individual requiring a comprehensive history, a comprehensive examination, the identification of risk factors, and the ordering of appropriate laboratory/diagnostic procedures, new patient; infant (age under 1 year)

99382 early childhood (age 1 through 4 years)

99383 late childhood (age 5 through 11 years)

99384 adolescent (age 12 through 17 years)

99385 18-39 years

99386 40-64 years

99387 65 years and over

ESTABLISHED PATIENT

99391 Periodic reevaluation and management of a healthy individual requiring a comprehensive history, comprehensive examination, the identification of risk factors and the ordering of appropriate laboratory/diagnostic procedures, established patient; infant (age under 1 year)

99392 early childhood (age 1 through 4 years)

99393 late childhood (age 5 through 11 years)

99394 adolescent (age 12 through 17 years)

99395 18-39 years

99396 40-64 years

99397 65 years and over

COUNSELING AND/OR RISK FACTOR REDUCTION INTERVENTION

NEW OR ESTABLISHED PATIENT

These codes are used to report services provided to healthy individuals for the purpose of promoting health and preventing illness or injury. Counseling and risk factor reduction interventions provided in conjunction with an initial or periodic preventive medicine visit will vary with age and should address such issues as family problems, diet and exercise, substance abuse, sexual practices, injury prevention and dental health.

These codes are not to be used to report counseling and risk factor reduction interventions provided to patients with symptoms or established illness. For counseling individual patients with symptoms or established illness, use the appropriate office, hospital or consultation or other evaluation and management codes. For counseling groups of patients with symptoms or established illness, use 99078.

PREVENTIVE MEDICINE, INDIVIDUAL COUNSELING

99401 Counseling and/or risk factor reduction intervention(s) provided to a healthy individual; approximately 15 minutes

99402 approximately 30 minutes

99403 approximately 45 minutes

99404 approximately 60 minutes

PREVENTIVE MEDICINE, GROUP COUNSELING

99411 Counseling and/or risk factor reduction intervention(s) provided to healthy individuals in a group setting; approximately 30 minutes

99412 approximately 60 minutes

OTHER PREVENTIVE MEDICINE SERVICES

99420 Administration and interpretation of health risk assessment instrument (eg, health hazard appraisal)

99429 Unlisted preventive medicine service

Newborn Care

The following codes are used to report the services provided to normal or high risk newborns in several different settings. For hospital discharge services, use 99238.

99431 History and examination of the normal newborn infant, initiation of diagnostic and treatment programs and preparation of hospital records. (This code should also be used for birthing room deliveries.)

99432 Normal newborn care in other than hospital or birthing room setting, including physical examination of baby and conference(s) with parent(s)

99433 Subsequent hospital care, for the evaluation and management of a normal newborn, per day

(99438 has been deleted)

99440 Newborn resuscitation: care of the high risk newborn at delivery, including, for example, inhalation therapy, aspiration, administration of medication for initial stabilization

Other Evaluation and Management Services

99499 Unlisted evaluation and management service

Anesthesia

Guidelines

Services involving administration of anesthesia are reported by the use of the anesthesia five-digit procedure code (00100-01999) plus modifier codes (defined under "Anesthesia Modifiers" later in these Guidelines).

The reporting of anesthesia services is appropriate by or under the responsible supervision of a physician. These services may include but are not limited to general, regional, supplementation of local anesthesia, or other supportive services in order to afford the patient the anesthesia care deemed optimal by the anesthesiologist during any procedure. These services include the usual preoperative and postoperative visits, the anesthesia care during the procedure, the administration of fluids and/or blood and the usual monitoring services (eg, ECG, temperature, blood pressure, oximetry, capnography and mass spectrometry). Unusual forms of monitoring (eg, intra-arterial, central venous and Swan-Ganz) are not included.

Items used by all physicians in reporting their services are presented in the **INTRODUCTION.** Some of the commonalities are repeated here for the convenience of those physicians referring to this section on **ANESTHESIA.** Other definitions and items unique to anesthesia are also listed.

1. **TIME REPORTING:** Time for anesthesia procedures may be reported as is customary in the local area. Anesthesia time begins when the anesthesiologist begins to prepare the patient for the induction of anesthesia in the operating room or in an equivalent area and ends when the anesthesiologist is no longer in personal attendance, that is, when the patient may be safely placed under postoperative supervision.

2. **PHYSICIAN'S SERVICES** rendered in the office, home, or hospital, consultation and other medical services are listed in the section entitled **EVALUATION AND MANAGEMENT SERVICES** (99200 series) found in the front of the book, beginning on page 1. "Special Services and Reporting" (99000 series) are presented in the **MEDICINE** section.

3. **MATERIALS SUPPLIED BY PHYSICIAN:** Supplies and materials provided by the physician (eg, sterile trays, drugs) over and above those usually included with the office visit or other services rendered may be listed separately. List drugs, tray supplies, and materials provided. Identify as 99070.

4. **SEPARATE OR MULTIPLE PROCEDURES:** It is appropriate to designate multiple procedures that are rendered on the same date by separate entries. This can be reported by using the multiple procedure modifier (-51 or 09951). See item 6 for modifier definitions.

5. **SPECIAL REPORT:** A service that is rarely provided, unusual, variable, or new may require a special report in determining medical appropriateness of the service. Pertinent information should include an adequate definition or description of the nature, extent, and need for the procedure; and the time, effort and equipment necessary to provide the service. Additional items which may be included are:

   Complexity of symptoms, final diagnosis, pertinent physical findings, diagnostic and therapeutic procedures, concurrent problems, and follow-up care.

6. **ANESTHESIA MODIFIERS:** All anesthesia services are reported by use of the anesthesia five-digit procedure code (00100-01999) plus the addition of a physical status modifier. The use of other optional modifiers may be appropriate.

   A. Physical Status modifiers are represented by the initial letter P followed by a single digit from 1 to 6 defined below.

      P1—A normal healthy patient.
      P2—A patient with mild systemic disease.
      P3—A patient with severe systemic disease.
      P4—A patient with severe systemic disease that is a constant threat to life.
      P5—A moribund patient who is not expected to survive without the operation.
      P6—A declared brain-dead patient whose organs are being removed for donor purposes.

The above six levels are consistent with the American Society of Anesthesiologists (ASA) ranking of patient physical status. Physical status is included in CPT to distinguish between various levels of complexity of the anesthesia service provided.

Example: 00100-P1

B. Other Modifiers (optional): Under certain circumstances, medical services and procedures may need to be further modified. Other modifiers commonly used in **ANESTHESIA** are included below. A complete list of modifiers and their respective codes are listed in Appendix A.

-22 Unusual Procedural Services: When the service(s) provided is greater than that usually required for the listed procedure, it may be identified by adding modifier '-22' to the usual procedure number or by use of the separate five digit modifier code 09922. A report may also be appropriate.

-23 Unusual Anesthesia: Occasionally, a procedure, which usually requires either no anesthesia or local anesthesia, because of unusual circumstances must be done under general anesthesia. This circumstance may be reported by adding the modifier '-23' to the procedure code of the basic service or by use of the separate five digit modifier code 09923.

Note: Modifier -47, Anesthesia by Surgeon, (See Appendix A) would not be used as a modifier for the anesthesia procedures 00100-01999.

-32 Mandated Services: Services related to *mandated* consultation and/or related services (eg, PRO, 3rd party payor) may be identified by adding the modifier '-32' to the basic procedure or the service may be reported by use of the five digit modifier 09932.

-51 Multiple Procedures: When multiple procedures are performed on the same day or at the same session, the major procedure or service may be reported as listed. The secondary additional, or lesser procedure(s) or service(s) may be identified by adding the modifier '-51' to the secondary procedure or service code(s) or by use of the separate five digit modifier code 09951. This modifier may be used to report multiple medical procedures performed at the same session, as well as a combination of medical and surgical procedures, or several surgical procedures performed at the same operative session.

7. **QUALIFYING CIRCUMSTANCES:** (More than one may be selected.)

Many anesthesia services are provided under particularly difficult circumstances depending on factors such as extraordinary condition of patient, notable operative conditions, unusual risk factors. This section includes a list of important qualifying circumstances that significantly impact on the character of the anesthesia service provided. These procedures would not be reported alone but would be reported as additional procedure numbers qualifying an anesthesia procedure or service.

99100 Anesthesia for patient of extreme age, under one year and over seventy

99116 Anesthesia complicated by utilization of total body hypothermia

99135 Anesthesia complicated by utilization of controlled hypotension

99140 Anesthesia complicated by emergency conditions (specify)

(An emergency is defined as existing when delay in treatment of the patient would lead to a significant increase in the threat to life or body part.)

Anesthesia
00100 - 01999

ANESTHESIA

Procedures

HEAD

00100 Anesthesia for procedures on integumentary system of head and/or salivary glands, including biopsy; not otherwise specified

00102 plastic repair of cleft lip

00104 Anesthesia for electroconvulsive therapy

00120 Anesthesia for procedures on external, middle, and inner ear including biopsy; not otherwise specified

(00122 has been deleted. To report, use 00120)

00124 otoscopy

00126 tympanotomy

00140 Anesthesia for procedures on eye; not otherwise specified

00142 lens surgery

00144 corneal transplant

00145 vitrectomy

(00146 has been deleted. To report, use 00140)

00147 iridectomy

00148 ophthalmoscopy

00160 Anesthesia for procedures on nose and accessory sinuses; not otherwise specified

00162 radical surgery

00164 biopsy, soft tissue

00170 Anesthesia for intraoral procedures, including biopsy; not otherwise specified

00172 repair of cleft palate

00174 excision of retropharyngeal tumor

00176 radical surgery

00190 Anesthesia for procedures on facial bones; not otherwise specified

00192 radical surgery (including prognathism)

00210 Anesthesia for intracranial procedures; not otherwise specified

00212 subdural taps

00214 burr holes

(For burr holes for ventriculography, see 01902)

00216 vascular procedures

00218 procedures in sitting position

00220 spinal fluid shunting procedures

00222 electrocoagulation of intracranial nerve

NECK

00300 Anesthesia for all procedures on integumentary system of neck, including subcutaneous tissue

00320 Anesthesia for all procedures on esophagus, thyroid, larynx, trachea and lymphatic system of neck; not otherwise specified

00322 needle biopsy of thyroid

(For procedures on cervical spine and cord, see 00600, 00604, 00670)

00350 Anesthesia for procedures on major vessels of neck; not otherwise specified

00352 simple ligation

(For arteriography, see 01916)

THORAX (CHEST WALL AND SHOULDER GIRDLE)

00400 Anesthesia for procedures on anterior integumentary system of chest, including subcutaneous tissue; not otherwise specified

00402 reconstructive procedures on breast (eg, reduction or augmentation mammoplasty, muscle flaps)

00404 radical or modified radical procedures on breast

00406 radical or modified radical procedures on breast with internal mammary node dissection

00410 electrical conversion of arrhythmias

00420 Anesthesia for procedures on posterior integumentary system of chest, including subcutaneous tissue

00450 Anesthesia for procedures on clavicle and scapula; not otherwise specified

00452 radical surgery

00454 biopsy of clavicle

00470 Anesthesia for partial rib resection; not otherwise specified

00472 thoracoplasty (any type)

00474 radical procedures (eg, pectus excavatum)

(00476 has been deleted. To report, use 00470)

INTRATHORACIC

00500 Anesthesia for all procedures on esophagus

00520 Anesthesia for closed chest procedures (including esophagoscopy, bronchoscopy, thoracoscopy); not otherwise specified

00522 needle biopsy of pleura

00524 pneumocentesis

(00526 has been deleted. To report, use 00520)

00528 mediastinoscopy

00530 Anesthesia for transvenous pacemaker insertion

00532 Anesthesia for access to central venous circulation

• **00534** Anesthesia for transvenous insertion or replacement of cardioverter/defibrillator

(For transthoracic approach, use 00560)

00540 Anesthesia for thoracotomy procedures involving lungs, pleura, diaphragm, and mediastinum; not otherwise specified

00542 decortication

00544 pleurectomy

00546 pulmonary resection with thoracoplasty

00548 intrathoracic repair of trauma to trachea and bronchi

00560 Anesthesia for procedures on heart, pericardium, and great vessels of chest; without pump oxygenator

00562 with pump oxygenator

00580 Anesthesia for heart transplant or heart/lung transplant

SPINE AND SPINAL CORD

00600 Anesthesia for procedures on cervical spine and cord; not otherwise specified

(For myelography and diskography, see radiological procedures 01906-01914)

00604 posterior cervical laminectomy in sitting position

00620 Anesthesia for procedures on thoracic spine and cord; not otherwise specified

00622 thoracolumbar sympathectomy

00630 Anesthesia for procedures in lumbar region; not otherwise specified

00632 lumbar sympathectomy

00634 chemonucleolysis

(00650 has been deleted. To report, use 00220)

00670 Anesthesia for extensive spine and spinal cord procedures (eg, Harrington rod technique)

UPPER ABDOMEN

00700 Anesthesia for procedures on upper anterior abdominal wall; not otherwise specified

00702 percutaneous liver biopsy

00730 Anesthesia for procedures on upper posterior abdominal wall

00740 Anesthesia for upper gastrointestinal endoscopic procedures

00750 Anesthesia for hernia repairs in upper abdomen; not otherwise specified

00752 lumbar and ventral (incisional) hernias and/or wound dehiscence

00754 omphalocele

00756 transabdominal repair of diaphragmatic hernia

00770 Anesthesia for all procedures on major abdominal blood vessels

00790 Anesthesia for intraperitoneal procedures in upper abdomen, including bowel shunts; not otherwise specified

00792 partial hepatectomy (excluding liver biopsy)

00794 pancreatectomy, partial or total (eg, Whipple procedure)

00796 liver transplant (recipient)

(For harvesting of liver, use 01990)

LOWER ABDOMEN

00800 Anesthesia for procedures on lower anterior abdominal wall; not otherwise specified

00802 panniculectomy

00806 Anesthesia for laparoscopic procedures

00810 Anesthesia for intestinal endoscopic procedures

00820 Anesthesia for procedures on lower posterior abdominal wall

00830 Anesthesia for hernia repairs in lower abdomen; not otherwise specified

00832 ventral and incisional hernias

00840 Anesthesia for intraperitoneal procedures in lower abdomen; not otherwise specified

00842 amniocentesis

00844 abdominoperineal resection

00846 radical hysterectomy

00848 pelvic exenteration

00850 cesarean section

00855 cesarean hysterectomy

00857 Continuous epidural analgesia, for labor and cesarean section

00860 Anesthesia for extraperitoneal procedures in lower abdomen, including urinary tract; not otherwise specified

00862 renal procedures, including upper 1/3 of ureter, or donor nephrectomy

00864 total cystectomy

00866 adrenalectomy

00868 renal transplant (recipient)

(For donor nephrectomy, use 00862)

(For harvesting kidney from brain-dead patient, use 01990)

00870 cystolithotomy

00872 Anesthesia for lithotripsy, extracorporeal shock wave; with water bath

00873 without water bath

00880 Anesthesia for procedures on major lower abdominal vessels; not otherwise specified

00882 inferior vena cava ligation

00884 transvenous umbrella insertion

PERINEUM

00900 Anesthesia for procedures on perineal integumentary system (including biopsy of male genital system); not otherwise specified

00902 anorectal procedure (including endoscopy and/or biopsy)

00904 radical perineal procedure

00906 vulvectomy

00908 perineal prostatectomy

00910 Anesthesia for transurethral procedures (including urethrocystoscopy); not otherwise specified

00912 transurethral resection of bladder tumor(s)

00914 transurethral resection of prostate

00916 post-transurethral resection bleeding

00918 with fragmentation and/or removal of ureteral calculus

00920 Anesthesia for procedures on male external genitalia; not otherwise specified

00922 seminal vesicles

00924 undescended testis, unilateral or bilateral

00926 radical orchiectomy, inguinal

00928 radical orchiectomy, abdominal

00930 orchiopexy, unilateral or bilateral

00932 complete amputation of penis

00934 radical amputation of penis with bilateral inguinal lymphadenectomy

00936 radical amputation of penis with bilateral inguinal and iliac lymphadenectomy

00938 insertion of penile prosthesis (perineal approach)

00940 Anesthesia for vaginal procedures (including biopsy of labia, vagina, cervix or endometrium); not otherwise specified

00942 colpotomy, colpectomy, colporrhaphy

00944 vaginal hysterectomy

00946 vaginal delivery

00948 cervical cerclage

00950 culdoscopy

00952 hysteroscopy

00955 Continuous epidural analgesia, for labor and vaginal delivery

PELVIS (EXCEPT HIP)

01000 Anesthesia for procedures on anterior integumentary system of pelvis (anterior to iliac crest), except external genitalia

01110 Anesthesia for procedures on posterior integumentary system of pelvis (posterior to iliac crest), except perineum

01120 Anesthesia for procedures on bony pelvis

(01122 has been deleted. To report, use 01120)

01130 Anesthesia for body cast application or revision

01140 Anesthesia for interpelviabdominal (hindquarter) amputation

01150 Anesthesia for radical procedures for tumor of pelvis, except hindquarter amputation

01160 Anesthesia for closed procedures involving symphysis pubis or sacroiliac joint

01170 Anesthesia for open procedures involving symphysis pubis or sacroiliac joint

01180 Anesthesia for obturator neurectomy; extrapelvic

01190 intrapelvic

UPPER LEG (EXCEPT KNEE)

01200 Anesthesia for all closed procedures involving hip joint

01202 Anesthesia for arthroscopic procedures of hip joint

01210 Anesthesia for open procedures involving hip joint; not otherwise specified

01212 hip disarticulation

01214 total hip replacement or revision

01220 Anesthesia for all closed procedures involving upper 2/3 of femur

01230 Anesthesia for open procedures involving upper 2/3 of femur; not otherwise specified

01232 amputation

01234 radical resection

01240 Anesthesia for all procedures on integumentary system of upper leg

01250 Anesthesia for all procedures on nerves, muscles, tendons, fascia, and bursae of upper leg

01260 Anesthesia for all procedures involving veins of upper leg, including exploration

01270 Anesthesia for procedures involving arteries of upper leg, including bypass graft; not otherwise specified

01272 femoral artery ligation

01274 femoral artery embolectomy

(01276 has been deleted. To report, use 00880)

KNEE AND POPLITEAL AREA

01300 Anesthesia for all procedures on integumentary system of knee and/or popliteal area

01320 Anesthesia for all procedures on nerves, muscles, tendons, fascia, and bursae of knee and/or popliteal area

01340 Anesthesia for all closed procedures on lower 1/3 of femur

01360 Anesthesia for all open procedures on lower 1/3 of femur

01380 Anesthesia for all closed procedures on knee joint

01382 Anesthesia for arthroscopic procedures of knee joint

01390 Anesthesia for all closed procedures on upper ends of tibia, fibula, and/or patella

01392 Anesthesia for all open procedures on upper ends of tibia, fibula, and/or patella

01400 Anesthesia for open procedures on knee joint; not otherwise specified

01402 total knee replacement

01404 disarticulation at knee

01420 Anesthesia for all cast applications, removal, or repair involving knee joint

01430 Anesthesia for procedures on veins of knee and popliteal area; not otherwise specified

01432 arteriovenous fistula

01440 Anesthesia for procedures on arteries of knee and popliteal area; not otherwise specified

01442 popliteal thromboendarterectomy, with or without patch graft

01444 popliteal excision and graft or repair for occlusion or aneurysm

LOWER LEG (BELOW KNEE)

(Includes ankle and foot)

01460 Anesthesia for all procedures on integumentary system of lower leg, ankle, and foot

01462 Anesthesia for all closed procedures on lower leg, ankle, and foot

01464 Anesthesia for arthroscopic procedures of ankle joint

01470 Anesthesia for procedures on nerves, muscles, tendons, and fascia of lower leg, ankle, and foot; not otherwise specified

01472 repair of ruptured Achilles tendon, with or without graft

01474 gastrocnemius recession (eg, Strayer procedure)

01480 Anesthesia for open procedures on bones of lower leg, ankle, and foot; not otherwise specified

01482 radical resection

01484 osteotomy or osteoplasty of tibia and/or fibula

01486 total ankle replacement

01490 Anesthesia for lower leg cast application, removal, or repair

01500 Anesthesia for procedures on arteries of lower leg, including bypass graft; not otherwise specified

01502 embolectomy, direct or catheter

01520 Anesthesia for procedures on veins of lower leg; not otherwise specified

01522 venous thrombectomy, direct or catheter

SHOULDER AND AXILLA

(Includes humeral head and neck, sternoclavicular joint, acromioclavicular joint, and shoulder joint)

01600 Anesthesia for all procedures on integumentary system of shoulder and axilla

01610 Anesthesia for all procedures on nerves, muscles, tendons, fascia, and bursae of shoulder and axilla

01620 Anesthesia for all closed procedures on humeral head and neck, sternoclavicular joint, acromioclavicular joint, and shoulder joint

01622 Anesthesia for arthroscopic procedures of shoulder joint

01630 Anesthesia for open procedures on humeral head and neck, sternoclavicular joint, acromioclavicular joint, and shoulder joint; not otherwise specified

01632 radical resection

01634 shoulder disarticulation

01636 interthoracoscapular (forequarter) amputation

01638 total shoulder replacement

01650 Anesthesia for procedures on arteries of shoulder and axilla; not otherwise specified

01652 axillary-brachial aneurysm

01654 bypass graft

01656 axillary-femoral bypass graft

01670 Anesthesia for all procedures on veins of shoulder and axilla

01680 Anesthesia for shoulder cast application, removal or repair; not otherwise specified

01682 shoulder spica

UPPER ARM AND ELBOW

01700 Anesthesia for all procedures on integumentary system of upper arm and elbow

01710 Anesthesia for procedures on nerves, muscles, tendons, fascia, and bursae of upper arm and elbow; not otherwise specified

01712 tenotomy, elbow to shoulder, open

01714 tenoplasty, elbow to shoulder

01716 tenodesis, rupture of long tendon of biceps

01730 Anesthesia for all closed procedures on humerus and elbow

01732 Anesthesia for arthroscopic procedures of elbow joint

01740 Anesthesia for open procedures on humerus and elbow; not otherwise specified

01742 osteotomy of humerus

01744 repair of nonunion or malunion of humerus

01756 radical procedures

01758 excision of cyst or tumor of humerus

01760 total elbow replacement

01770 Anesthesia for procedures on arteries of upper arm and elbow; not otherwise specified

01772 embolectomy

01780 Anesthesia for procedures on veins of upper arm and elbow; not otherwise specified

01782 phleborrhaphy

01784 Anesthesia for repair of arterio-venous (A-V) fistula, congenital or acquired

FOREARM, WRIST AND HAND

01800 Anesthesia for all procedures on integumentary system of forearm, wrist, and hand

01810 Anesthesia for all procedures on nerves, muscles, tendons, fascia, and bursae of forearm, wrist, and hand

01820 Anesthesia for all closed procedures on radius, ulna, wrist, or hand bones

01830 Anesthesia for open procedures on radius, ulna, wrist, or hand bones; not otherwise specified

01832 total wrist replacement

01840 Anesthesia for procedures on arteries of forearm, wrist, and hand; not otherwise specified

01842 embolectomy

01844 Anesthesia for vascular shunt, or shunt revision, any type (eg, dialysis)

01850 Anesthesia for procedures on veins of forearm, wrist, and hand; not otherwise specified

01852 phleborrhaphy

01860 Anesthesia for forearm, wrist, or hand cast application, removal, or repair

RADIOLOGICAL PROCEDURES

01900 Anesthesia for injection procedure for hysterosalpingography

01902 Anesthesia for burr hole(s) for ventriculography

01904 Anesthesia for injection procedure for pneumoencephalography

01906 Anesthesia for injection procedure for myelography; lumbar

01908 cervical

01910 posterior fossa

01912 Anesthesia for injection procedure for diskography; lumbar

01914 cervical

01916 Anesthesia for arteriograms, needle; carotid, or vertebral

01918 retrograde, brachial or femoral

01920 Anesthesia for cardiac catheterization including coronary arteriography and ventriculography (not to include Swan-Ganz catheter)

01921 Anesthesia for angioplasty

01922 Anesthesia for computerized axial tomography scanning or magnetic resonance imaging

MISCELLANEOUS PROCEDURE(S)

01990 Physiological support for harvesting of organ(s) from brain-dead patient

01995 Regional IV administration of local anesthetic agent (upper or lower extremity)

(For intra-arterial or intravenous therapy for pain management, see 90783, 90784)

01996 Daily management of epidural or subarachnoid drug administration

01999 Unlisted anesthesia procedure(s)

Surgery

Guidelines

Items used by all physicians in reporting their services are presented in the **INTRODUCTION.** Some of the commonalities are repeated here for the convenience of those physicians referring to this section on **SURGERY.** Other definitions and items unique to Surgery are also listed.

1. **PHYSICIANS' SERVICES** rendered in the office, home, or hospital, consultations and other medical services are listed in the section entitled **"EVALUATION AND MANAGEMENT SERVICES"** (99200 series) found in the front of the book, beginning on page 1. "Special Services and Reports" (99000 series) is presented in the **MEDICINE** section.

2. **LISTED SURGICAL PROCEDURES** includes the operation per se, local infiltration, metacarpal/digital block or topical anesthesia when used, and the normal, uncomplicated follow-up care. This concept is referred to as a "package" for surgical procedures. To report a postoperative follow-up visit for documentation purposes only, use 99024.

3. **FOLLOW-UP CARE FOR DIAGNOSTIC PROCEDURES** (eg, endoscopy, arthroscopy, injection procedures for radiography), includes only that care related to recovery from the diagnostic procedure itself. Care of the condition for which the diagnostic procedure was performed or of other concomitant conditions is not included and may be listed separately.

4. **FOLLOW-UP CARE FOR THERAPEUTIC SURGICAL PROCEDURES** includes only that care which is usually a part of the surgical service. Complications, exacerbations, recurrence or the presence of other diseases or injuries requiring additional services should be reported with the identification of appropriate procedures.

5. **MATERIALS SUPPLIED BY PHYSICIAN:** Supplies and materials provided by the physician (eg, sterile trays/drugs), over and above those usually included with the office visit or other services rendered may be listed separately. List drugs, trays, supplies, and materials provided. Identify as 99070.

6. **MULTIPLE PROCEDURES:** It is appropriate to designate multiple procedures that are rendered on the same date by separate entries. This can be reported by using the multiple procedure modifier (-51 or 09951). See item 11 below for modifier definitions.

7. **SEPARATE PROCEDURE:** Some of the listed procedures are commonly carried out as an integral part of a total service, and as such do not warrant a separate identification. When, however, such a procedure is performed independently of, and is not immediately related to, other services, it may be listed as a "separate procedure." Thus, when a procedure that is ordinarily a component of a larger procedure is performed alone for a specific purpose, it may be considered to be a separate procedure.

8. **SUBSECTION INFORMATION:** Several of the subheadings or subsections have special needs or instructions unique to that section. Where these are indicated (eg, "Maternity Care and Delivery"), special **"NOTES"** will be presented preceding those procedural terminology listings, referring to that subsection specifically. If there is an "Unlisted Procedure" code number (see item 9 below) for the individual subsection, it will also be shown. Those subsections within the **SURGERY** section that have **"NOTES"** are as follows:

Subsection	**Code Numbers**
Musculoskeletal	20000-29909
Cardiovascular System	36000-37799

9. **UNLISTED SERVICE OR PROCEDURE:** A service or procedure may be provided that is not listed in this edition of CPT. When reporting such a service, the appropriate "Unlisted Procedure" code may be used to indicate the service, identifying it by "Special Report" as discussed in item 10 below. The "Unlisted Procedures" and accompanying codes for **SURGERY** are as follows:

   15999 Unlisted procedure, excision pressure ulcer
   17999 Unlisted procedure, skin, mucous membrane and subcutaneous tissue

19499	Unlisted procedure, breast
20999	Unlisted procedure, musculoskeletal system, general
21299	Unlisted craniofacial and maxillofacial procedure
21499	Unlisted musculoskeletal procedure, head
21899	Unlisted procedure, neck or thorax
22899	Unlisted procedure, spine
22999	Unlisted procedure, abdomen, musculoskeletal system
23929	Unlisted procedure, shoulder
24999	Unlisted procedure, humerus or elbow
25999	Unlisted procedure, forearm or wrist
26989	Unlisted procedure, hands or fingers
27299	Unlisted procedure, pelvis or hip joint
27599	Unlisted procedure, femur or knee
27899	Unlisted procedure, leg or ankle
28899	Unlisted procedure, foot or toes
29799	Unlisted procedure, casting or strapping
29909	Unlisted procedure, arthroscopy
30999	Unlisted procedure, nose
31299	Unlisted procedure, accessory sinuses
31599	Unlisted procedure, larynx
31899	Unlisted procedure, trachea, bronchi
32999	Unlisted procedure, lungs and pleura
33999	Unlisted procedure, cardiac surgery
36299	Unlisted procedure, vascular injection
37799	Unlisted procedure, vascular surgery
38999	Unlisted procedure, hemic or lymphatic system
39499	Unlisted procedure, mediastinum
39599	Unlisted procedure, diaphragm
40799	Unlisted procedure, lips
40899	Unlisted procedure, vestibule of mouth
41599	Unlisted procedure, tongue, floor of mouth
41899	Unlisted procedure, dentoalveolar structures
42299	Unlisted procedure, palate, uvula
42699	Unlisted procedure, salivary glands or ducts
42999	Unlisted procedure, pharynx, adenoids, or tonsils
43499	Unlisted procedure, esophagus
43999	Unlisted procedure, stomach
44799	Unlisted procedure, intestine
44899	Unlisted procedure, Meckel's diverticulum and the mesentery
45999	Unlisted procedure, rectum

46999 Unlisted procedure, anus
47399 Unlisted procedure, liver
47999 Unlisted procedure, biliary tract
48999 Unlisted procedure, pancreas
49999 Unlisted procedure, abdomen, peritoneum and omentum
53899 Unlisted procedure, urinary system
55899 Unlisted procedure, male genital system
58999 Unlisted procedure, female genital system nonobstetrical
59899 Unlisted procedure, maternity care and delivery
60699 Unlisted procedure, endocrine system
64999 Unlisted procedure, nervous system
66999 Unlisted procedure, anterior segment of eye
67299 Unlisted procedure, posterior segment
67399 Unlisted procedure, ocular muscle
67599 Unlisted procedure, orbit
67999 Unlisted procedure, eyelids
68399 Unlisted procedure, conjunctiva
68899 Unlisted procedure, lacrimal system
69399 Unlisted procedure, external ear
69799 Unlisted procedure, middle ear
69949 Unlisted procedure, inner ear
69979 Unlisted procedure, temporal bone, middle fossa approach

10. **SPECIAL REPORT:** A service that is rarely provided, unusual, variable, or new may require a special report in determining medical appropriateness of the service. Pertinent information should include an adequate definition or description of the nature, extent, and need for the procedure, and the time, effort, and equipment necessary to provide the service. Additional items which may be included are:

    Complexity of symptoms, final diagnosis, pertinent physical findings (such as size, locations, and number of lesion(s), if appropriate), diagnostic and therapeutic procedures (including major and supplementary surgical procedures, if appropriate), concurrent problems, and follow-up care.

11. **MODIFIERS:** Listed services and procedures may be modified under certain circumstances. When applicable, the modifying circumstance should be identified by the addition of the appropriate modifier code, which may be reported in either of two ways. The modifier may be reported by a two digit number placed after the usual procedure number from which it is separated by a hyphen. Or the modifier may be reported by a separate five digit code that is used in addition to the procedure code. If more than one modifier is used, place the "Multiple Modifiers" code immediately after the procedure code. This indicates that one or more additional modifier codes will follow. Modifiers commonly used in **SURGERY** are as follows:

-20 Microsurgery: When the surgical services are performed using the techniques of microsurgery, requiring the use of an operating microscope, modifier '-20' may be added to the surgical procedure or the separate five digit modifier code 09920 may be used. Modifier '-20' is not to be used when a magnifying surgical loupe is used, whether attached to the eyeglasses or on a headband. A special report may be appropriate to document the necessity of the microsurgical approach.

-22 Unusual Procedural Services: When the service(s) provided is greater than that usually required for the listed procedure, it may be identified by adding modifier '-22' to the usual procedure number or by use of the separate five digit modifier code 09922. A report may also be appropriate.

-26 Professional Component: Certain procedures are a combination of a physician component and a technical component. When the physician component is reported separately, the service may be identified by adding the modifier '-26' to the usual procedure number or the service may be reported by use of the five digit modifier code 09926.

-32 Mandated Services: Services related to *mandated* consultation and/or related services (eg, PRO, 3rd party payor) may be identified by adding the modifier '-32' to the basic procedure or the service may be reported by use of the five digit modifier 09932.

-47 Anesthesia by Surgeon: Regional or general anesthesia provided by the surgeon may be reported by adding the modifier '-47' to the basic service or by use of the separate five digit modifier code 09947. (This does not include local anesthesia)

Note: Modifier -47 or 09947 would not be used as a modifier for the anesthesia procedures 00100-01999.

-50 Bilateral Procedure: Unless otherwise identified in the listings, bilateral procedures that are performed at the same operative session, should be identified by the appropriate five digit code describing the first procedure. The second (bilateral) procedure is identified either by adding modifier '-50' to the procedure number or by use of the separate five digit modifier code 09950.

-51 Multiple Procedures: When multiple procedures are performed on the same day or at the same session, the major procedure or service may be reported as listed. The secondary additional, or lesser procedure(s) or service(s) may be identified by adding the modifier '-51' to the secondary procedure or service code(s) or by use of the separate five digit modifier code 09951. This modifier may be used to report multiple medical procedures performed at the same session, as well as a combination of medical and surgical procedures, or several surgical procedures performed at the same operative session.

-52 Reduced Services: Under certain circumstances a service or procedure is partially reduced or eliminated at the physician's election. Under these circumstances the service provided can be identified by its usual procedure number and the addition of the modifier '-52,' signifying that the service is reduced. This provides a means of reporting reduced services without disturbing the identification of the basic service. Modifier code 09952 may be used as an alternative to modifier '-52.'

-54 Surgical Care Only: When one physician performs a surgical procedure and another provides preoperative and/or postoperative management, surgical services may be identified by adding the modifier '-54' to the usual procedure number or by use of the separate five digit modifier code 09954.

-55 Postoperative Management Only: When one physician performs the postoperative management and another physician has performed the surgical procedure, the postoperative component may be identified by adding the modifier '-55' to the usual procedure number or by use of the separate five digit modifier code 09955.

-56 Preoperative Management Only: When one physician performs the preoperative care and evaluation and another physician performs the surgical procedure, the preoperative component may be identified by adding the modifier '-56' to the usual procedure number or by use of the separate five digit modifier code 09956.

-62 Two Surgeons: Under certain circumstances the skills of two surgeons (usually with different skills) may be required in the management of a specific surgical procedure. Under such circumstances the separate services may be identified by adding the modifier '-62' to the procedure number used by each surgeon for reporting his services. Modifier code 09962 may be used as an alternative to modifier '-62.'

-66 Surgical Team: Under some circumstances, highly complex procedures (requiring the concomitant services of several physicians, often of different specialties, plus other highly skilled, specially trained personnel and various types of complex equipment) are carried out under the "surgical team" concept. Such circumstances may be identified by each participating physician with the addition of the modifier '-66' to the basic procedure number used for reporting services. Modifier code 09966 may be used as an alternative to modifier '-66'.

-76 Repeat Procedure by Same Physician: The physician may need to indicate that a procedure or service was repeated subsequent to the original service. This circumstance may be reported by adding the modifier '-76' to the repeated service or the separate five digit modifier code 09976 may be used.

-77 Repeat Procedure by Another Physician: The physician may need to indicate that a basic procedure performed by another physician had to be repeated. This situation may be reported by adding modifier '-77' to the repeated service or the separate five digit modifier code 09977 may be used.

-78 Return to the Operating Room for a Related Procedure During the Postoperative Period: The physician may need to indicate that another procedure was performed during the postoperative period of the initial procedure. When this subsequent procedure is related to the first, and requires the use of the operating room, it may be reported by adding the modifier '-78' to the related procedure, or by using the separate five digit modifier 09978. (For repeat procedures on the same day, see -76).

-79 Unrelated Procedure or Service by the Same Physician During the Postoperative Period: The physician may need to indicate that the performance of a procedure or service during the postoperative period was unrelated to the original procedure. This circumstance may be reported by using the modifier '-79' or by using the separate five digit modifier 09979. (For repeat procedures on the same day, see -76).

-80 Assistant Surgeon: Surgical assistant services may be identified by adding the modifier '-80' to the usual procedure number(s) or by use of the separate five digit modifier code 09980.

-81 Minimum Assistant Surgeon: Minimum surgical assistant services are identified by adding the modifier '-81' to the usual procedure number or by use of the separate five digit modifier code 09981.

-82 Assistant Surgeon (when qualified resident surgeon not available): The unavailability of a qualified resident surgeon is a prerequisite for use of modifier '-82' appended to the usual procedure code number(s) or by use of the separate five digit modifier code 09982.

-90 Reference (Outside) Laboratory: When laboratory procedures are performed by a party other than the treating or reporting physician, the procedure may be identified by adding the modifier '-90' to the usual procedure number or by using the separate five digit modifier code 09990.

-99 Multiple Modifiers: Under certain circumstances two or more modifiers may be necessary to completely delineate a service. In such situations modifier '-99' should be added to the basic procedure, and other applicable modifiers may be listed as part of the description of the service. Modifier code 09999 may be used as an alternative to modifier '-99.'

12. **STARRED (⋆) PROCEDURES OR ITEMS:** Certain relatively small surgical services involve a readily identifiable surgical procedure but include variable preoperative and postoperative services (eg, incision and drainage of an abscess, injection of a tendon sheath, manipulation of a joint under anesthesia, dilation of the urethra). Because of the indefinite pre- and postoperative services the usual "package" concept for surgical services (see above) cannot be applied. Such procedures are identified by a star (⋆) following the procedure code number.

When a star (⋆) follows a surgical procedure code number, the following rules apply:

a. The service as listed includes the surgical procedure only. Associated pre- and postoperative services are not included in the service as listed.

b. Preoperative services are considered as one of the following:

1) When the starred (⋆) procedure is carried out at the time of an initial visit (new patient) and this procedure constitutes the major service at that visit, procedure number 99025 is listed in lieu of the usual initial visit as an additional service.

2) When the starred (⋆) procedure is carried out at the time of an initial or other visit involving significant identifiable services (eg, removal of a small skin lesion at the time of a comprehensive history and physical examination), the appropriate visit is listed in addition to the starred (⋆) procedure and its follow-up care.

3) When the starred (⋆) procedure is carried out at the time of a follow-up (established patient) visit and this procedure constitutes the major service at that visit, the service visit is usually not added.

4) When the starred (⋆) procedure requires hospitalization, an appropriate hospital visit is listed in addition to the starred (⋆) procedure and its follow-up care.

c. All postoperative care is added on a service-by-service basis (eg, office or hospital visit, cast change).

d. Complications are added on a service-by-service basis (as with all surgical procedures).

13. **SURGICAL DESTRUCTION** is a part of a surgical procedure and different methods of destruction are not ordinarily listed separately unless the technique substantially alters the standard management of a problem or condition. Exceptions under special circumstances are provided for by separate code numbers.

Integumentary
10040 - 19499

SURGERY

Procedures

Integumentary System

SKIN, SUBCUTANEOUS AND ACCESSORY STRUCTURES

INCISION AND DRAINAGE

(10000-10020 have been deleted. To report, see 10060, 10061)

10040* Acne surgery (eg, marsupialization, opening or removal of multiple milia, comedones, cysts, pustules)

10060* Incision and drainage of abscess (eg, carbuncle, suppurative hidradenitis, cutaneous or subcutaneous abscess, cyst, furuncle, or paronychia); simple or single

10061 complicated or multiple

10080* Incision and drainage of pilonidal cyst; simple

10081 complicated

(For excision of pilonidal cyst, see 11770-11772)

(10100, 10101 have been deleted. To report, see 10060, 10061)

10120* Incision and removal of foreign body, subcutaneous tissues; simple

10121 complicated

▲**10140*** Incision and drainage of hematoma, seroma or fluid collection

(10141 has been deleted. To report, see 10140)

10160* Puncture aspiration of abscess, hematoma, bulla, or cyst

10180 Incision and drainage, complex, postoperative wound infection

(For secondary closure of surgical wound, see 12020, 12021, 13160)

EXCISION—DEBRIDEMENT

(For dermabrasions, see 15780-15791)

(For nail debridement, see 11700-11711)

(For burn(s), see 16000-16042)

11000* Debridement of extensive eczematous or infected skin; up to 10% of body surface

11001 each additional 10% of the body surface

11040 Debridement; skin, partial thickness

11041 skin, full thickness

11042 skin, and subcutaneous tissue

11043 skin, subcutaneous tissue, and muscle

11044 skin, subcutaneous tissue, muscle, and bone

PARING OR CURETTEMENT

11050* Paring or curettement of benign hyperkeratotic skin lesion with or without chemical cauterization (such as verrucae or clavi) not extending through the stratum corneum (eg, callus or wart) with or without local anesthesia; single lesion

11051 two to four lesions

11052 more than four lesions

(11060-11062 have been deleted. To report, see 11300-11313)

BIOPSY

▲11100 Biopsy of skin, subcutaneous tissue and/or mucous membrane (including simple closure), unless otherwise listed (separate procedure); single lesion

▲11101 each separate/additional lesion

(For biopsy of conjunctiva, see 68100; eyelid, see 67810)

REMOVAL OF SKIN TAGS

Removal by scissoring, or any sharp method or ligature strangulation including chemical or electrocauterization of wound, with or without local anesthesia.

▲ **11200*** Removal of skin tags, multiple fibrocutaneous tags, any area; up to and including 15 lesions

11201 each additional ten lesions

(For electrosurgical destruction, see 17200, 17201)

SHAVING OF EPIDERMAL OR DERMAL LESIONS

Shaving is the sharp removal by transverse incision or horizontal slicing to remove epidermal and dermal lesions without a full-thickness dermal excision. This includes local anesthesia, chemical or electrocauterization of the wound. The wound does not require suture closure.

● **11300*** Shaving of epidermal or dermal lesion, single lesion, trunk, arms or legs; lesion diameter 0.5 cm or less

● **11301** lesion diameter 0.6 to 1.0 cm

● **11302** lesion diameter 1.1 to 2.0 cm

● **11303** lesion diameter over 2.0 cm

● **11305*** Shaving of epidermal or dermal lesion, single lesion, scalp, neck, hands, feet, genitalia; lesion diameter 0.5 cm or less

● **11306** lesion diameter 0.6 to 1.0 cm

● **11307** lesion diameter 1.1 to 2.0 cm

● **11308** lesion diameter over 2.0 cm

● **11310*** Shaving of epidermal or dermal lesion, single lesion, face, ears, eyelids, nose, lips, mucous membrane; lesion diameter 0.5 cm or less

● **11311** lesion diameter 0.6 to 1.0 cm

● **11312** lesion diameter 1.1 to 2.0 cm

● **11313** lesion diameter over 2.0 cm

EXCISION—BENIGN LESIONS

Excision (including simple closure) of benign lesions of skin or subcutaneous tissues (eg, cicatricial, fibrous, inflammatory, congenital, cystic lesions), including local anesthesia. See appropriate size and area below.

Excision is defined as full-thickness (through the dermis) removal of the following lesions and includes simple (non-layered) closure. The closure of defects created by incision, excision, or trauma may require intermediate (layered) closure. Layered closure involves dermal closure with separate suture closure of at least one of the deeper layers of subcutaneous and non-muscle fascial tissues. See pages 101 and following for repair codes.

(For excision of lesions requiring more than simple closure, ie, requiring intermediate, complex or reconstructive closure, see 12031-12057, 13100-13300, 14000-14300, 15000-15261, 15570-15770)

(For electrosurgical and other methods, see 17000 et seq)

11400 Excision, benign lesion, except skin tag (unless listed elsewhere), trunk, arms or legs; lesion diameter 0.5 cm or less

11401 lesion diameter 0.6 to 1.0 cm

11402 lesion diameter 1.1 to 2.0 cm

11403 lesion diameter 2.1 to 3.0 cm

11404 lesion diameter 3.1 to 4.0 cm

11406 lesion diameter over 4.0 cm

(For unusual or complicated excision, add modifier -22 or 09922)

11420 Excision, benign lesion, except skin tag (unless listed elsewhere), scalp, neck, hands, feet, genitalia; lesion diameter 0.5 cm or less

11421 lesion diameter 0.6 to 1.0 cm

11422 lesion diameter 1.1 to 2.0 cm

11423 lesion diameter 2.1 to 3.0 cm

11424 lesion diameter 3.1 to 4.0 cm

11426 lesion diameter over 4.0 cm

(For unusual or complicated excision, add modifier -22 or 09922)

11440 Excision, other benign lesion (unless listed elsewhere), face, ears, eyelids, nose, lips, mucous membrane; lesion diameter 0.5 cm or less

11441 lesion diameter 0.6 to 1.0 cm

11442 lesion diameter 1.1 to 2.0 cm

11443 lesion diameter 2.1 to 3.0 cm

11444 lesion diameter 3.1 to 4.0 cm

11446 lesion diameter over 4.0 cm

(For unusual or complicated excision, add modifier -22 or 09922)

(For eyelids involving more than skin, see also 67800 et seq)

▲**11450** Excision of skin and subcutaneous tissue for hidradenitis, axillary; with simple or intermediate repair

▲**11451** with complex repair

▲**11462** Excision of skin and subcutaneous tissue for hidradenitis, inguinal; with simple or intermediate repair

▲**11463** with complex repair

▲**11470** Excision of skin and subcutaneous tissue for hidradenitis, perianal, perineal, or umbilical; with simple or intermediate repair

▲**11471** with complex repair

(When skin graft or flap is used for closure, use appropriate procedure code in addition)

(For bilateral procedure, add modifier -50 or 09950)

EXCISION—MALIGNANT LESIONS

Excision (including simple closure) of malignant lesion of skin or subcutaneous tissues including local anesthesia, each lesion. For removal of malignant lesions of skin by any method other than excision, as defined above, see destruction codes 17000-17999.

Excision is defined as full-thickness (through the dermis) removal of the following lesions and includes simple (non-layered) closure. The closure of defects created by incision, excision, or trauma may require intermediate (layered) closure. Layered closure involves dermal closure with separate suture closure of at least one of the deeper layers of subcutaneous and non-muscle fascial tissues.

(For excision of lesions requiring more than simple closure, ie, requiring intermediate, complex or reconstructive repair, see 12031-12057, 13100-13300, 14000-14300, 15000-15261, 15570-15770)

11600 Excision, malignant lesion, trunk, arms, or legs; lesion diameter 0.5 cm or less

11601 lesion diameter 0.6 to 1.0 cm

11602 lesion diameter 1.1 to 2.0 cm

11603 lesion diameter 2.1 to 3.0 cm

11604 lesion diameter 3.1 to 4.0 cm

11606 lesion diameter over 4.0 cm

11620 Excision, malignant lesion, scalp, neck, hands, feet, genitalia; lesion diameter 0.5 cm or less

11621 lesion diameter 0.6 to 1.0 cm

11622 lesion diameter 1.1 to 2.0 cm

11623 lesion diameter 2.1 to 3.0 cm

11624 lesion diameter 3.1 to 4.0 cm

11626 lesion diameter over 4.0 cm

11640 Excision, malignant lesion, face, ears, eyelids, nose, lips; lesion diameter 0.5 cm or less

11641 lesion diameter 0.6 to 1.0 cm

11642 lesion diameter 1.1 to 2.0 cm

11643 lesion diameter 2.1 to 3.0 cm

11644 lesion diameter 3.1 to 4.0 cm

11646 lesion diameter over 4.0 cm

(For eyelids involving more than skin, see also 67800 et seq)

NAILS

(For drainage of paronychia or onychia, see 10060, 10061)

11700* Debridement of nails, manual; five or less

11701 each additional, five or less

11710* Debridement of nails, electric grinder; five or less

11711 each additional, five or less

11730* Avulsion of nail plate, partial or complete, simple; single

11731 second nail plate

11732 each additional nail plate

11740 Evacuation of subungual hematoma

11750 Excision of nail and nail matrix, partial or complete, (eg, ingrown or deformed nail) for permanent removal;

11752 with amputation of tuft of distal phalanx

(For skin graft, if used, see 15050)

11760 Repair of nail bed

11762 Reconstruction of nail bed with graft

11765 Wedge excision of skin of nail fold (eg, for ingrown toenail)

MISCELLANEOUS

(For incision of pilonidal cyst, see 10080, 10081)

11770 Excision of pilonidal cyst or sinus; simple

11771 extensive

11772 complicated

INTRODUCTION

11900* Injection, intralesional; up to and including seven lesions

11901* more than seven lesions

(For veins, see 36470, 36471)

11920 Tattooing, intradermal introduction of insoluble opaque pigments to correct color defects of skin, including micropigmentation; 6.0 sq cm or less

11921 6.1 to 20.0 sq cm

11922 each additional 20.0 sq cm

11950 Subcutaneous injection of "filling" material (eg, collagen); 1 cc or less

11951 1.1 to 5.0 cc

11952 5.1 to 10.0 cc

11954 over 10.0 cc

11960 Insertion of tissue expander(s) for other than breast, including subsequent expansion

(For breast reconstruction with tissue expander(s), see 19357)

11970 Replacement of tissue expander with permanent prosthesis

11971 Removal of tissue expander(s) without insertion of prosthesis

▲ **11975** Insertion, implantable contraceptive capsules

▲ **11976** Removal, implantable contraceptive capsules

● **11977** Removal with reinsertion, implantable contraceptive capsules

REPAIR (CLOSURE)

The repair of wounds may be classified as Simple, Intermediate or Complex.

SIMPLE REPAIR is used when the wound is superficial; ie, involving primarily epidermis or dermis, or subcutaneous tissues without significant involvement of deeper structures, and requires simple one layer closure/suturing. This includes local anesthesia and chemical or electrocauterization of wounds not closed.

(Closure with adhesive strips is included in appropriate E/M service)

INTERMEDIATE REPAIR includes the repair of wounds that, in addition to the above, require layered closure of one or more of the subcutaneous tissue and superficial (non-muscle) fascia, in addition to the skin (epidermal and dermal) closure. Single-layer closure of heavily contaminated wounds that have required extensive cleaning or removal of particulate matter also constitutes intermediate repair.

COMPLEX REPAIR includes the repair of wounds requiring more than layered closure, viz., scar revision, debridement, (eg, traumatic lacerations or avulsions), extensive undermining, stents or retention sutures. It may include creation of the defect and necessary preparation for repairs or the debridement and repair of complicated lacerations or avulsions.

Instructions for listing services at time of wound repair:

1. The repaired wound(s) should be measured and recorded in centimeters, whether curved, angular or stellate.

2. When multiple wounds are repaired, add together the lengths of those in the same classification (see above) and report as a single item. When more than one classification of wounds is repaired, list the more complicated as the primary procedure and the less complicated as the secondary procedure, using either modifier '-51' or 09951.

3. Decontamination and/or debridement: Debridement is considered a separate procedure only when gross contamination requires prolonged cleansing, when appreciable amounts of devitalized or contaminated tissue are removed, or when debridement is carried out separately without immediate primary closure. (For extensive debridement of soft tissue and/or bone, see 11040-11044.)

4. Involvement of nerves, blood vessels and tendons: Report under appropriate system (Nervous, Cardiovascular, Musculoskeletal) for repair of these structures. The repair of these associated wounds is included in the primary procedure unless it qualifies as a complex wound, in which case either modifier '-51' or 09951 applies.

Simple ligation of vessels in an open wound is considered as part of any wound closure.

Simple "exploration" of nerves, blood vessels or tendons exposed in an open wound is also considered part of the essential treatment of the wound and is not a separate procedure unless appreciable dissection is required.

REPAIR—SIMPLE

(Sum of lengths of repairs)

12001* Simple repair of superficial wounds of scalp, neck, axillae, external genitalia, trunk and/or extremities (including hands and feet); 2.5 cm or less

12002* 2.6 cm to 7.5 cm

12004* 7.6 cm to 12.5 cm

12005 12.6 cm to 20.0 cm

12006 20.1 cm to 30.0 cm

12007 over 30.0 cm

12011* Simple repair of superficial wounds of face, ears, eyelids, nose, lips and/or mucous membranes; 2.5 cm or less

12013* 2.6 cm to 5.0 cm

12014 5.1 cm to 7.5 cm

12015 7.6 cm to 12.5 cm

12016 12.6 cm to 20.0 cm

12017 20.1 cm to 30.0 cm

12018 over 30.0 cm

12020 Treatment of superficial wound dehiscence; simple closure

12021 with packing

(For extensive or complicated secondary wound closure, see 13160)

REPAIR—INTERMEDIATE

(Sum of lengths of repairs)

12031* Layer closure of wounds of scalp, axillae, trunk and/or extremities (excluding hands and feet); 2.5 cm or less

12032* 2.6 cm to 7.5 cm

12034 7.6 cm to 12.5 cm

12035 12.6 cm to 20.0 cm

12036 20.1 cm to 30.0 cm

12037 over 30.0 cm

12041* Layer closure of wounds of neck, hands, feet and/or external genitalia; 2.5 cm or less

12042 2.6 cm to 7.5 cm

12044 7.6 cm to 12.5 cm

12045 12.6 cm to 20.0 cm

12046 20.1 cm to 30.0 cm

12047 over 30.0 cm

12051* Layer closure of wounds of face, ears, eyelids, nose, lips and/or mucous membranes; 2.5 cm or less

12052 2.6 cm to 5.0 cm

12053 5.1 cm to 7.5 cm

12054 7.6 cm to 12.5 cm

12055 12.6 cm to 20.0 cm

12056 20.1 cm to 30.0 cm

12057 over 30.0 cm

REPAIR—COMPLEX

(Reconstructive procedures, complicated wound closure)

(Sum of lengths of repairs)

(For full thickness repair of lip or eyelid, see respective anatomical subsections)

13100 Repair, complex, trunk; 1.1 cm to 2.5 cm

(For 1.0 cm or less, see simple or intermediate repairs)

13101 2.6 cm to 7.5 cm

13120 Repair, complex, scalp, arms, and/or legs; 1.1 cm to 2.5 cm

(For 1.0 cm or less, see simple or intermediate repairs)

13121 2.6 cm to 7.5 cm

13131 Repair, complex, forehead, cheeks, chin, mouth, neck, axillae, genitalia, hands and/or feet; 1.1 cm to 2.5 cm

(For 1.0 cm or less, see simple or intermediate repairs)

13132 2.6 cm to 7.5 cm

13150 Repair, complex, eyelids, nose, ears and/or lips; 1.0 cm or less

(See also 40650-40654, 67961-67975)

13151 1.1 cm to 2.5 cm

13152 2.6 cm to 7.5 cm

13160 Secondary closure of surgical wound or dehiscence, extensive or complicated

(For packing or simple secondary wound closure, see 12020, 12021)

13300 Repair, unusual, complicated, over 7.5 cm, any area

ADJACENT TISSUE TRANSFER OR REARRANGEMENT

(For full thickness repair of lip or eyelid, see respective anatomical subsections)

Excision (including lesion) and/or repair by adjacent tissue transfer or rearrangement (eg, Z-plasty, W-plasty, V-Y plasty, rotation flap, advancement flap, double pedicle flap). When applied in repairing lacerations, the procedures listed must be developed by the surgeon to accomplish the repair. They do not apply when direct closure or rearrangement of traumatic wounds incidentally result in these configurations.

(Skin graft necessary to close secondary defect is considered an additional procedure)

14000 Adjacent tissue transfer or rearrangement, trunk; defect 10 sq cm or less

14001 defect 10.1 sq cm to 30.0 sq cm

14020 Adjacent tissue transfer or rearrangement, scalp, arms and/or legs; defect 10 sq cm or less

14021 defect 10.1 sq cm to 30.0 sq cm

14040 Adjacent tissue transfer or rearrangement, forehead, cheeks, chin, mouth, neck, axillae, genitalia, hands and/or feet; defect 10 sq cm or less

14041 defect 10.1 sq cm to 30.0 sq cm

14060 Adjacent tissue transfer or rearrangement, eyelids, nose, ears and/or lips; defect 10 sq cm or less

14061 defect 10.1 sq cm to 30.0 sq cm

(For eyelid, full thickness, see 67961 et seq)

14300 Adjacent tissue transfer or rearrangement, more than 30 sq cm, unusual or complicated, any area

14350 Filleted finger or toe flap, including preparation of recipient site

FREE SKIN GRAFTS

Identify by size and location of the defect (recipient area) and the type of graft; includes simple debridement of granulations or recent avulsion.

When a primary procedure such as orbitectomy, radical mastectomy or deep tumor removal requires skin graft for definitive closure, see appropriate anatomical subsection for primary procedure and this section for skin graft.

(Repair of donor site requiring skin graft or local flaps is to be added as an additional procedure)

15000 Excisional preparation or creation of recipient site by excision of essentially intact skin (including subcutaneous tissues), scar, or other lesion prior to repair with free skin graft (list as separate service in addition to skin graft)

(For appropriate skin grafts, see 15050-15261; list the free graft separately by its procedure number when the graft, immediate or delayed, is applied)

15050 Pinch graft, single or multiple, to cover small ulcer, tip of digit, or other minimal open area (except on face), up to defect size 2 cm diameter

(For tissue-cultured skin grafts, use 15100-15121. These codes include harvesting of keratinocytes. Procedures are coded by recipient site.)

15100 Split graft, trunk, scalp, arms, legs, hands, and/or feet (except multiple digits); 100 sq cm or less, or each one percent of body area of infants and children (except 15050)

15101 each additional 100 sq cm, or each one percent of body area of infants and children, or part thereof

15120 Split graft, face, eyelids, mouth, neck, ears, orbits, genitalia, and/or multiple digits; 100 sq cm or less, or each one percent of body area of infants and children (except 15050)

15121 each additional 100 sq cm, or each one percent of body area of infants and children, or part thereof

(For eyelids, see also 67961 et seq)

15200 Full thickness graft, free, including direct closure of donor site, trunk; 20 sq cm or less

15201 each additional 20 sq cm

15220 Full thickness graft, free, including direct closure of donor site, scalp, arms, and/or legs; 20 sq cm or less

15221 each additional 20 sq cm

15240 Full thickness graft, free, including direct closure of donor site, forehead, cheeks, chin, mouth, neck, axillae, genitalia, hands, and/or feet; 20 sq cm or less

(For finger tip graft, see 15050)

(For repair of syndactyly, fingers, see 26560-26562)

15241 each additional 20 sq cm

15260 Full thickness graft, free, including direct closure of donor site, nose, ears, eyelids, and/or lips; 20 sq cm or less

15261 each additional 20 sq cm

(For eyelids, see also 67961 et seq)

(Repair of donor site requiring skin graft or local flaps, to be added as additional separate procedure)

15350 Application of allograft, skin

15400 Application of xenograft, skin

(15410-15416 have been deleted. To report, use 15755)

FLAPS (SKIN AND/OR DEEP TISSUES)

Regions listed refer to recipient area (not donor site) when flap is being attached in transfer or to final site.

Regions listed refer to donor site when tube is formed for later or when "delay" of flap is prior to transfer.

Procedures 15570-15738 do not include extensive immobilization (eg, large plaster casts and other immobilizing devices are considered additional separate procedures).

(Repair of donor site requiring skin graft or local flaps is considered an additional separate procedure)

(15500-15515 have been deleted. To report, see 15570-15576)

(15540-15555 have been deleted. To report, see 15570-15576)

15570 Formation of direct or tubed pedicle, with or without transfer; trunk

15572 scalp, arms, or legs

15574 forehead, cheeks, chin, mouth, neck, axillae, genitalia, hands or feet

15576 eyelids, nose, ears, lips, or intraoral

15580 Cross finger flap, including free graft to donor site

(For major debridement or excisional preparation of recipient area at the time of attachment of pedicle flap, see 15570-15576)

15600 Delay of flap or sectioning of flap (division and inset); at trunk

15610 at scalp, arms, or legs

15620 at forehead, cheeks, chin, neck, axillae, genitalia, hands (except 15625), or feet

15625 section pedicle of cross finger flap

15630 at eyelids, nose, ears, or lips

15650 Transfer, intermediate, of any pedicle flap (eg, abdomen to wrist, "Walking" tube), any location

(15700-15730 have been deleted. To report, see 15570-15576)

(For eyelids, nose, ears, or lips, see also anatomical area)

(For revision, defatting or rearranging of transferred pedicle flap or skin graft, see 13100-14300)

(Procedures 15732-15738 are described by donor site of the muscle, myocutaneous, or fasciocutaneous flap)

15732 Muscle, myocutaneous, or fasciocutaneous flap; head and neck (eg, temporalis, masseter, sternocleidomastoid, levator scapulae)

15734 trunk

15736 upper extremity

15738 lower extremity

OTHER FLAPS AND GRAFTS

(Repair of donor site requiring skin graft or local flaps should be reported as an additional procedure)

15740 Flap; island pedicle

(15745 has been deleted. To report, see 15732-15738)

15750 neurovascular pedicle

15755 Free flap (microvascular transfer)

15760 Graft; composite (full thickness of external ear or nasal ala), including primary closure, donor area

15770 derma-fat-fascia

15775 Punch graft for hair transplant; 1 to 15 punch grafts

15776 more than 15 punch grafts

(For strip transplant, use 15220)

MISCELLANEOUS PROCEDURES

15780 Dermabrasion; total face (eg, for acne scarring, fine wrinkling, rhytids, general keratosis)

15781 segmental, face

15782 regional, other than face

15783 superficial, any site, (eg, tattoo removal)

(15785 has been deleted. To report, see 15781, 15782)

15786* Abrasion; single lesion (eg, keratosis, scar)

15787 each additional four lesions or less

15790 Chemical peel (chemexfoliation); total face

15791 regional, face, hand, or elsewhere

(15800 has been deleted)

15810 Salabrasion; 20 sq cm or less

15811 over 20 sq cm

15819 Cervicoplasty

15820 Blepharoplasty, lower eyelid;

15821 with extensive herniated fat pad

15822 Blepharoplasty, upper eyelid;

15823 with excessive skin weighting down lid

(For bilateral blepharoplasty, add modifier -50 or 09950)

(See also 67916, 67917, 67923, 67924)

15824 Rhytidectomy; forehead

15825 neck with platysmal tightening (platysmal flap, "P-flap")

15826 glabellar frown lines

(15827 has been deleted. To report, use 15838)

15828 cheek, chin, and neck

15829 superficial musculoaponeurotic system (SMAS) flap

(For bilateral rhytidectomy, add modifier -50 or 09950)

15831 Excision, excessive skin and subcutaneous tissue (including lipectomy); abdomen (abdominoplasty)

15832 thigh

15833 leg

15834 hip

15835 buttock

15836 arm

15837 forearm or hand

15838 submental fat pad

15839 other area

(For bilateral procedure, add modifier -50 or 09950)

15840 Graft for facial nerve paralysis; free fascia graft (including obtaining fascia)

(For bilateral procedure, add modifier -50 or 09950)

15841 free muscle graft (including obtaining graft)

15842 free muscle graft by microsurgical technique

15845 regional muscle transfer

(For intravenous fluorescein examination of blood flow in graft or flap, see 15860)

(For nerve transfers, decompression, or repair, see 64830-64876, 64905, 64907, 69720, 69725, 69740, 69745, 69955)

15850 Removal of sutures under anesthesia (other than local), same surgeon

15851 Removal of sutures under anesthesia (other than local), other surgeon

15852 Dressing change (for other than burns) under anesthesia (other than local)

15860 Intravenous injection of agent (eg, fluorescein) to test blood flow in flap or graft

(15875 has been deleted. To report, see 15876-15879)

15876 Suction assisted lipectomy; head and neck

15877 trunk

15878 upper extremity

15879 lower extremity

PRESSURE ULCERS (DECUBITUS ULCERS)

15920 Excision, coccygeal pressure ulcer, with coccygectomy; with primary suture

15922 with flap closure

(15930 has been deleted. To report, use 15934)

15931 Excision, sacral pressure ulcer, with primary suture;

(15932 has been deleted)

15933 with ostectomy

15934 Excision, sacral pressure ulcer, with skin flap closure;

15935 with ostectomy

15936 Excision, sacral pressure ulcer, with muscle or myocutaneous flap closure;

15937 with ostectomy

(To identify muscle or myocutaneous flap closure, use also code number for specific flap)

15940 Excision, ischial pressure ulcer, with primary suture;

15941 with ostectomy (ischiectomy)

(15942, 15943 have been deleted. To report, use 15944-15946)

15944 Excision, ischial pressure ulcer, with skin flap closure;

15945 with ostectomy

15946 Excision, ischial pressure ulcer, with ostectomy, with muscle or myocutaneous flap closure

(To identify muscle or myocutaneous flap closure, use also code number for specific flap)

15950 Excision, trochanteric pressure ulcer, with primary suture;

15951 with ostectomy

15952 Excision, trochanteric pressure ulcer, with skin flap closure;

15953 with ostectomy

(15954 and 15955 have been deleted. To report, use appropriate debridement, closure or flap codes)

15956 Excision, trochanteric pressure ulcer, with muscle or myocutaneous flap closure;

15958 with ostectomy

(To identify muscle or myocutaneous flap closure, use also code number for specific flap)

(15960-15983 have been deleted. To report, use appropriate debridement, closure or flap codes)

15999 Unlisted procedure, excision pressure ulcer

(For free skin graft to close ulcer or donor site, see 15000 et seq)

BURNS, LOCAL TREATMENT

Procedures 16000-16042 refer to local treatment of burned surface only.

List percentage of body surface involved and depth of burn.

(For skin graft, see 15100-15650)

(For necessary related medical services (eg, hospital visits, detention) in management of burned patients, see appropriate services in Evaluation and Management and Medicine Sections)

16000 Initial treatment, first degree burn, when no more than local treatment is required

16010 Dressings and/or debridement, initial or subsequent; under anesthesia, small

16015 under anesthesia, medium or large, or with major debridement

16020* without anesthesia, office or hospital, small

16025* without anesthesia, medium (eg, whole face or whole extremity)

16030 without anesthesia, large (eg, more than one extremity)

16035 Escharotomy

● **16040** Excision burn wound, without skin grafting, employing alloplastic dressing (eg, synthetic mesh), any anatomic site; less than one percent total body surface area

● **16041** greater than one percent and less than nine percent total body surface area

● **16042** each additional nine percent total body surface area, or part thereof

(For debridement, curettement of burn wound, see 16010-16030)

DESTRUCTION

Destruction means the ablation of benign, pre-malignant or malignant tissues by any method, with or without curettement, including local anesthesia, and not usually requiring closure. Any method includes electrocautery, electrodesiccation, cryosurgery, laser and chemical treatment. Lesions include condylomata, papillomata, molluscum contagiosum, herpetic lesions, flat (plane, juvenile) warts, milia, or other benign, pre-malignant, or malignant lesions.

(For sharp removal of skin tags and fibrocutaneous lesions, see codes 11200, 11201)

(For electrosurgical destruction of skin tags, see codes 17200, 17201)

(For destruction of malignant skin lesions, see 17260-17286)

DESTRUCTION, BENIGN OR PREMALIGNANT LESIONS

17000* Destruction by any method, including laser, with or without surgical curettement, all benign facial lesions or premalignant lesions in any location, or benign lesions other than cutaneous vascular proliferative lesions, including local anesthesia; one lesion

17001 second and third lesions, each

17002 over three lesions, each additional lesion

17010 complicated lesion(s)

17100* Destruction by any method, including laser, of benign skin lesions other than cutaneous vascular proliferative lesions on any area other than the face, including local anesthesia; one lesion

17101 second lesion

17102 over two lesions, each additional lesion up to 15 lesions

17104 15 or more lesions

▲**17105** complicated or extensive lesions

17106 Destruction of cutaneous vascular proliferative lesions (eg, laser technique); less than 10 sq cm

17107 10.0 - 50.0 sq cm

17108 over 50.0 sq cm

17110* Destruction by any method of flat (plane, juvenile) warts or molluscum contagiosum, milia, up to 15 lesions

(Retreatment same as office visit)

17200* Electrosurgical destruction of multiple fibrocutaneous tags; up to 15 lesions

17201 each additional ten lesions

(For excision of fibrocutaneous tags, see 11200, 11201)

▲**17250*** Chemical cauterization of granulation tissue (proud flesh, sinus or fistula)

(17250 is not to be used with removal or excision codes)

DESTRUCTION, MALIGNANT LESIONS, ANY METHOD

17260* Destruction, malignant lesion, any method, trunk, arms or legs; lesion diameter 0.5 cm or less

17261 lesion diameter 0.6 to 1.0 cm

17262 lesion diameter 1.1 to 2.0 cm

17263 lesion diameter 2.1 to 3.0 cm

17264 lesion diameter 3.1 to 4.0 cm

17266 lesion diameter over 4.0 cm

17270* Destruction, malignant lesion, any method, scalp, neck, hands, feet, genitalia; lesion diameter 0.5 cm or less

17271 lesion diameter 0.6 to 1.0 cm

17272 lesion diameter 1.1 to 2.0 cm

17273 lesion diameter 2.1 to 3.0 cm

17274 lesion diameter 3.1 to 4.0 cm

17276 lesion diameter over 4.0 cm

17280* Destruction, malignant lesion, any method, face, ears, eyelids, nose, lips, mucous membrane; lesion diameter 0.5 cm or less

17281 lesion diameter 0.6 to 1.0 cm

17282 lesion diameter 1.1 to 2.0 cm

17283 lesion diameter 2.1 to 3.0 cm

17284 lesion diameter 3.1 to 4.0 cm

17286 lesion diameter over 4.0 cm

MOHS' MICROGRAPHIC SURGERY

Mohs' micrographic surgery, for the removal of complex or ill-defined skin cancer, requires a single physician to act in two integrated, but separate and distinct capacities: surgeon and pathologist. If either of these responsibilities are delegated to another physician who reports his services separately, these codes are not appropriate. Mohs' micrographic surgery does not routinely require wound repair.

(17300-17302 have been deleted. To report, use 17304-17310)

(17303 has been deleted)

17304 Chemosurgery (Mohs' micrographic technique); first stage, fresh tissue technique, including removal of all gross tumor, surgical excision of tissue specimens, mapping, color coding of specimens, and microscopic examination of specimens by the surgeon, of up to 5 specimens

17305 second stage, fixed or fresh tissue, up to 5 specimens

17306 third stage, fixed or fresh tissue, up to 5 specimens

17307 additional stage(s), up to 5 specimens, each stage

17310 more than 5 specimens, fixed or fresh tissue, any stage

(For initiation or follow-up care of topical chemotherapy (eg, 5-FU or similar agents), see appropriate office visits)

MISCELLANEOUS PROCEDURES

17340* Cryotherapy (CO_2 slush, liquid N_2)

17360* Chemical exfoliation for acne (eg, acne paste, acid)

17380* Electrolysis epilation, each 1/2 hour

(For actinotherapy, see 96900)

17999 Unlisted procedure, skin, mucous membrane and subcutaneous tissue

BREAST

INCISION

19000* Puncture aspiration of cyst of breast;

19001 each additional cyst

19020 Mastotomy with exploration or drainage of abscess, deep

19030 Injection procedure only for mammary ductogram or galactogram

(For radiological supervision and interpretation, see 76086, 76088)

EXCISION

(All codes for bilateral procedures have been deleted. To report, add modifier -50 or 09950)

19100* Biopsy of breast; needle (separate procedure)

19101 incisional

19110 Nipple exploration, with or without excision of a solitary lactiferous duct or a papilloma lactiferous duct

19112 Excision of lactiferous duct fistula

19120 Excision of cyst, fibroadenoma, or other benign or malignant tumor aberrant breast tissue, duct lesion or nipple lesion (except 19140), male or female, one or more lesions

19140 Mastectomy for gynecomastia through circumareolar or other incision

19160 Mastectomy, partial;

19162 with axillary lymphadenectomy

19180 Mastectomy, simple, complete

(For immediate or delayed insertion of implant, use 19340 or 19342)

(For gynecomastia, see 19140)

19182 Mastectomy, subcutaneous

(19184-19187 have been deleted. To report, use 19182 with 19340 or 19342)

19200 Mastectomy, radical, including pectoral muscles, axillary lymph nodes

(19211-19216 have been deleted. To report, use 19200 with 19340 or 19342)

19220 Mastectomy, radical, including pectoral muscles, axillary and internal mammary lymph nodes (Urban type operation)

(19224-19229 have been deleted. To report, use 19220 with 19340 or 19342)

▲ **19240** Mastectomy, modified radical, including axillary lymph nodes, with or without pectoralis minor muscle, but excluding pectoralis major muscle

(19250-19255 have been deleted. To report, use 19240 with 19340 or 19342)

19260 Excision of chest wall tumor including ribs

19271 Excision of chest wall tumor involving ribs, with plastic reconstruction; without mediastinal lymphadenectomy

19272 with mediastinal lymphadenectomy

INTRODUCTION

● **19290** Preoperative placement of needle localization wire, breast;

● **19291** each additional lesion

(For radiological supervision and interpretation, see 76096)

REPAIR AND RECONSTRUCTION

(19300-19304 have been deleted. To report, see 19316, 19318)

(19310, 19311 have been deleted. To report, use 19325)

(All codes for bilateral procedures have been deleted. To report, add modifier -50 or 09950)

19316 Mastopexy

19318 Reduction mammaplasty

19324 Mammaplasty, augmentation; without prosthetic implant

19325 with prosthetic implant

(For flap or graft, use also appropriate number)

19328 Removal of intact mammary implant

19330 Removal of mammary implant material

19340 Immediate insertion of breast prosthesis following mastopexy, mastectomy or in reconstruction

19342 Delayed insertion of breast prosthesis following mastopexy, mastectomy or in reconstruction

(For supply of implant, use 99070)

(For preparation of custom breast implant, see 19396)

19350 Nipple/areola reconstruction

19355 Correction of inverted nipples

19357 Breast reconstruction, immediate or delayed, with tissue expander, including subsequent expansion

(19360 has been deleted)

19361 Breast reconstruction with latissimus dorsi flap, with or without prosthetic implant

19362 Breast reconstruction with transverse rectus abdominis flap (TRAM), including closure of donor site, single or double pedicle, with or without microvascular anastomosis

19364 Breast reconstruction with free flap

(Use also code number for specific flap)

19366 Breast reconstruction with other technique

(For microsurgical technique, add modifier -20 or 09920)

(For insertion of prosthesis, use also 19340 or 19342)

19370 Open periprosthetic capsulotomy, breast

19371 Periprosthetic capsulectomy, breast

19380 Revision of reconstructed breast

19396 Preparation of moulage for custom breast implant

19499 Unlisted procedure, breast

Musculoskeletal System

Cast and strapping procedures appear at the end of this section. The services listed below include the application and removal of the first cast or traction device only. Subsequent replacement of cast and/or traction device may require an additional listing.

The terms "closed treatment," "open treatment" and "percutaneous skeletal fixation" have been carefully chosen to accurately reflect current orthopaedic procedural treatments.

CLOSED TREATMENT

"Closed treatment" specifically means that the fracture site is not surgically opened (exposed to the external environment and directly visualized). This terminology is used to describe procedures that treat fractures by three methods:

1) without manipulation

2) with manipulation

3) with or without traction

OPEN TREATMENT

"Open treatment" is used when the fracture is surgically opened (exposed to the external environment). In this instance, the fracture (bone ends) is visualized and internal fixation may be used.

PERCUTANEOUS SKELETAL FIXATION

"Percutaneous skeletal fixation" describes fracture treatment which is neither open nor closed. In this procedure, the fracture fragments are not visualized, but fixation (eg, pins) is placed across the fracture site, usually under x-ray imaging.

The type of fracture (eg, open, compound, closed) does not have any coding correlation with the type of treatment (eg, closed, open or percutaneous) provided.

The codes for treatment of fractures and joint injuries (dislocations) are categorized by the type of manipulation (reduction) and stabilization (fixation or immobilization). These codes can apply to either open (compound) or closed fractures or joint injuries.

Skeletal traction is the application of a force (distracting or traction force) to a limb segment through a wire, pin, screw or clamp that is attached (eg, penetrates) to bone.

Skin traction is the application of a force (longitudinal) to a limb using felt or strapping applied directly to skin only.

External fixation is the usage of skeletal pins plus an attaching mechanism/device used for temporary or definitive treatment of acute or chronic bony deformity.

Codes for obtaining autogenous bone grafts, cartilage, tendon fascia lata grafts or other tissues, through separate incisions are to be used only when the graft is not already listed as part of the basic procedure.

Re-reduction of a fracture and/or dislocation performed by the primary physician may be identified by either the addition of the modifier '-76' to the usual procedure number or by use of modifier code 09976 to indicate "Repeat Procedure by Same Physician". (See Guidelines.)

Codes for external fixation are to be used only when external fixation is not already listed as part of the basic procedure.

All codes for suction irrigation have been deleted. To report, list only the primary surgical procedure performed (eg, sequestrectomy, deep incision).

GENERAL

INCISION

20000* Incision of soft tissue abscess (eg, secondary to osteomyelitis); superficial

20005 deep or complicated

(20010 has been deleted)

EXCISION

(For aspiration of bone marrow, see 85095)

20200 Biopsy, muscle; superficial

20205 deep

20206* Biopsy, muscle, percutaneous needle

(For radiological supervision and interpretation, see 76360, 76942)

(For fine needle aspiration, preparation, and interpretation of smears, see 88170-88173)

(For excision of muscle tumor, deep, see specific anatomic section)

20220 Biopsy, bone, trocar or needle; superficial (eg, ilium, sternum, spinous process, ribs)

20225 deep (vertebral body, femur)

(For bone marrow biopsy, use 85102)

20240 Biopsy, excisional; superficial (eg, ilium, sternum, spinous process, ribs, trochanter of femur)

20245 deep (eg, humerus, ischium, femur)

20250 Biopsy, vertebral body, open; thoracic

20251 lumbar or cervical

(For sequestrectomy, osteomyelitis or drainage of bone abscess, see anatomical area)

INTRODUCTION OR REMOVAL

(For injection procedure for arthrography, see anatomical area)

20500* Injection of sinus tract; therapeutic (separate procedure)

20501* diagnostic (sinogram)

(For radiological supervision and interpretation, see 76080)

20520* Removal of foreign body in muscle or tendon sheath; simple

20525 deep or complicated

20550* Injection, tendon sheath, ligament, trigger points or ganglion cyst

20600* Arthrocentesis, aspiration and/or injection; small joint, bursa or ganglion cyst (eg, fingers, toes)

20605* intermediate joint, bursa or ganglion cyst (eg, temporomandibular, acromioclavicular, wrist, elbow or ankle, olecranon bursa)

20610* major joint or bursa (eg, shoulder, hip, knee joint, subacromial bursa)

20615 Aspiration and injection for treatment of bone cyst

20650* Insertion of wire or pin with application of skeletal traction, including removal (separate procedure)

20660 Application of cranial tongs, caliper, or stereotactic frame, including removal (separate procedure)

20661 Application of halo, including removal; cranial

20662 pelvic

20663 femoral

20665* Removal of tongs or halo applied by another physician

20670* Removal of implant; superficial, (eg, buried wire, pin or rod) (separate procedure)

20680 deep (eg, buried wire, pin, screw, metal band, nail, rod or plate)

20690 Application of a uniplane (pins or wires in one plane), unilateral, external fixation system

(List 20690 in addition to code for treatment of the fracture or joint injury unless listed as part of basic procedure)

(20691 has been deleted. To report, use 20690)

20692 Application of a multiplane (pins or wires in more than one plane), unilateral, external fixation system (eg, Ilizarov, Monticelli type)

(List 20692 in addition to code for treatment of fracture or joint injury unless listed as part of basic procedure)

▲**20693** Adjustment or revision of external fixation system requiring anesthesia (eg, new pin(s) or wire(s) and/or new ring(s) or bar(s))

20694 Removal, under anesthesia, of external fixation system

REPAIR

(For debridement as a separate procedure (eg, in traumatic wound) involving soft tissue and/or bone, see 11042-11044)

REPLANTATION

20802 Replantation, arm (includes surgical neck of humerus through elbow joint); complete amputation

20804 incomplete amputation (devascularized extremity with soft tissue pedicle)

20805 Replantation, forearm (includes radius and ulna to radial carpal joint); complete amputation

20806 incomplete amputation (devascularized extremity with soft tissue pedicle)

20808 Replantation, hand (includes hand through metacarpophalangeal joints); complete amputation

20812 incomplete amputation (devascularized extremity with soft tissue pedicle)

20816 Replantation, digit, excluding thumb (includes metacarpophalangeal joint to insertion of flexor sublimis tendon); complete amputation

20820 incomplete amputation (devascularized extremity with soft tissue pedicle)

20822 Replantation, digit, excluding thumb (includes distal tip to sublimis tendon insertion); complete amputation

20823 incomplete amputation (devascularized extremity with soft tissue pedicle)

20824 Replantation, thumb (includes carpometacarpal joint to MP joint); complete amputation

20826 incomplete amputation (devascularized extremity with soft tissue pedicle)

20827 Replantation, thumb (includes distal tip to MP joint); complete amputation

20828 incomplete amputation (devascularized extremity with soft tissue pedicle)

20832 Replantation, leg; complete amputation

20834 incomplete amputation (devascularized extremity with soft tissue pedicle)

20838 Replantation, foot; complete amputation

20840 incomplete amputation (devascularized extremity with soft tissue pedicle)

GRAFTS (OR IMPLANTS)

Codes for obtaining autogenous bone, cartilage, tendon, fascia lata grafts, or other tissues, through separate incisions are to be used only when graft is not already listed as part of basic procedure.

20900 Bone graft, any donor area; minor or small (eg, dowel or button)

20902 major or large

20910 Cartilage graft; costochondral

20912 nasal septum

(For ear cartilage, see 21235)

20920 Fascia lata graft; by stripper

20922 by incision and area exposure, complex or sheet

20924 Tendon graft, from a distance (eg, palmaris, toe extensor, plantaris)

20926 Tissue grafts, other (eg, paratenon, fat, dermis)

MISCELLANEOUS

20950 Monitoring of interstitial fluid pressure (includes insertion of device, eg, wick catheter technique, needle manometer technique) in detection of muscle compartment syndrome

20955 Bone graft with microvascular anastomosis; fibula

20960 rib

20962 other bone graft (specify)

20969 Free osteocutaneous flap with microvascular anastomosis; other than iliac crest, rib, metatarsal, or great toe

20970 Free osteocutaneous flap with microvascular anastomosis; iliac crest

20971 rib

20972 metatarsal

20973 great toe with web space

20974 Electrical stimulation to aid bone healing; noninvasive (nonoperative)

(Use 20974 in addition to code for appropriate bony procedure, when applicable)

20975 invasive (operative)

(Use 20975 in addition to code for appropriate bony procedure, when applicable)

(20976 has been deleted)

20999 Unlisted procedure, musculoskeletal system, general

HEAD

(Skull, facial bones and temporomandibular joint)

INCISION

(For drainage of superficial abscess and hematoma, see 20000)

(For removal of embedded foreign body from dentoalveolar structure, see 41805, 41806)

21010 Arthrotomy, temporomandibular joint

(21011 has been deleted. To report, use 21010 with modifier -50 or 09950)

EXCISION

(For biopsy, see 20220, 20240)

(21020 has been deleted. To report, use 61501)

21015 Radical resection of tumor (eg, malignant neoplasm), soft tissue of face or scalp

21025 Excision of bone (eg, for osteomyelitis or bone abscess); mandible

21026 facial bone(s)

21029 Removal by contouring of benign tumor of facial bone (eg, fibrous dysplasia)

21030 Excision of benign tumor or cyst of facial bone other than mandible

21031 Excision of torus mandibularis

21032 Excision of maxillary torus palatinus

21034 Excision of malignant tumor of facial bone other than mandible

21040 Excision of benign cyst or tumor of mandible; simple

21041 complex

21044 Excision of malignant tumor of mandible;

21045 radical resection

(For bone graft, see 21215)

21050 Condylectomy, temporomandibular joint (separate procedure)

(21051 has been deleted. To report, use 21050 with modifier -50 or 09950)

21060 Meniscectomy, partial or complete, temporomandibular joint (separate procedure)

(21061 has been deleted. To report, use 21060 with modifier -50 or 09950)

21070 Coronoidectomy (separate procedure)

(21071 has been deleted. To report, use 21070 with modifier -50 or 09950)

INTRODUCTION OR REMOVAL

(For application or removal of caliper or tongs, see 20660, 20665)

21079-21089 describe professional services for the rehabilitation of patients with oral, facial or other anatomical deficiencies by means of prostheses such as an artificial eye, ear, or nose or intraoral obturator to close a cleft. Codes 21079-21089 should only be used when the physician actually designs and prepares the prosthesis (ie, not prepared by an outside laboratory).

21079 Impression and custom preparation; interim obturator prosthesis

21080 definitive obturator prosthesis

21081 mandibular resection prosthesis

21082 palatal augmentation prosthesis

21083 palatal lift prosthesis

21084 speech aid prosthesis

21085 oral surgical splint

21086 auricular prosthesis

21087 nasal prosthesis

21088 facial prosthesis

21089 Unlisted maxillofacial prosthetic procedure

21100* Application of halo type appliance for maxillofacial fixation, includes removal (separate procedure)

21110 Application of interdental fixation device for conditions other than fracture or dislocation, includes removal

(For removal of interdental fixation by another physician, see 20670-20680)

21116 Injection procedure for temporomandibular joint arthrography

(For radiological supervision and interpretation, see 70332)

REPAIR, REVISION, OR RECONSTRUCTION

(For cranioplasty, see 21179, 21180 and 62116, 62120, 62140-62147)

21120 Genioplasty; augmentation (autograft, allograft, prosthetic material)

21121 sliding osteotomy, single piece

21122 sliding osteotomies, two or more osteotomies (eg, wedge excision or bone wedge reversal for asymmetrical chin)

21123 sliding, augmentation with interpositional bone grafts (includes obtaining autografts)

21125 Augmentation, mandibular body or angle; prosthetic material

21127 with bone graft, onlay or interpositional (includes obtaining autograft)

21137 Reduction forehead; contouring only

21138 contouring and application of prosthetic material or bone graft (includes obtaining autograft)

21139 contouring and setback of anterior frontal sinus wall

21144 Reconstruction midface, LeFort I; intrusion, single piece (eg, for Long Face Syndrome)

21145 single piece, any direction, requiring bone grafts (includes obtaining autografts)

21146 two pieces, any direction, requiring bone grafts (includes obtaining autografts) (eg, ungrafted unilateral alveolar cleft)

21147 three or more pieces, any direction, requiring bone grafts (includes obtaining autografts) (eg, ungrafted bilateral alveolar cleft or multiple osteotomies)

21150 Reconstruction midface, LeFort II; anterior intrusion (eg, Treacher-Collins Syndrome)

21151 any direction, requiring bone grafts (includes obtaining autografts)

21154 Reconstruction midface, LeFort III (extracranial), any type, requiring bone grafts (includes obtaining autografts); without LeFort I

21155 with LeFort I

21159 Reconstruction midface, LeFort III (extra and intracranial) with forehead advancement (eg, mono bloc), requiring bone grafts (includes obtaining autografts); without LeFort I

21160 with LeFort I

21172 Reconstruction superior-lateral orbital rim and lower forehead, advancement or alteration, with or without grafts (includes obtaining autografts)

(For frontal or parietal craniotomy performed for craniosynostosis, see 61556)

21175 Reconstruction, bifrontal, superior-lateral orbital rims and lower forehead, advancement or alteration (eg, plagiocephaly, trigonocephaly, brachycephaly), with or without grafts (includes obtaining autografts)

(For bifrontal craniotomy performed for craniosynostosis, see 61557)

21179 Reconstruction, entire or majority of forehead and/or supraorbital rims; with grafts (allograft or prosthetic material)

21180 with autograft (includes obtaining grafts)

(For extensive craniectomy for multiple suture craniosynostosis, use only 61558 or 61559)

21181 Reconstruction by contouring of benign tumor of cranial bones (eg, fibrous dysplasia), extracranial

21182 Reconstruction of orbital walls, rims, forehead, nasoethmoid complex following intra and extracranial excision of benign tumor of cranial bone (eg, fibrous dysplasia), with multiple autografts (includes obtaining grafts); total area of bone grafting less than 40 cm^2

21183 total area of bone grafting greater than 40 cm^2 but less than 80 cm^2

21184 total area of bone grafting greater than 80 cm^2

(For excision of benign tumor of cranial bones, see 61563, 61564)

21188 Reconstruction midface, osteotomies (other than LeFort type) and bone grafts (includes obtaining autografts)

21193 Reconstruction of mandibular ramus, horizontal, vertical, "C", or "L" osteotomy; without bone graft

21194 with bone graft (includes obtaining graft)

21195 Reconstruction of mandibular ramus, sagittal split; without internal rigid fixation

21196 with internal rigid fixation

21198 Osteotomy, mandible, segmental

(21200, 21202, 21203 have been deleted. To report, see 21193-21198)

(21204 has been deleted. To report, see 21144-21160)

21206 Osteotomy, maxilla, segmental (eg, Wassmund or Schuchard)

(21207 has been deleted. To report, use 21209)

21208 Osteoplasty, facial bones; augmentation (autograft, allograft, or prosthetic implant)

21209 reduction

21210 Graft, bone; nasal, maxillary or malar areas (includes obtaining graft)

(For cleft palate repair, see 42200-42225)

21215 mandible (includes obtaining graft)

21230 Graft; rib cartilage, autogenous, to face, chin, nose or ear (includes obtaining graft)

21235 ear cartilage, autogenous, to nose or ear (includes obtaining graft)

(21239 has been deleted. To report, use 21208)

21240 Arthroplasty, temporomandibular joint, with or without autograft (includes obtaining graft)

(21241 has been deleted. To report, use 21240 with modifier -50 or 09950)

(If bone or cartilage graft is used for temporomandibular joint arthroplasty, use 20900-20910)

21242 Arthroplasty, temporomandibular joint, with allograft

21243 Arthroplasty, temporomandibular joint, with prosthetic joint replacement

21244 Reconstruction of mandible, extraoral, with transosteal bone plate (eg, mandibular staple bone plate)

21245 Reconstruction of mandible or maxilla, subperiosteal implant; partial

21246 complete

21247 Reconstruction of mandibular condyle with bone and cartilage autografts (includes obtaining grafts) (eg, for hemifacial microsomia)

21248 Reconstruction of mandible or maxilla, endosteal implant (eg, blade, cylinder); partial

21249 complete

(21250, 21254 have been deleted. To report, see 21144-21160)

21255 Reconstruction of zygomatic arch and glenoid fossa with bone and cartilage (includes obtaining autografts)

21256 Reconstruction of orbit with osteotomies (extracranial) and with bone grafts (includes obtaining autografts) (eg, microophthalmia)

21260 Periorbital osteotomies for orbital hypertelorism, with bone grafts; extracranial approach

21261 combined intra- and extracranial approach

21263 with forehead advancement

21267 Orbital repositioning, periorbital osteotomies, unilateral, with bone grafts; extracranial approach

21268 combined intra- and extracranial approach

21270 Malar augmentation, prosthetic material

(For malar augmentation with bone graft, see 21210)

21275 Secondary revision of orbitocraniofacial reconstruction

21280 Medial canthopexy (separate procedure)

(For medial canthoplasty, see 67950)

21282 Lateral canthopexy

21295 Reduction of masseter muscle and bone (eg, for treatment of benign masseteric hypertrophy); extraoral approach

21296 intraoral approach

21299 Unlisted craniofacial and maxillofacial procedure

FRACTURE AND/OR DISLOCATION

▲**21300** Closed treatment of skull fracture without operation

(For operative repair, see 62000-62010)

▲**21310** Closed treatment of nasal bone fracture without manipulation

▲**21315*** Closed treatment, nasal bone fracture; without stabilization

21320 with stabilization

21325 Open treatment of nasal fracture; uncomplicated

21330 complicated, with internal and/or external skeletal fixation

21335 with concomitant open treatment of fractured septum

● **21336** Open treatment of nasal septal fracture, with or without stabilization

▲21337 Closed treatment of nasal septal fracture, with or without stabilization

21338 Open treatment of nasoethmoid fracture; without external fixation

21339 with external fixation

▲21340 Percutaneous treatment of nasoethmoid complex fracture, with splint, wire or headcap fixation, including repair of canthal ligaments and/or the nasolacrimal apparatus

▲21343 Open treatment of depressed frontal sinus fracture

● 21344 Open treatment of complicated (eg, comminuted or involving posterior wall) frontal sinus fracture, via coronal or multiple approaches

▲21345 Closed treatment of nasomaxillary complex fracture (LeFort II type), with interdental wire fixation or fixation of denture or splint

21346 Open treatment of nasomaxillary complex fracture (LeFort II type); with wiring and/or local fixation

▲21347 requiring multiple open approaches

● 21348 with bone grafting (includes obtaining graft)

(21350 has been deleted. If necessary to report, use appropriate medical encounter code)

▲21355* Percutaneous treatment of fracture of malar area, including zygomatic arch and malar tripod, with manipulation

● 21356 Open treatment of depressed zygomatic arch fracture (eg, Gilles approach)

▲21360 Open treatment of depressed malar fracture, including zygomatic arch and malar tripod

▲21365 Open treatment of complicated (eg, comminuted or involving cranial nerve foramina) fracture(s) of malar area, including zygomatic arch and malar tripod; with internal fixation and multiple surgical approaches

● 21366 with bone grafting (includes obtaining graft)

(21380 has been deleted. If necessary to report, use appropriate evaluation and management code)

21385 Open treatment of orbital floor "blowout" fracture; transantral approach (Caldwell-Luc type operation)

21386 periorbital approach

21387 combined approach

21390 periorbital approach, with alloplastic or other implant

21395 periorbital approach with bone graft (includes obtaining graft)

▲**21400** Closed treatment of fracture of orbit, except "blowout"; without manipulation

21401 with manipulation

21406 Open treatment of fracture of orbit, except "blowout"; without implant

21407 with implant

● **21408** with bone grafting (includes obtaining graft)

(21420 has been deleted. If necessary to report, use appropriate evaluation and management code)

▲**21421** Closed treatment of palatal or maxillary fracture (LeFort I type), with interdental wire fixation or fixation of denture or splint

▲**21422** Open treatment of palatal or maxillary fracture (LeFort I type);

● **21423** complicated (comminuted or involving cranial nerve foramina), multiple approaches

▲**21431** Closed treatment of craniofacial separation (LeFort III type) using interdental wire fixation of denture or splint

▲**21432** Open treatment of craniofacial separation (LeFort III type); with wiring and/or internal fixation

▲**21433** complicated (eg, comminuted or involving cranial nerve foramina), multiple surgical approaches

▲**21435** complicated, utilizing internal and/or external fixation techniques (eg, head cap, halo device, and/or intermaxillary fixation

(For removal of internal or external fixation device, see 20670)

● **21436** complicated, multiple surgical approaches, internal fixation, with bone grafting (includes obtaining graft)

▲**21440** Closed treatment of mandibular or maxillary alveolar ridge fracture (separate procedure)

▲**21445** Open treatment of mandibular or maxillary alveolar ridge fracture (separate procedure)

▲**21450** Closed treatment of mandibular fracture; without manipulation

▲**21451** with manipulation

▲**21452** Percutaneous treatment of mandibular fracture, with external fixation

▲**21453** Closed treatment of mandibular fracture with interdental fixation

▲**21454** Open treatment of mandibular fracture with external fixation

(21455 has been deleted. To report, see 21453)

▲**21461** Open treatment of mandibular fracture; without interdental fixation

21462 with interdental fixation

21465 Open treatment of mandibular condylar fracture

▲**21470** Open treatment of complicated mandibular fracture by multiple surgical approaches including internal fixation, interdental fixation, and/or wiring of dentures or splints

▲**21480** Closed treatment of temporomandibular dislocation, initial or subsequent

▲**21485** complicated (eg, recurrent requiring intermaxillary fixation or splinting), initial or subsequent

21490 Open treatment of temporomandibular dislocation

(For interdental wire fixation, see 21462)

▲**21493** Closed treatment of hyoid fracture; without manipulation

21494 with manipulation

▲**21495** Open treatment of hyoid fracture

(For treatment of fracture of larynx, see 31584-31586)

21497 Interdental wiring, for condition other than fracture

21499 Unlisted musculoskeletal procedure, head

NECK (SOFT TISSUES) AND THORAX

(For cervical spine, see 22010 et seq)

(For injection of fracture site or trigger point, see 20550)

INCISION

(For incision and drainage of abscess or hematoma, superficial, see 10060, 10140)

21501 Incision and drainage, deep abscess or hematoma, soft tissues of neck or thorax;

21502 with partial rib ostectomy

21510 Incision, deep, with opening of bone cortex (eg, for osteomyelitis or bone abscess), thorax

(21511 has been deleted)

EXCISION

(For bone biopsy, see 20220-20251)

21550 Biopsy, soft tissue of neck or thorax

(For needle biopsy of soft tissue, see 20206)

21555 Excision tumor, soft tissue of neck or thorax; subcutaneous

21556 deep, subfascial, intramuscular

21557 Radical resection of tumor (eg, malignant neoplasm), soft tissue of neck or thorax

21600 Excision of rib, partial

(For radical resection of chest wall and rib cage for tumor, see 19260)

(For radical debridement of chest wall and rib cage for injury, see 11040-11044)

21610 Costotransversectomy (separate procedure)

21615 Excision first and/or cervical rib for outlet compression syndrome or other cause;

21616 with sympathectomy

21620 Ostectomy of sternum, partial

21627 Sternal debridement

(For debridement and closure, see 21750)

21630 Radical resection of sternum; for tumor

21632 with mediastinal lymphadenectomy

21633 for osteomyelitis

REPAIR, REVISION OR RECONSTRUCTION

(For superficial wound, see Integumentary System Section under Repair-Simple)

21700 Division of scalenus anticus; without resection of cervical rib

21705 with resection of cervical rib

21720 Division of sternocleidomastoid for torticollis, open operation; without cast application

(For transection of spinal accessory and cervical nerves, see 63191, 64722)

21725 with cast application

21740 Reconstructive repair of pectus excavatum or carinatum

(21741 has been deleted. To report, use 21899)

21750 Closure of sternotomy separation with or without debridement (separate procedure)

FRACTURE AND/OR DISLOCATION

▲21800 Closed treatment of rib fracture, uncomplicated, each

▲21805 Open treatment of rib fracture without fixation, each

▲21810 Treatment of rib fracture requiring external fixation ("flail chest")

▲21820 Closed treatment of sternum fracture

▲21825 Open treatment of sternum fracture with or without skeletal fixation

(For sternoclavicular dislocation, see 23520-23532)

MISCELLANEOUS

21899 Unlisted procedure, neck or thorax

BACK AND FLANK

EXCISION

21920 Biopsy, soft tissue of back or flank; superficial

21925 deep

(For needle biopsy of soft tissue, use 20206)

21930 Excision, tumor, soft tissue of back or flank

21935 Radical resection of tumor (eg, malignant neoplasm), soft tissue of back or flank

SPINE (VERTEBRAL COLUMN)

(Cervical, thoracic, and lumbar spine)

EXCISION

(For bone biopsy, see 20220-20251)

(22010 has been deleted. To report, use 21920)

(22011 has been deleted. To report, use 21925)

(22012 has been deleted. To report, use 20206)

(22030-22033 have been deleted. To report, use 21930)

22100 Partial resection of vertebral component, spinous processes; cervical

22101 thoracic

22102 lumbar

22105 Partial resection of vertebral component for tumor (eg, partial facetectomy, without primary grafting); cervical

22106 thoracic

22107 lumbar

22110 Partial excision of vertebrae (eg, for osteomyelitis); cervical

(22111 has been deleted)

22112 thoracic

(22113 has been deleted)

22114 lumbar

(22115 has been deleted)

INTRODUCTION

(For injection procedure for myelography, use 62284)

(For injection procedure for diskography, see 62290, 62291)

(For injection procedure, chemonucleolysis, single or multiple levels, use 62292)

(For injection procedure for facet joints, see 64442, 64443, 64622, 64623)

(For needle or trocar biopsy, see 20220-20225)

REPAIR, REVISION AND RECONSTRUCTION

(22120-22130 have been deleted. For radical resection of vertebral body, see vertebral corpectomy, 63081-63091)

(For prosthetic replacement of vertebrae, see 22150-22152)

22140 Reconstruction of spine with bone graft (autograft, allograft) and/or methylmethacrylate following resection of single vertebral body; cervical

22141 thoracic

22142 lumbar

22145 Reconstruction of spine following vertebral body resection, each additional vertebral body

22148 Harvesting of bone autograft for vertebral reconstruction following vertebral corpectomy

(List separately in addition to codes 22140-22145)

22150 Reconstruction of spine with prefabricated prosthetic replacement following resection of one or more vertebral bodies; cervical

22151 thoracic

22152 lumbar

(22200-22207 have been deleted. For osteotomy of spine, see 22210-22230)

22210 Osteotomy of spine, posterior approach, for correction of deformity, single segment; cervical

22212 thoracic

22214 lumbar

22220 Osteotomy of spine, anterior approach, for correction of deformity, single segment; cervical

22222 thoracic

22224 lumbar

22230 Osteotomy of spine for correction of deformity, each additional segment

(22250, 22251 have been deleted. For vertebral corpectomy, see 63081-63091. For spinal instrumentation, see 22840-22845. For reconstruction following vertebral corpectomy, see 22140-22152)

FRACTURE AND/OR DISLOCATION

22305 Closed treatment of vertebral process fracture(s)

22310 Closed treatment of vertebral body fracture(s), without manipulation

22315 Closed treatment of vertebral fracture and/or dislocation, with or without anesthesia, by manipulation or traction, each

22325 Open treatment of vertebral fracture and/or dislocation; lumbar, each

22326 cervical, each

22327 thoracic, each

(22330-22379 have been deleted. For decompression of spine following fracture, see 63001-63091; for arthrodesis of spine following fracture, see 22548-22650)

MANIPULATION

(22500 has been deleted. To report, use 97260)

22505 Manipulation of spine requiring anesthesia, any region

ARTHRODESIS

(Spinal arthrodesis procedures, 22548-22812, include either an allograft or an autograft. When an autograft is taken through a separate incision, use procedure code 22820 for the harvesting of autograft in addition to the code for the arthrodesis)

ARTHRODESIS, ANTERIOR OR ANTEROLATERAL APPROACH TECHNIQUE

Procedure codes 22554-22558 are for SINGLE interspace arthrodesis (2 adjacent vertebral segments); for additional interspaces or segments, use 22585.

22548 Arthrodesis, anterior transoral or extraoral technique, clivus-C1-C2 (atlas-axis), with bone graft, with or without excision of odontoid process

(22550, 22552, 22555, 22560, 22561, 22565 have been deleted. For intervertebral disk excision by laminotomy or laminectomy, see 63020-63042. For arthrodesis, see 22548-22650)

22554 Arthrodesis, anterior interbody technique; cervical below C2, with bone graft

22556 thoracic, with local bone (eg, rib) and/or bone allograft

22558 lumbar, with bone graft

22585 Arthrodesis, anterior or anterolateral, each additional interspace (list separately in addition to single level arthrodesis)

(Procedure codes 22548-22585 exclude reconstruction following vertebral corpectomy)

ARTHRODESIS, POSTERIOR, POSTEROLATERAL OR LATERAL TRANSVERSE PROCESS TECHNIQUE

Procedure codes 22590-22630 are for SINGLE interspace arthrodesis (2 adjacent vertebral segments); for additional interspaces or segments, see 22650.

22590 Arthrodesis, posterior technique, craniocervical (occiput-C2), with bone graft and/or internal fixation

22595 Arthrodesis, posterior technique, atlas-axis (C1-C2) with bone graft and/or internal fixation

22600 Arthrodesis, posterior technique, cervical below C2 segment, local bone or bone allograft and/or internal fixation

(22605 has been deleted. To report, use 22600)

22610 Arthrodesis, posterior or posterolateral technique, with local bone or bone allograft and/or internal fixation; thoracic

22612 lumbar

(22615 has been deleted. To report, use 22554 and 22820)

(22617 has been deleted. To report, use 22548 and 22820)

(22620 has been deleted. To report, use 22590 and 22820)

22625 Arthrodesis, lateral transverse process technique, with local bone or bone allograft and/or internal wire fixation, lumbar

22630 Arthrodesis, posterior interbody technique, with local bone or bone allograft and/or internal wire fixation, lumbar

(22640-22645 have been deleted. To report, see 22610, 22612, 22820)

22650 Arthrodesis, posterior, posterolateral or lateral transverse process technique, each additional interspace

(List separately in addition to code for single level arthrodesis, 22590-22630)

(22655 has been deleted. To report, use 22630 and 22820)

(22670 has been deleted. To report, use 22625 and 22820)

(22680 has been deleted. To report, see 22556-22585, 22820)

(22700 has been deleted. To report, use 22558 and 22820)

(22720 has been deleted. To report, use 22612 and 22820)

(22730 has been deleted. To report, see 22585, 22650)

(22735 has been deleted. To report, see 22585, 22650)

ARTHRODESIS FOR SPINE DEFORMITY (eg, SCOLIOSIS, KYPHOSIS)

22800 Arthrodesis, posterior, for spinal deformity, with or without cast, with bone graft; 6 or less vertebrae

(22801 has been deleted. To report, use 22800)

22802 7 or more vertebrae

(22803 has been deleted. To report, use 22802)

22810 Arthrodesis, anterior, for spinal deformity, with or without cast, with bone graft; 4 to 7 vertebrae

22812 8 or more vertebrae

(For spinal instrumentation, see 22840-22855)

ARTHRODESIS, MISCELLANEOUS

22820 Harvesting of bone autograft through separate incision (eg, ilium, fibula) for spinal arthrodesis

(Use code 22820 once regardless of number of levels of arthrodesis)

(List separately in addition to codes 22548-22650)

22830 Exploration of spinal fusion

SPINAL INSTRUMENTATION

(List separately, in addition to code for fracture, dislocation or arthrodesis of the spine, 22305-22812)

22840 Posterior instrumentation; without segmental fixation (eg, single Harrington rod technique)

22842 segmental fixation (eg, pedicle fixation, dual rods with multiple hooks and sublaminal wires)

22845 Anterior instrumentation

22849 Reinsertion of spinal fixation device

22850 Removal of posterior nonsegmental instrumentation (eg, Harrington rod)

22852 Removal of posterior segmental instrumentation

22855 Removal of anterior instrumentation

(For spinal cord monitoring, use 95925)

MISCELLANEOUS

22899 Unlisted procedure, spine

ABDOMEN

EXCISION

22900 Excision, abdominal wall tumor, subfascial (eg, desmoid)

(22910 has been deleted. To report, use 22999)

MISCELLANEOUS

22999 Unlisted procedure, abdomen, musculoskeletal system

SHOULDER

(Clavicle, scapula, humerus head and neck, sternoclavicular joint, acromioclavicular joint and shoulder joint)

INCISION

23000 Removal of subdeltoid (or intratendinous) calcareous deposits, open method

23020 Capsular contracture release (Sever type procedure) for Erb's palsy

(For incision and drainage procedures, superficial, see 10040-10160)

23030 Incision and drainage, shoulder area; deep abscess or hematoma

23031 infected bursa

23035 Incision, deep, with opening of cortex (eg, for osteomyelitis or bone abscess), shoulder area

(23036 has been deleted)

23040 Arthrotomy, glenohumeral joint, for infection, with exploration, drainage or removal of foreign body

(23042 has been deleted)

23044 Arthrotomy, acromioclavicular, sternoclavicular joint, for infection, with exploration, drainage or removal of foreign body

EXCISION

23065 Biopsy, soft tissue of shoulder area; superficial

23066 deep

(For needle biopsy of soft tissue, use 20206)

23075 Excision, tumor, shoulder area; subcutaneous

23076 deep, subfascial or intramuscular

23077 Radical resection of tumor (eg, malignant neoplasm), soft tissue of shoulder area

23100 Arthrotomy for biopsy, glenohumeral joint

23101 Arthrotomy for biopsy or for excision of torn cartilage, acromioclavicular, sternoclavicular joint

23105 Arthrotomy for synovectomy; glenohumeral joint

23106 sternoclavicular joint

23107 Arthrotomy, glenohumeral joint, with joint exploration, with or without removal of loose or foreign body

(23110 has been deleted. To report, use 23929)

23120 Claviculectomy; partial

23125 total

23130 Acromioplasty or acromionectomy, partial

23140 Excision or curettage of bone cyst or benign tumor of clavicle or scapula;

23145 with autograft (includes obtaining graft)

23146 with allograft

23150 Excision or curettage of bone cyst or benign tumor of proximal humerus;

23155 with autograft (includes obtaining graft)

23156 with allograft

23170 Sequestrectomy (eg, for osteomyelitis or bone abscess), clavicle

(23171 has been deleted)

23172 Sequestrectomy (eg, for osteomyelitis or bone abscess), scapula

(23173 has been deleted)

23174 Sequestrectomy (eg, for osteomyelitis or bone abscess), humeral head to surgical neck

(23175 has been deleted)

23180 Partial excision (craterization, saucerization, or diaphysectomy) of bone (eg, for osteomyelitis), clavicle

(23181 has been deleted)

23182 Partial excision (craterization, saucerization, or diaphysectomy) of bone (eg, for osteomyelitis), scapula

(23183 has been deleted)

23184 Partial excision (craterization, saucerization, or diaphysectomy) of bone (eg, for osteomyelitis), proximal humerus

(23185 has been deleted)

23190 Ostectomy of scapula, partial (eg, superior medial angle)

23195 Resection humeral head

(For replacement with implant, see 23470)

23200 Radical resection for tumor; clavicle

23210 scapula

23220 Radical resection for tumor, proximal humerus;

23221 with autograft (includes obtaining graft)

23222 with prosthetic replacement

INTRODUCTION OR REMOVAL

(For arthrocentesis or needling of bursa, see 20610)

(For K-wire or pin insertion or removal, see 20650, 20670, 20680)

23330 Removal of foreign body, shoulder; subcutaneous

23331 deep (eg, Neer prosthesis removal)

23332 complicated, including "total shoulder"

23350 Injection procedure for shoulder arthrography

(For radiological supervision and interpretation, see 73040)

(23355-23358 have been deleted. To report, see 29815-29825)

REPAIR, REVISION OR RECONSTRUCTION

23395 Muscle transfer, any type for paralysis of shoulder or upper arm; single

23397 multiple

23400 Scapulopexy (eg, Sprengel's deformity or for paralysis)

23405 Tenomyotomy, shoulder area; single

23406 multiple through same incision

23410 Repair of ruptured supraspinatus tendon (rotator cuff) or musculotendinous cuff; acute

23412 chronic

23415 Coracoacromial ligament release, with or without acromioplasty

23420 Repair of complete shoulder (rotator) cuff avulsion, chronic (includes acromioplasty)

23430 Tenodesis for rupture of long tendon of biceps

23440 Resection or transplantation of long tendon of biceps, for chronic tenosynovitis

23450 Capsulorrhaphy for recurrent dislocation, anterior; Putti-Platt procedure or Magnuson type operation

23455 Bankart type operation with or without stapling

23460 Capsulorrhaphy for recurrent dislocation, anterior, any type; with bone block

23462 with coracoid process transfer

23465 Capsulorrhaphy for recurrent dislocation, posterior, with or without bone block

(For sternoclavicular and acromioclavicular reconstruction, see 23530, 23550)

23466 Capsulorrhaphy for recurrent dislocation with any type multi-directional instability

23470 Arthroplasty with proximal humeral implant (eg, Neer type operation)

23472 Arthroplasty with glenoid and proximal humeral replacement (eg, total shoulder)

(For removal of total shoulder implants, see 23331, 23332)

(For osteotomy, proximal humerus, see 24400)

23480 Osteotomy, clavicle, with or without internal fixation;

23485 with bone graft for nonunion or malunion (includes obtaining graft and/or necessary fixation)

23490 Prophylactic treatment (nailing, pinning, plating or wiring) with or without methylmethacrylate; clavicle

23491 proximal humerus and humeral head

FRACTURE AND/OR DISLOCATION

▲23500 Closed treatment of clavicular fracture; without manipulation

23505 with manipulation

(23510 has been deleted. To report, see 23500, 23505, 23515)

▲23515 Open treatment of clavicular fracture, with or without internal or external fixation

▲23520 Closed treatment of sternoclavicular dislocation; without manipulation

23525 with manipulation

▲23530 Open treatment of sternoclavicular dislocation, acute or chronic;

23532 with fascial graft (includes obtaining graft)

▲23540 Closed treatment of acromioclavicular dislocation; without manipulation

23545 with manipulation

▲23550 Open treatment of acromioclavicular dislocation, acute or chronic;

23552 with fascial graft (includes obtaining graft)

▲23570 Closed treatment of scapular fracture; without manipulation

▲23575 with manipulation, with or without skeletal traction (with or without shoulder joint involvement)

(23580 has been deleted. To report, see 23570, 23575, 23585)

▲23585 Open treatment of scapular fracture (body, glenoid or acromion) with or without internal fixation

▲23600 Closed treatment of proximal humeral (surgical or anatomical neck) fracture; without manipulation

▲23605 with manipulation, with or without skeletal traction

(23610 has been deleted. To report, see 23600, 23605, 23615)

▲23615 Open treatment of proximal humeral (surgical or anatomical neck) fracture, with or without internal or external fixation, with or without repair of tuberosity(-ies);

● 23616 with proximal humeral prosthetic replacement

▲23620 Closed treatment of greater tuberosity fracture; without manipulation

23625 with manipulation

▲23630 Open treatment of greater tuberosity fracture, with or without internal or external fixation

▲23650 Closed treatment of shoulder dislocation, with manipulation; without anesthesia

23655 requiring anesthesia

(23658 has been deleted. To report, see 23650, 23655, 23660, 23665, 23670)

▲23660 Open treatment of acute shoulder dislocation

(Repairs for recurrent dislocations, see 23450-23466)

▲23665 Closed treatment of shoulder dislocation, with fracture of greater tuberosity, with manipulation

▲23670 Open treatment of shoulder dislocation, with fracture of greater tuberosity, with or without internal or external fixation

▲23675 Closed treatment of shoulder dislocation, with surgical or anatomical neck fracture, with manipulation

▲23680 Open treatment of shoulder dislocation, with surgical or anatomical neck fracture, with or without internal or external fixation

MANIPULATION

23700* Manipulation under anesthesia, shoulder joint, including application of fixation apparatus (dislocation excluded)

ARTHRODESIS

23800 Arthrodesis, shoulder joint; with or without local bone graft

23802 with primary autogenous graft (includes obtaining graft)

AMPUTATION

23900 Interthoracoscapular amputation (forequarter)

23920 Disarticulation of shoulder;

23921 secondary closure or scar revision

MISCELLANEOUS

23929 Unlisted procedure, shoulder

HUMERUS (UPPER ARM) AND ELBOW

(Elbow area includes head and neck of radius and olecranon process)

INCISION

(For incision and drainage procedures, superficial, see 10040-10160)

23930 Incision and drainage, upper arm or elbow area; deep abscess or hematoma

23931 infected bursa

23935 Incision, deep, with opening of bone cortex (eg, for osteomyelitis or bone abscess), humerus or elbow

(23936 has been deleted)

24000 Arthrotomy, elbow, for infection, with exploration, drainage or removal of foreign body

(24001 has been deleted)

● **24006** Arthrotomy of the elbow, with capsular excision for capsular release (separate procedure)

EXCISION

24065 Biopsy, soft tissue of upper arm or elbow area; superficial

24066 deep

(For needle biopsy of soft tissue, use 20206)

24075 Excision, tumor, upper arm or elbow area; subcutaneous

24076 deep, subfascial or intramuscular

24077 Radical resection of tumor (eg, malignant neoplasm), soft tissue of upper arm or elbow area

24100 Arthrotomy, elbow; for synovial biopsy only

24101 with joint exploration, with or without biopsy, with or without removal of loose or foreign body

24102 for synovectomy

24105 Excision, olecranon bursa

24110 Excision or curettage of bone cyst or benign tumor, humerus;

24115 with autograft (includes obtaining graft)

24116 with allograft

24120 Excision or curettage of bone cyst or benign tumor of head or neck of radius or olecranon process;

24125 with autograft (includes obtaining graft)

24126 with allograft

24130 Excision, radial head

(For replacement with implant, see 24366)

24134 Sequestrectomy (eg, for osteomyelitis or bone abscess), shaft or distal humerus

(24135 has been deleted)

24136 Sequestrectomy (eg, for osteomyelitis or bone abscess), radial head or neck

(24137 has been deleted)

24138 Sequestrectomy (eg, for osteomyelitis or bone abscess), olecranon process

(24139 has been deleted)

24140 Partial excision (craterization, saucerization or diaphysectomy) of bone (eg, for osteomyelitis), humerus

(24144 has been deleted)

24145 Partial excision (craterization, saucerization or diaphysectomy) of bone (eg, for osteomyelitis), radial head or neck

(24146 has been deleted)

24147 Partial excision (craterization, saucerization or diaphysectomy) of bone (eg, for osteomyelitis), olecranon process

(24148 has been deleted)

24150 Radical resection for tumor, shaft or distal humerus;

24151 with autograft (includes obtaining graft)

24152 Radical resection for tumor, radial head or neck;

24153 with autograft (includes obtaining graft)

24155 Resection of elbow joint (arthrectomy)

INTRODUCTION OR REMOVAL

(For K-wire or pin insertion or removal, see 20650, 20670, 20680)

(For arthrocentesis or needling of bursa or joint, see 20605)

24160 Implant removal; elbow joint

24164 radial head

24200 Removal of foreign body, upper arm or elbow area; subcutaneous

24201 deep

24220 Injection procedure for elbow arthrography

(For radiological supervision and interpretation, see 73085)

(For injection of tennis elbow, see 20550)

REPAIR, REVISION AND RECONSTRUCTION

24301 Muscle or tendon transfer, any type, upper arm or elbow, single (excluding 24320-24331)

24305 Tendon lengthening, upper arm or elbow, single, each

24310 Tenotomy, open, elbow to shoulder, single, each

24320 Tenoplasty, with muscle transfer, with or without free graft, elbow to shoulder, single (Seddon-Brookes type procedure)

24330 Flexor-plasty, elbow (eg, Steindler type advancement);

24331 with extensor advancement

24340 Tenodesis for rupture of biceps tendon at elbow

24342 Reinsertion of ruptured biceps tendon, distal, with or without tendon graft (includes obtaining graft)

24350 Fasciotomy, lateral or medial (eg, "tennis elbow" or epicondylitis);

24351 with extensor origin detachment

24352 with annular ligament resection

24354 with stripping

24356 with partial ostectomy

24360 Arthroplasty, elbow; with membrane

24361 with distal humeral prosthetic replacement

24362 with implant and fascia lata ligament reconstruction

24363 with distal humerus and proximal ulnar prosthetic replacement ("total elbow")

24365 Arthroplasty, radial head;

24366 with implant

24400 Osteotomy, humerus, with or without internal fixation

24410 Multiple osteotomies with realignment on intramedullary rod, humeral shaft (Sofield type procedure)

24420 Osteoplasty, humerus (eg, shortening or lengthening) (excluding 64876)

24430 Repair of nonunion or malunion, humerus; without graft (eg, compression technique)

24435 with iliac or other autograft (includes obtaining graft)

(For proximal radius and/or ulna, see 25400-25420)

24470 Hemiepiphyseal arrest (eg, for cubitus varus or valgus, distal humerus)

24495 Decompression fasciotomy, forearm, with brachial artery exploration

24498 Prophylactic treatment (nailing, pinning, plating or wiring), with or without methylmethacrylate, humerus

FRACTURE AND/OR DISLOCATION

▲24500 Closed treatment of humeral shaft fracture; without manipulation

▲24505 with manipulation, with or without skeletal traction

(24506 has been deleted. To report, see 24516)

(24510 has been deleted. To report, see 24500, 24505, 24515, 24516)

▲24515 Open treatment of humeral shaft fracture with plate/screws, with or without cerclage

● 24516 Open treatment of humeral shaft fracture, with insertion of intramedullary implant, with or without cerclage and/or locking screws

▲24530 Closed treatment of supracondylar or transcondylar humeral fracture, with or without intercondylar extension; without manipulation

(24531 has been deleted. To report, see 24535)

▲24535 with manipulation, with or without skin or skeletal traction

(24536 has been deleted. To report, see 24535)

▲24538 Percutaneous skeletal fixation of supracondylar or transcondylar humeral fracture, with or without intercondylar extension

(24540 and 24542 have been deleted. To report, see 24530, 24535, 24538, 24545, 24546)

▲24545 Open treatment of humeral supracondylar or transcondylar fracture, with or without internal or external fixation; without intercondylar extension

● 24546 with intercondylar extension

▲24560 Closed treatment of humeral epicondylar fracture, medial or lateral; without manipulation

24565 with manipulation

(24570 has been deleted. To report, see 24560, 24565, 24575)

▲24575 Open treatment of humeral epicondylar fracture, medial or lateral, with or without internal or external fixation

▲**24576** Closed treatment of humeral condylar fracture, medial or lateral; without manipulation

24577 with manipulation

(24578 has been deleted. To report, see 24576, 24577, 24579)

▲**24579** Open treatment of humeral condylar fracture, medial or lateral, with or without internal or external fixation

(24580 has been deleted. To report, see 24530, 24560, 24576, 24650, 24670)

(24581 has been deleted. To report, see 24535, 24565, 24577, 24675)

(24583 has been deleted. To report, see 24535, 24538, 24545, 24560, 24565, 24577)

(24585 has been deleted. To report, see 24538, 24545, 24575, 24579, 24665, 24666, 24685)

▲**24586** Open treatment of periarticular fracture and/or dislocation of the elbow (fracture distal humerus and proximal ulna and/or proximal radius);

▲**24587** with implant arthroplasty

(See also 24361)

(24588 has been deleted. To report, see 24586, 24587)

24600 Treatment of closed elbow dislocation; without anesthesia

24605 requiring anesthesia

(24610 has been deleted. To report, see 24586, 24600, 24605, 24615)

▲**24615** Open treatment of acute or chronic elbow dislocation

▲**24620** Closed treatment of Monteggia type of fracture dislocation at elbow (fracture proximal end of ulna with dislocation of radial head), with manipulation

(24625 has been deleted. To report, see 24620, 24635)

▲**24635** Open treatment of Monteggia type of fracture dislocation at elbow (fracture proximal end of ulna with dislocation of radial head), with or without internal or external fixation

▲**24640*** Closed treatment of radial head subluxation in child, "nursemaid elbow", with manipulation

▲**24650** Closed treatment of radial head or neck fracture; without manipulation

24655 with manipulation

(24660 has been deleted. To report, see 24650, 24655, 24665, 24666)

▲**24665** Open treatment of radial head or neck fracture, with or without internal fixation or radial head excision;

▲**24666** with radial head prosthetic replacement

▲**24670** Closed treatment of ulnar fracture, proximal end (olecranon process); without manipulation

24675 with manipulation

(24680 has been deleted. To report, see 24670, 24675, 24685)

▲**24685** Open treatment of ulnar fracture proximal end (olecranon process), with or without internal or external fixation

MANIPULATION

(24700 has been deleted. To report, use 24999)

ARTHRODESIS

24800 Arthrodesis, elbow joint; with or without local autograft or allograft

24802 with autograft (includes obtaining graft other than locally obtained)

AMPUTATION

24900 Amputation, arm through humerus; with primary closure

24920 open, circular (guillotine)

24925 secondary closure or scar revision

24930 re-amputation

24931 with implant

24935 Stump elongation, upper extremity

24940 Cineplasty, upper extremity, complete procedure

MISCELLANEOUS

24999 Unlisted procedure, humerus or elbow

FOREARM AND WRIST

(Radius, ulna, carpal bones and joints)

INCISION

25000 Tendon sheath incision; at radial styloid for deQuervain's disease

25005 at wrist for other stenosing tenosynovitis

(For decompression median nerve or for carpal tunnel syndrome, see 64721)

▲**25020** Decompression fasciotomy, forearm and/or wrist; flexor or extensor compartment

25023 with debridement of nonviable muscle and/or nerve

(For decompression fasciotomy with brachial artery exploration, see 24495)

(For incision and drainage procedures, superficial, see 10040-10160)

(For debridement, see also 11000-11044)

25028 Incision and drainage, forearm and/or wrist; deep abscess or hematoma

25031 infected bursa

25035 Incision, deep, with opening of bone cortex (eg, for osteomyelitis or bone abscess), forearm and/or wrist

(25036 has been deleted)

25040 Arthrotomy, radiocarpal or mediocarpal joint, for infection, with exploration, drainage, or removal of foreign body

(25041 has been deleted)

EXCISION

25065 Biopsy, soft tissue of forearm and/or wrist; superficial

25066 deep

(For needle biopsy of soft tissue, use 20206)

25075 Excision, tumor, forearm and/or wrist area; subcutaneous

25076 deep, subfascial or intramuscular

25077 Radical resection of tumor (eg, malignant neoplasm), soft tissue of forearm and/or wrist area

25085 Capsulotomy, wrist (eg, for contracture)

25100 Arthrotomy, wrist joint; for biopsy

25101 with joint exploration, with or without biopsy, with or without removal of loose or foreign body

25105 for synovectomy

25107 Arthrotomy, distal radioulnar joint for repair of triangular cartilage complex

25110 Excision, lesion of tendon sheath, forearm and/or wrist

25111 Excision of ganglion, wrist (dorsal or volar); primary

25112 recurrent

(For hand or finger, see 26160)

25115 Radical excision of bursa, synovia of wrist, or forearm tendon sheaths (eg, tenosynovitis, fungus, Tbc, or other granulomas, rheumatoid arthritis); flexors

25116 extensors, with or without transposition of dorsal retinaculum

(For finger synovectomies, see 26145)

25118 Synovectomy, extensor tendon sheath, wrist, single compartment;

25119 with resection of distal ulna

25120 Excision or curettage of bone cyst or benign tumor of radius or ulna (excluding head or neck of radius and olecranon process);

(For head or neck of radius or olecranon process, see 24120-24126)

25125 with autograft (includes obtaining graft)

25126 with allograft

25130 Excision or curettage of bone cyst or benign tumor of carpal bones;

25135 with autograft (includes obtaining graft)

25136 with allograft

25145 Sequestrectomy (eg, for osteomyelitis or bone abscess), forearm and/or wrist

(25146 has been deleted)

25150 Partial excision (craterization, saucerization or diaphysectomy) of bone (eg, for osteomyelitis); ulna

25151 radius

(25153 has been deleted)

(For head or neck of radius or olecranon process, see 24145, 24147)

25170 Radical resection for tumor, radius or ulna

25210 Carpectomy; one bone

(For carpectomy with implant, see 25441-25445)

25215 all bones of proximal row

25230 Radial styloidectomy (separate procedure)

25240 Excision distal ulna (Darrach type procedure)

(For implant replacement, distal ulna, see 25442)

(For obtaining fascia for interposition, see 20920, 20922)

INTRODUCTION OR REMOVAL

(For K-wire, pin or rod insertion or removal, see 20650, 20670, 20680)

25246 Injection procedure for wrist arthrography

(For radiological supervision and interpretation, see 73115)

(For foreign body removal, superficial see 20520)

25248 Exploration for removal of deep foreign body, forearm or wrist

25250 Removal of wrist prosthesis; (separate procedure)

25251 complicated, including "total wrist"

REPAIR, REVISION OR RECONSTRUCTION

25260 Repair, tendon or muscle, flexor, forearm and/or wrist; primary, single, each tendon or muscle

25263 secondary, single, each tendon or muscle

25265 secondary, with free graft (includes obtaining graft), each tendon or muscle

25270 Repair, tendon or muscle, extensor, forearm and/or wrist; primary, single, each tendon or muscle

25272 secondary, single, each tendon or muscle

25274 Repair, tendon or muscle, extensor, secondary, with tendon graft (includes obtaining graft), forearm and/or wrist, each tendon or muscle

25280 Lengthening or shortening of flexor or extensor tendon, forearm and/or wrist, single, each tendon

25290 Tenotomy, open, flexor or extensor tendon, forearm and/or wrist, single, each tendon

25295 Tenolysis, flexor or extensor tendon, forearm and/or wrist, single, each tendon

25300 Tenodesis at wrist; flexors of fingers

25301 extensors of fingers

25310 Tendon transplantation or transfer, flexor or extensor, forearm and/or wrist, single; each tendon

25312 with tendon graft(s) (includes obtaining graft), each tendon

25315 Flexor origin slide for cerebral palsy, forearm and/or wrist;

25316 with tendon(s) transfer

25317 Flexor origin slide for Volkmann contracture;

25318 with tendon(s) transfer

25320 Capsulorrhaphy or reconstruction, capsulectomy, wrist (includes synovectomy, resection of capsule, tendon insertions)

25330 Arthroplasty, wrist;

25331 with implant

25332 pseudarthrosis type with internal fixation

(For obtaining fascia for interposition, see 20920, 20922)

25335 Centralization of wrist on ulna (eg, radial club hand)

25350 Osteotomy, radius; distal third

25355 middle or proximal third

25360 Osteotomy; ulna

25365 radius and ulna

25370 Multiple osteotomies, with realignment on intramedullary rod (Sofield type procedure); radius OR ulna

25375 radius AND ulna

25390 Osteoplasty, radius OR ulna; shortening

25391 lengthening with autograft

25392 Osteoplasty, radius AND ulna; shortening (excluding 64876)

25393 lengthening with autograft

25400 Repair of nonunion or malunion, radius OR ulna; without graft (eg, compression technique)

25405 with iliac or other autograft (includes obtaining graft)

25415 Repair of nonunion or malunion, radius AND ulna; without graft (eg, compression technique)

25420 with iliac or other autograft (includes obtaining graft)

25425 Repair of defect with autograft; radius OR ulna

25426 radius AND ulna

25440 Repair of nonunion, scaphoid (navicular) bone, with or without radial styloidectomy (includes obtaining graft and necessary fixation)

25441 Arthroplasty with prosthetic replacement; distal radius

25442 distal ulna

25443 scaphoid (navicular)

25444 lunate

25445 trapezium

25446 distal radius and partial or entire carpus ("total wrist")

25447 Interposition arthroplasty, intercarpal or carpometacarpal joints

25449 Revision of arthroplasty, including removal of implant, wrist joint

25450 Epiphyseal arrest by epiphysiodesis or stapling; distal radius OR ulna

25455 distal radius AND ulna

25490 Prophylactic treatment (nailing, pinning, plating or wiring) with or without methylmethacrylate; radius

25491 ulna

25492 radius AND ulna

FRACTURE AND/OR DISLOCATION

▲**25500** Closed treatment of radial shaft fracture; without manipulation

25505 with manipulation

(25510 has been deleted. To report, see 25500, 25505, 25515)

▲**25515** Open treatment of radial shaft fracture, with or without internal or external fixation

● **25520** Closed treatment of radial shaft fracture, with dislocation of distal radioulnar joint (Galeazzi fracture/dislocation)

● **25525** Open treatment of radial shaft fracture, with internal and/or external fixation and closed treatment of dislocation of distal radioulnar joint (Galeazzi fracture/dislocation), with or without percutaneous skeletal fixation

● **25526** Open treatment of radial shaft fracture, with internal and/or external fixation and open treatment, with or without internal or external fixation of distal radioulnar joint (Galeazzi fracture/dislocation), includes repair of triangular cartilage

▲**25530** Closed treatment of ulnar shaft fracture; without manipulation

25535 with manipulation

(25540 has been deleted. To report, see 25530, 25535, 25545)

▲**25545** Open treatment of ulnar shaft fracture, with or without internal or external fixation

▲**25560** Closed treatment of radial and ulnar shaft fractures; without manipulation

25565 with manipulation

(25570 has been deleted. To report, see 25560, 25565, 25574, 25575)

● **25574** Open treatment of radial and ulnar shaft fractures, with internal or external fixation; of radius or ulna

▲**25575** of radius and ulna

▲**25600** Closed treatment of distal radial fracture (eg, Colles or Smith type) or epiphyseal separation, with or without fracture of ulnar styloid; without manipulation

25605 with manipulation

(25610 has been deleted. To report, see 25605)

▲**25611** Percutaneous skeletal fixation of distal radial fracture (eg, Colles or Smith type) or epiphyseal separation, with or without fracture of ulnar styloid, requiring manipulation, with or without external fixation

(25615 has been deleted. To report, see 25600, 25605, 25611, 25620)

▲**25620** Open treatment of distal radial fracture (eg, Colles or Smith type) or epiphyseal separation, with or without fracture of ulnar styloid, with or without internal or external fixation

▲**25622** Closed treatment of carpal scaphoid (navicular) fracture; without manipulation

25624 with manipulation

(25626 has been deleted. To report, see 25622, 25624, 25628)

▲**25628** Open treatment of carpal scaphoid (navicular) fracture, with or without internal or external fixation

▲**25630** Closed treatment of carpal bone fracture (excluding carpal scaphoid (navicular)); without manipulation, each bone

25635 with manipulation, each bone

(25640 has been deleted. To report, see 25630, 25635, 25645)

▲**25645** Open treatment of carpal bone fracture (excluding carpal scaphoid (navicular)), each bone

▲**25650** Closed treatment of ulnar styloid fracture

▲**25660** Closed treatment of radiocarpal or intercarpal dislocation, one or more bones, with manipulation

(25665 has been deleted. To report, see 25650, 25660, 25670)

▲**25670** Open treatment of radiocarpal or intercarpal dislocation, one or more bones

▲**25675** Closed treatment of distal radioulnar dislocation with manipulation

▲**25676** Open treatment of distal radioulnar dislocation, acute or chronic

▲**25680** Closed treatment of trans-scaphoperilunar type of fracture dislocation, with manipulation

▲**25685** Open treatment of trans-scaphoperilunar type of fracture dislocation

▲**25690** Closed treatment of lunate dislocation, with manipulation

25695 Open treatment of lunate dislocation

MANIPULATION

(25700 has been deleted. To report, use 25999)

ARTHRODESIS

25800 Arthrodesis, wrist joint (including radiocarpal and/or ulnocarpal fusion); without bone graft

25805 with sliding graft

25810 with iliac or other autograft (includes obtaining graft)

(25815 has been deleted. To report, see 25820, 25825)

25820 Intercarpal fusion; without bone graft

25825 with autograft (includes obtaining graft)

AMPUTATION

25900 Amputation, forearm, through radius and ulna;

25905 open, circular (guillotine)

25907 secondary closure or scar revision

25909 re-amputation

25915 Krukenberg procedure

25920 Disarticulation through wrist;

25922 secondary closure or scar revision

25924 re-amputation

25927 Transmetacarpal amputation;

25929 secondary closure or scar revision

25931 re-amputation

MISCELLANEOUS

25999 Unlisted procedure, forearm or wrist

HAND AND FINGERS

INCISION

26010* Drainage of finger abscess; simple

26011* complicated (eg, felon)

26020 Drainage of tendon sheath, one digit and/or palm

26025 Drainage of palmar bursa; single, ulnar or radial

26030 multiple or complicated

(26032 has been deleted)

26034 Incision, deep, with opening of bone cortex (eg, for osteomyelitis or bone abscess), hand or finger

26035 Decompression fingers and/or hand, injection injury (eg, grease gun)

26037 Decompressive fasciotomy, hand (excludes 26035)

(For injection injury, see 26035)

26040 Fasciotomy, palmar, for Dupuytren's contracture; closed (subcutaneous)

26045 open, partial

(For fasciectomy, see 26121-26125)

26055 Tendon sheath incision for trigger finger

26060 Tenotomy, subcutaneous, single, each digit

26070 Arthrotomy, for infection, with exploration, drainage or removal of foreign body; carpometacarpal joint

26075 metacarpophalangeal joint

26080 interphalangeal joint, each

EXCISION

26100 Arthrotomy for synovial biopsy; carpometacarpal joint

26105 metacarpophalangeal joint

26110 interphalangeal joint, each

26115 Excision, tumor or vascular malformation, hand or finger; subcutaneous

26116 deep, subfascial, intramuscular

26117 Radical resection of tumor (eg, malignant neoplasm), soft tissue of hand or finger

(26120 has been deleted. To report, use 26121-26125)

26121 Fasciectomy, palmar only, with or without z-plasty, other local tissue rearrangement, or skin grafting (includes obtaining graft);

(26122 has been deleted. To report, use 26121-26125)

26123 partial palmar excision with release of single digit including proximal interphalangeal joint

(26124 has been deleted. To report, use 26121-26125)

26125 partial excision with release of each additional digit, including proximal interphalangeal joint

(26126, 26128 have been deleted. To report, use 26121-26125)

(For fasciotomy, see 26040, 26045)

26130 Synovectomy, carpometacarpal joint

26135 Synovectomy, metacarpophalangeal joint including intrinsic release and extensor hood reconstruction, each digit

26140 Synovectomy, proximal interphalangeal joint, including extensor reconstruction, each interphalangeal joint

26145 Synovectomy tendon sheath, radical (tenosynovectomy), flexor, palm or finger, single, each digit

(For tendon sheath synovectomies at wrist, see 25115, 25116)

26160 Excision of lesion of tendon sheath or capsule (eg, cyst, mucous cyst, or ganglion), hand or finger

(For wrist ganglion, see 25111, 25112)

(For trigger digit, see 26055)

26170 Excision of tendon, palm, flexor, single (separate procedure), each

26180 Excision of tendon, finger, flexor (separate procedure)

26200 Excision or curettage of bone cyst or benign tumor of metacarpal;

26205 with autograft (includes obtaining graft)

(26206 has been deleted. To report, use 26989)

26210 Excision or curettage of bone cyst or benign tumor of proximal, middle or distal phalanx of finger;

26215 with autograft (includes obtaining graft)

(26216 has been deleted. To report, use 26989)

26230 Partial excision (craterization, saucerization, or diaphysectomy) of bone (eg, for osteomyelitis); metacarpal

26235 proximal or middle phalanx of finger

26236 distal phalanx of finger

26250 Radical resection (ostectomy) for tumor, metacarpal;

26255 with autograft (includes obtaining graft)

26260 Radical resection (ostectomy) for tumor, proximal or middle phalanx of finger;

26261 with autograft (includes obtaining graft)

26262 Radical resection (ostectomy) for tumor, distal phalanx of finger

INTRODUCTION OR REMOVAL

26320 Removal of implant from finger or hand

(For removal of foreign body in hand or finger, see 20520, 20525)

REPAIR, REVISION OR RECONSTRUCTION

26350 Flexor tendon repair or advancement, single, not in "no man's land"; primary or secondary without free graft, each tendon

26352 secondary with free graft (includes obtaining graft), each tendon

26356 Flexor tendon repair or advancement, single, in "no man's land"; primary, each tendon

26357 secondary, each tendon

26358 secondary with free graft (includes obtaining graft), each tendon

26370 Profundus tendon repair or advancement, with intact sublimis; primary

26372 secondary with free graft (includes obtaining graft)

26373 secondary without free graft

26390 Flexor tendon excision, implantation of plastic tube or rod for delayed tendon graft, hand or finger

26392 Removal of tube or rod and insertion of flexor tendon graft (includes obtaining graft), hand or finger

26410 Extensor tendon repair, dorsum of hand, single, primary or secondary; without free graft, each tendon

26412 with free graft (includes obtaining graft), each tendon

26415 Extensor tendon excision, implantation of plastic tube or rod for delayed extensor tendon graft, hand or finger

26416 Removal of tube or rod and insertion of extensor tendon graft (includes obtaining graft), hand or finger

26418 Extensor tendon repair, dorsum of finger, single, primary or secondary; without free graft, each tendon

26420 with free graft (includes obtaining graft) each tendon

26426 Extensor tendon repair, central slip repair, secondary (boutonniere deformity); using local tissues

26428 with free graft (includes obtaining graft)

26432 Extensor tendon repair, distal insertion (''mallet finger''), closed, splinting with or without percutaneous pinning

26433 Extensor tendon repair, distal insertion (''mallet finger''), open, primary or secondary repair; without graft

26434 with free graft (includes obtaining graft)

(For tenovaginotomy for trigger finger, see 26055)

26437 Extensor tendon realignment, hand

26440 Tenolysis, simple, flexor tendon; palm OR finger, single, each tendon

26442 palm AND finger, each tendon

26445 Tenolysis, extensor tendon, dorsum of hand or finger; each tendon

26449 Tenolysis, complex, extensor tendon, dorsum of hand or finger, including hand and forearm

26450 Tenotomy, flexor, single, palm, open, each

26455 Tenotomy, flexor, single, finger, open, each

26460 Tenotomy, extensor, hand or finger, single, open, each

26471 Tenodesis; for proximal interphalangeal joint stabilization

26474 for distal joint stabilization

26476 Tendon lengthening, extensor, hand or finger, single, each

26477 Tendon shortening, extensor, hand or finger, single, each

26478 Tendon lengthening, flexor, hand or finger, single, each

26479 Tendon shortening, flexor, hand or finger, single, each

26480 Tendon transfer or transplant, carpometacarpal area or dorsum of hand, single; without free graft, each

26483 with free tendon graft (includes obtaining graft), each tendon

26485 Tendon transfer or transplant, palmar, single, each tendon; without free tendon graft

26489 with free tendon graft (includes obtaining graft), each tendon

26490 Opponensplasty; sublimis tendon transfer type

26492 tendon transfer with graft (includes obtaining graft)

26494 hypothenar muscle transfer

26496 other methods

(For thumb fusion in opposition, see 26820)

26497 Tendon transfer to restore intrinsic function; ring and small finger

26498 all four fingers

26499 Correction claw finger, other methods

26500 Tendon pulley reconstruction; with local tissues (separate procedure)

26502 with tendon or fascial graft (includes obtaining graft) (separate procedure)

26504 with tendon prosthesis (separate procedure)

26508 Thenar muscle release for thumb contracture

26510 Cross intrinsic transfer

26516 Capsulodesis for M-P joint stabilization; single digit

26517 two digits

26518 three or four digits

26520 Capsulectomy or capsulotomy for contracture; metacarpophalangeal joint, single, each

26525 interphalangeal joint, single, each

26527 Arthroplasty, carpometacarpal joint

26530 Arthroplasty, metacarpophalangeal joint; single, each

26531 with prosthetic implant, single, each

26535 Arthroplasty interphalangeal joint; single, each

26536 with prosthetic implant, single, each

26540 Primary repair of collateral ligament, metacarpophalangeal joint;

26541 with tendon or fascial graft (includes obtaining graft)

26542 with local tissue (eg, adductor advancement)

26545 Reconstruction, collateral ligament, interphalangeal joint, single, including graft, each joint

26548 Repair and reconstruction, finger, volar plate, interphalangeal joint

26550 Pollicization of a digit

26552 Reconstruction thumb with toe

26555 Positional change of other finger

26557 Toe to finger transfer; first stage

26558 each delay

26559 second stage

26560 Repair of syndactyly (web finger) each web space; with skin flaps

26561 with skin flaps and grafts

26562 complex (eg, involving bone, nails)

26565 Osteotomy for correction of deformity; metacarpal

26567 phalanx of finger

26568 Osteoplasty for lengthening of metacarpal or phalanx

(26570, 26574 have been deleted. To report, use 26989)

26580 Repair cleft hand

26585 Repair bifid digit

26587 Reconstruction of supernumerary digit, soft tissue and bone

(For excision of supernumerary digit, soft tissue only, use 11200)

26590 Repair macrodactylia

26591 Repair, intrinsic muscles of hand (specify)

(For microsurgical technique, use modifier -20 or 09920)

26593 Release, intrinsic muscles of hand (specify)

(For microsurgical technique, use modifier -20 or 09920)

26596 Excision of constricting ring of finger, with multiple Z-plasties

26597 Release of scar contracture, flexor or extensor, with skin grafts, rearrangement flaps, or Z-plasties, hand and/or finger

FRACTURES AND/OR DISLOCATIONS

▲**26600** Closed treatment of metacarpal fracture, single; without manipulation, each bone

26605 with manipulation, each bone

▲**26607** Closed treatment of metacarpal fracture, with manipulation, with internal or external fixation, each bone

● **26608** Percutaneous skeletal fixation of metacarpal fracture, each bone

(26610 has been deleted. To report, see 26605, 26607, 26608)

▲**26615** Open treatment of metacarpal fracture, single, with or without internal or external fixation, each bone

▲**26641** Closed treatment of carpometacarpal dislocation, thumb, with manipulation

▲**26645** Closed treatment of carpometacarpal fracture dislocation, thumb (Bennett fracture), with manipulation

▲**26650** Percutaneous skeletal fixation of carpometacarpal fracture dislocation, thumb (Bennett fracture), with manipulation, with or without external fixation

(26655 has been deleted. To report, see 26645, 26650, 26665)

(26660 has been deleted. To report, see 26650, 26665)

▲**26665** Open treatment of carpometacarpal fracture dislocation, thumb (Bennett fracture), with or without internal or external fixation

▲**26670** Closed treatment of carpometacarpal dislocation, other than thumb (Bennett fracture), single, with manipulation; without anesthesia

26675 requiring anesthesia

▲26676 Percutaneous skeletal fixation of carpometacarpal dislocation, other than thumb (Bennett fracture), single, with manipulation

(26680 has been deleted. To report, see 26670, 26675, 26676, 26685)

▲26685 Open treatment of carpometacarpal dislocation, other than thumb (Bennett fracture); single, with or without internal or external fixation

26686 complex, multiple or delayed reduction

▲26700 Closed treatment of metacarpophalangeal dislocation, single, with manipulation; without anesthesia

26705 requiring anesthesia

▲26706 Percutaneous skeletal fixation of metacarpophalangeal dislocation, single, with manipulation

(26710 has been deleted. To report, see 26700, 26705, 26706, 26715)

▲26715 Open treatment of metacarpophalangeal dislocation, single, with or without internal or external fixation

▲26720 Closed treatment of phalangeal shaft fracture, proximal or middle phalanx, finger or thumb; without manipulation, each

▲26725 with manipulation, with or without skin or skeletal traction, each

▲26727 Percutaneous skeletal fixation of unstable phalangeal shaft fracture, proximal or middle phalanx, finger or thumb, with manipulation, each

(26730 has been deleted. To report, see 26720, 26725, 26727, 26735)

▲26735 Open treatment of phalangeal shaft fracture, proximal or middle phalanx, finger or thumb, with or without internal or external fixation, each

▲26740 Closed treatment of articular fracture, involving metacarpophalangeal or proximal interphalangeal joint; without manipulation, each

26742 with manipulation, each

(26743 has been deleted. To report, use 26989)

(26744 has been deleted. To report, see 26740, 26742, 26743, 26746)

▲26746 Open treatment of articular fracture, involving metacarpophalangeal or proximal interphalangeal joint, with or without internal or external fixation, each

▲26750 Closed treatment of distal phalangeal fracture, finger or thumb; without manipulation, each

26755 with manipulation, each

▲26756 Percutaneous skeletal fixation of distal phalangeal fracture, finger or thumb, each

(26760 has been deleted. To report, see 26750, 26755, 26756, 26765)

▲26765 Open treatment of distal phalangeal fracture, finger or thumb, with or without internal or external fixation, each

▲26770 Closed treatment of interphalangeal joint dislocation, single, with manipulation; without anesthesia

26775 requiring anesthesia

▲26776 Percutaneous skeletal fixation of interphalangeal joint dislocation, single, with manipulation

(26780 has been deleted. To report, see 26770, 26775, 26776, 26785)

▲26785 Open treatment of interphalangeal joint dislocation, with or without internal or external fixation, single

ARTHRODESIS

26820 Fusion in opposition, thumb, with autogenous graft (includes obtaining graft)

26841 Arthrodesis, carpometacarpal joint, thumb, with or without internal fixation;

26842 with autograft (includes obtaining graft)

26843 Arthrodesis, carpometacarpal joint, digits, other than thumb;

26844 with autograft (includes obtaining graft)

26850 Arthrodesis, metacarpophalangeal joint, with or without internal fixation;

26852 with autograft (includes obtaining graft)

26860 Arthrodesis, interphalangeal joint, with or without internal fixation;

26861 each additional interphalangeal joint

26862 with autograft (includes obtaining graft)

26863 with autograft (includes obtaining graft), each additional joint

AMPUTATION

(For hand through metacarpal bones, see 25927)

26910 Amputation, metacarpal, with finger or thumb (ray amputation), single, with or without interosseous transfer

(For repositioning, see 26550, 26555)

26951 Amputation, finger or thumb, primary or secondary, any joint or phalanx, single, including neurectomies; with direct closure

26952 with local advancement flaps (V-Y, hood)

(For repair of soft tissue defect requiring split or full thickness graft or other pedicle flaps, see 15050-15755)

MISCELLANEOUS

26989 Unlisted procedure, hands or fingers

PELVIS AND HIP JOINT

(Including head and neck of femur)

INCISION

(For incision and drainage procedures, superficial, see 10040-10160)

26990 Incision and drainage, pelvis or hip joint area; deep abscess or hematoma

26991 infected bursa

26992 Incision, deep, with opening of bone cortex (eg, for osteomyelitis or bone abscess), pelvis and/or hip joint

(26995 has been deleted)

27000 Tenotomy, adductor of hip, subcutaneous, closed (separate procedure)

27001 Tenotomy, adductor of hip, subcutaneous, open

(27002 has been deleted. To report, use 27001 with modifier -50 or 09950)

27003 Tenotomy, adductor, subcutaneous, open, with obturator neurectomy

(27004 has been deleted. To report, use 27003 with modifier -50 or 09950)

27005 Tenotomy, iliopsoas, open (separate procedure)

27006 Tenotomy, abductors of hip, open (separate procedure)

(27010, 27015 have been deleted. To report, see 27025)

27025 Fasciotomy, hip or thigh, any type

(27026 has been deleted. To report, use 27025 with modifier -50 or 09950)

27030 Arthrotomy, hip, for infection, with drainage

(27031 has been deleted)

27033 Arthrotomy, hip, for exploration or removal of loose or foreign body

27035 Hip joint denervation, intrapelvic or extrapelvic intra-articular branches of sciatic, femoral or obturator nerves

(For obturator neurectomy, see 64763, 64766)

EXCISION

27040 Biopsy, soft tissue of pelvis and hip area; superficial

27041 deep

(For needle biopsy of soft tissue, use 20206)

27047 Excision, tumor, pelvis and hip area; subcutaneous

27048 deep, subfascial, intramuscular

27049 Radical resection of tumor (eg, malignant neoplasm), soft tissue of pelvis and hip area

27050 Arthrotomy, for biopsy; sacroiliac joint

27052 hip joint

27054 Arthrotomy for synovectomy, hip joint

27060 Excision; ischial bursa

27062 trochanteric bursa or calcification

(For arthrocentesis or needling of bursa, see 20610)

27065 Excision of bone cyst or benign tumor; superficial (wing of ilium, symphysis pubis, or greater trochanter of femur) with or without autograft

27066 deep, with or without autograft

27067 with autograft requiring separate incision

27070 Partial excision (craterization, saucerization) (eg, for osteomyelitis); superficial (eg, wing of ilium, symphysis pubis or greater trochanter of femur)

27071 deep

27075 Radical resection for tumor or infection; wing of ilium, one pubic or ischial ramus or symphysis pubis

27076 ilium, including acetabulum, both pubic rami, or ischium and acetabulum

27077 innominate bone, total

27078 ischial tuberosity and greater trochanter of femur

27079 ischial tuberosity and greater trochanter of femur, with skin flaps

27080 Coccygectomy, primary

(For pressure (decubitus) ulcer, see 15920-15922 and 15931-15958)

INTRODUCTION AND/OR REMOVAL

27086* Removal of foreign body, pelvis or hip; subcutaneous tissue

27087 deep

(27088 has been deleted. To report, use 27087)

27090 Removal of hip prosthesis; (separate procedure)

27091 complicated, including "total hip" and methylmethacrylate, when applicable

27093 Injection procedure for hip arthrography; without anesthesia

(For radiological supervision and interpretation, see 73525)

27095 with anesthesia

(For radiological supervision and interpretation, see 73525)

REPAIR, REVISION OR RECONSTRUCTION

27097 Hamstring recession, proximal

27098 Adductor transfer to ischium

27100 Transfer external oblique muscle to greater trochanter including fascial or tendon extension (graft)

27105 Transfer paraspinal muscle to hip (includes fascial or tendon extension graft)

27110 Transfer iliopsoas; to greater trochanter

27111 to femoral neck

(27115 has been deleted. To report, use 27299)

27120 Acetabuloplasty; (eg, Whitman, Colonna, Haygroves, or cup type)

27122 resection femoral head (Girdlestone procedure)

27125 Partial hip replacement, prosthesis (eg, femoral stem prosthesis, bipolar arthroplasty)

(For prosthetic replacement following fracture of the hip, use 27236)

(27126, 27127 have been deleted. To report, use 27120)

27130 Arthroplasty, acetabular and proximal femoral prosthetic replacement (total hip replacement), with or without autograft or allograft

(27131 has been deleted. To report, use 27132)

27132 Conversion of previous hip surgery to total hip replacement, with or without autograft or allograft

27134 Revision of total hip arthroplasty; both components, with or without autograft or allograft

(27135 has been deleted. To report, see 27134, 27137, 27138)

27137 acetabular component only, with or without autograft or allograft

27138 femoral component only, with or without allograft

27140 Osteotomy and transfer of greater trochanter (separate procedure)

27146 Osteotomy, iliac, acetabular or innominate bone;

27147 with open reduction of hip

27151 with femoral osteotomy

27156 with femoral osteotomy and with open reduction of hip

(27157 has been deleted)

27158 Osteotomy, pelvis, bilateral for congenital malformation

27161 Osteotomy, femoral neck (separate procedure)

27165 Osteotomy, intertrochanteric or subtrochanteric including internal or external fixation and/or cast

27170 Bone graft, femoral head, neck, intertrochanteric or subtrochanteric area (includes obtaining bone graft)

27175 Treatment of slipped femoral epiphysis; by traction, without reduction

27176 by single or multiple pinning, in situ

27177 Open treatment of slipped femoral epiphysis; single or multiple pinning or bone graft (includes obtaining graft)

27178 closed manipulation with single or multiple pinning

27179 osteoplasty of femoral neck (Heyman type procedure)

27181 osteotomy and internal fixation

27185 Epiphyseal arrest by epiphysiodesis or stapling, greater trochanter

27187 Prophylactic treatment (nailing, pinning, plating or wiring) with or without methylmethacrylate, femoral neck and proximal femur

FRACTURES AND/OR DISLOCATIONS

(27190, 27191 have been deleted. To report, see 27193, 27194)

(27192 has been deleted. To report, see 27215, 27216)

• **27193** Closed treatment of pelvic ring fracture, dislocation, diastasis or subluxation; without manipulation

• **27194** with manipulation, requiring more than local anesthesia

(27195 has been deleted. To report, see 27193)

(27196 has been deleted. To report, see 27194)

▲ **27200** Closed treatment of coccygeal fracture

(27201 has been deleted. To report, see 27200, 27202)

▲ **27202** Open treatment of coccygeal fracture

(27210, 27211, 27212 have been deleted. To report, see 27193, 27194, 27215, 27216, 27217, 27218)

(27214 has been deleted. To report, see 27215, 27216, 27217, 27218)

• **27215** Open treatment of iliac spine(s), tuberosity avulsion, or iliac wing fracture(s) (eg, pelvic fracture(s) which do not disrupt the pelvic ring), with internal fixation

• **27216** Percutaneous skeletal fixation of posterior pelvic ring fracture and/or dislocation (includes ilium, sacroiliac joint and/or sacrum)

• **27217** Open treatment of anterior ring fracture and/or dislocation with internal fixation, (includes pubic symphysis and/or rami)

• **27218** Open treatment of posterior ring fracture and/or dislocation with internal fixation (includes ilium, sacroiliac joint and/or sacrum)

▲ **27220** Closed treatment of acetabulum (hip socket) fracture(s); without manipulation

27222 with manipulation, with or without skeletal traction

(27224 has been deleted. To report, see 27226, 27227)

(27225 has been deleted. To report, see 27227, 27228)

• **27226** Open treatment of posterior or anterior acetabular wall fracture, with internal fixation

• **27227** Open treatment of acetabular fracture(s) involving anterior or posterior (one) column, or a fracture running transversely across the acetabulum, with internal fixation

• **27228** Open treatment of acetabular fracture(s) involving anterior and posterior (two) columns, includes T-fracture and both column fracture with complete articular detachment, or single column or transverse fracture with associated acetabular wall fracture; with internal fixation

▲ **27230** Closed treatment of femoral fracture, proximal end, neck; without manipulation

▲ **27232** with manipulation, with or without skeletal traction

(27234 has been deleted. To report, see 27230, 27232, 27235, 27236)

▲ **27235** Percutaneous skeletal fixation of femoral fracture, proximal end, neck, undisplaced, mildly displaced, or impacted fracture

▲ **27236** Open treatment of femoral fracture, proximal end, neck, internal fixation or prosthetic replacement (direct fracture exposure)

▲ **27238** Closed treatment of intertrochanteric, pertrochanteric, or subtrochanteric femoral fracture; without manipulation

▲ **27240** with manipulation, with or without skin or skeletal traction

(27242 has been deleted. To report, see 27238, 27240, 27244, 27245)

▲ **27244** Open treatment of intertrochanteric, pertrochanteric or subtrochanteric femoral fracture; with plate/screw type implant, with or without cerclage

• **27245** with intramedullary implant, with or without interlocking screws and/or cerclage

▲ **27246** Closed treatment of greater trochanteric fracture, without manipulation

▲ **27248** Open treatment of greater trochanteric fracture, with or without internal or external fixation

▲ **27250** Closed treatment of hip dislocation, traumatic; without anesthesia

27252 requiring anesthesia

▲27253 Open treatment of hip dislocation, traumatic, without internal fixation

▲27254 Open treatment of hip dislocation, traumatic, with acetabular wall and femoral head fracture, with or without internal or external fixation

(27255 has been deleted. To report, see 27226, 27227, 27253, 27254)

▲27256* Treatment of spontaneous hip dislocation (developmental, including congenital or pathological), by abduction, splint or traction; without anesthesia, without manipulation

27257* with manipulation, requiring anesthesia

▲27258 Open treatment of spontaneous hip dislocation (developmental, including congenital or pathological), replacement of femoral head in acetabulum (including tenotomy, etc);

27259 with femoral shaft shortening

▲27265 Closed treatment of post hip arthroplasty dislocation; without anesthesia

▲27266 requiring regional or general anesthesia

MANIPULATION

27275* Manipulation, hip joint, requiring general anesthesia

ARTHRODESIS

27280 Arthrodesis, sacroiliac joint (including obtaining graft)

(27281 has been deleted. To report, use 27280 with modifier -50 or 09950)

27282 Arthrodesis, symphysis pubis (including obtaining graft)

27284 Arthrodesis, hip joint (includes obtaining graft);

27286 with subtrochanteric osteotomy

AMPUTATION

27290 Interpelviabdominal amputation (hindquarter amputation)

27295 Disarticulation of hip

MISCELLANEOUS

27299 Unlisted procedure, pelvis or hip joint

FEMUR (THIGH REGION) and KNEE JOINT

(Including tibial plateaus)

INCISION

(For incision and drainage of abscess or hematoma, superficial, see 10040-10160)

27301 Incision and drainage of deep abscess, infected bursa, or hematoma, thigh or knee region

27303 Incision, deep, with opening of bone cortex (eg, for osteomyelitis or bone abscess), femur or knee

(27304 has been deleted)

27305 Fasciotomy, iliotibial (tenotomy), open

(For combined Ober-Yount fasciotomy, see 27025)

27306 Tenotomy, subcutaneous, closed, adductor or hamstring, (separate procedure); single

27307 multiple

27310 Arthrotomy, knee, for infection, with exploration, drainage or removal of foreign body

(27311 has been deleted)

27315 Neurectomy, hamstring muscle

27320 Neurectomy, popliteal (gastrocnemius)

EXCISION

27323 Biopsy, soft tissue of thigh or knee area; superficial

27324 deep

(For needle biopsy of soft tissue, use 20206)

27327 Excision, tumor, thigh or knee area; subcutaneous

27328 deep, subfascial, or intramuscular

27329 Radical resection of tumor (eg, malignant neoplasm), soft tissue of thigh or knee area

27330 Arthrotomy, knee; for synovial biopsy only

27331 with joint exploration, with or without biopsy, with or without removal of loose or foreign bodies

27332 Arthrotomy, knee, for excision of semilunar cartilage (meniscectomy); medial OR lateral

27333 medial AND lateral

27334 Arthrotomy, knee, for synovectomy; anterior OR posterior

27335 anterior AND posterior including popliteal area

27340 Excision, prepatellar bursa

27345 Excision of synovial cyst of popliteal space (Baker's cyst)

27350 Patellectomy or hemipatellectomy

27355 Excision or curettage of bone cyst or benign tumor of femur;

27356 with allograft

27357 with autograft (includes obtaining graft)

27358 with internal fixation (list in addition to 27355, 27356, or 27357)

27360 Partial excision (craterization, saucerization, or diaphysectomy) of bone (eg, for osteomyelitis), femur, proximal tibia and/or tibula

(27361 has been deleted)

27365 Radical resection for tumor, femur or knee, bone

(For radical resection of tumor, soft tissue, use 27329)

INTRODUCTION AND/OR REMOVAL

27370 Injection procedure for knee arthrography

(For radiological supervision and interpretation, see 73580)

27372 Removal of foreign body, deep, thigh region or knee area

(For removal of knee prosthesis including "total knee", see 27488)

(27373-27379 have been deleted. To report, see 29870-29887)

REPAIR, REVISION OR RECONSTRUCTION

27380 Suture of infrapatellar tendon; primary

27381 secondary reconstruction, including fascial or tendon graft

27385 Suture of quadriceps or hamstring muscle rupture; primary

27386 secondary reconstruction, including fascial or tendon graft

27390 Tenotomy, open, hamstring, knee to hip; single

27391 multiple, one leg

27392 multiple, bilateral

27393 Lengthening of hamstring tendon; single

27394 multiple, one leg

27395 multiple, bilateral

27396 Transplant, hamstring tendon to patella; single

27397 multiple

27400 Tendon or muscle transfer, hamstrings to femur (Eggers type procedure)

27403 Arthrotomy with open meniscus repair

(For arthroscopic repair, use 29882)

27405 Repair, primary, torn ligament and/or capsule, knee; collateral

27407 cruciate

(27408 has been deleted. To report, use 27427)

27409 collateral and cruciate ligaments

(27410-27416 have been deleted. To report, see 27427-27429)

27418 Anterior tibial tubercleplasty for chondromalacia patellae (Maquet procedure)

27420 Reconstruction for recurrent dislocating patella; (Hauser type procedure)

27422 with extensor realignment and/or muscle advancement or release (Campbell, Goldwaite type procedure)

27424 with patellectomy

27425 Lateral retinacular release (any method)

27427 Ligamentous reconstruction (augmentation), knee; extra-articular

27428 intra-articular (open)

27429 intra-articular (open) and extra-articular

(When performed with primary repair, use in addition to the code for the primary repair)

27430 Quadricepsplasty (Bennett or Thompson type)

27435 Capsulotomy, knee, posterior capsular release

(27436 has been deleted. To report, use 29887)

27437 Arthroplasty, patella; without prosthesis

27438 with prosthesis

27440 Arthroplasty, knee, tibial plateau;

27441 with debridement and partial synovectomy

27442 Arthroplasty, knee, femoral condyles or tibial plateaus;

27443 with debridement and partial synovectomy

(27444 has been deleted. To report, see 27445-27447)

27445 Arthroplasty, knee, constrained prosthesis (eg, Walldius type)

27446 Arthroplasty, knee, condyle and plateau; medial OR lateral compartment

27447 medial AND lateral compartments with or without patella resurfacing ("total knee replacement")

(For revision of total knee arthroplasty, see 27487)

(For removal of total knee prosthesis, see 27488)

27448 Osteotomy, femur, shaft or supracondylar; without fixation

(27449 has been deleted. To report, use 27448 with modifier -50 or 09950)

27450 with fixation

(27452 has been deleted. To report, use 27450 with modifier -50 or 09950)

27454 Osteotomy, multiple, femoral shaft, with realignment on intramedullary rod (Sofield type procedure)

27455 Osteotomy, proximal tibia, including fibular excision or osteotomy (includes correction of genu varus (bowleg) or genu valgus (knock-knee)); before epiphyseal closure

27457 after epiphyseal closure

(27460 has been deleted. To report, use 27455 with modifier -50 or 09950)

(27462 has been deleted. To report, use 27457 with modifier -50 or 09950)

27465 Osteoplasty, femur; shortening (excluding 64876)

27466 lengthening

27468 combined, lengthening and shortening with femoral segment transfer

27470 Repair, nonunion or malunion, femur, distal to head and neck; without graft (eg, compression technique)

27472 with iliac or other autogenous bone graft (includes obtaining graft)

27475 Epiphyseal arrest by epiphysiodesis or stapling; distal femur

27477 tibia and fibula, proximal

27479 combined distal femur, proximal tibia and fibula

27485 Arrest, hemiepiphyseal, distal femur or proximal leg (eg, for genu varus or valgus)

27486 Revision of total knee arthroplasty, with or without allograft; one component

27487 all components

27488 Removal of knee prosthesis, including "total knee," methylmethacrylate and insertion of spacer, when applicable

(27490 has been deleted. To report, use 29882)

27495 Prophylactic treatment (nailing, pinning, plating or wiring) with or without methylmethacrylate, femur

● **27496** Decompression fasciotomy, thigh and/or knee, one compartment (flexor or extensor or adductor);

● **27497** with debridement of nonviable muscle and/or nerve

● **27498** Decompression fasciotomy, thigh and/or knee, multiple compartments;

● **27499** with debridement of nonviable muscle and/or nerve

FRACTURES AND/OR DISLOCATIONS

(For arthroscopic treatment of intercondylar spine(s) and tuberosity fracture(s) of the knee, see 29850, 29851)

(For arthroscopic treatment of tibial fracture, see 29855, 29856)

▲ **27500** Closed treatment of femoral shaft fracture, without manipulation

● **27501** Closed treatment of supracondylar or transcondylar femoral fracture with or without intercondylar extension, without manipulation

▲ **27502** Closed treatment of femoral shaft fracture, with manipulation, with or without skin or skeletal traction

● **27503** Closed treatment of supracondylar or transcondylar femoral fracture with or without intercondylar extension; with manipulation, with or without skin or skeletal traction

(27504 has been deleted. To report, see 27500, 27501, 27502, 27503, 27506, 27507, 27509, 27511, 27513)

▲ **27506** Open treatment of femoral shaft fracture, with or without external fixation, with insertion of intramedullary implant, with or without cerclage and/or locking screws

● **27507** Open treatment of femoral shaft fracture with plate/screws, with or without cerclage

▲ **27508** Closed treatment of femoral fracture, distal end, medial or lateral condyle, without manipulation

● **27509** Percutaneous skeletal fixation of supracondylar or transcondylar femoral fracture, with or without intercondylar extension

▲ **27510** Closed treatment of femoral fracture, distal end, medial or lateral condyle, with manipulation

● **27511** Open treatment of femoral supracondylar or transcondylar fracture without intercondylar extension, with or without internal or external fixation

(27512 has been deleted. To report, see 27508, 27510, 27514)

● **27513** Open treatment of femoral supracondylar or transcondylar fracture with intercondylar extension, with or without internal or external fixation

▲ **27514** Open treatment of femoral fracture, distal end, medial or lateral condyle, with or without internal or external fixation

▲ **27516** Closed treatment of distal femoral epiphyseal separation; without manipulation

▲ **27517** with manipulation, with or without skin or skeletal traction

(27518 has been deleted. To report, see 27516, 27517, 27519)

▲ **27519** Open treatment of distal femoral epiphyseal separation, with or without internal or external fixation

▲ **27520** Closed treatment of patellar fracture, without manipulation

(27522 has been deleted. To report, see 27520, 27524)

▲ **27524** Open treatment of patellar fracture, with internal fixation and/or partial or complete patellectomy and soft tissue repair

▲ **27530** Closed treatment of tibial fracture, proximal (plateau); without manipulation

▲ **27532** with or without manipulation, with skeletal traction

(27534 has been deleted. To report, see 27530, 27532, 27535, 27536)

(For arthroscopic treatment, see 29855, 29856)

● **27535** Open treatment of tibial fracture, proximal (plateau); unicondylar, with or without internal or external fixation

▲ **27536** bicondylar, with or without internal fixation

(For arthroscopic treatment, see 29855, 29856)

(27537 has been deleted. To report, see 27535, 27536)

▲ **27538** Closed treatment of intercondylar spine(s) and/or tuberosity fracture(s) of knee, with or without manipulation

(For arthroscopic treatment, see 29850, 29851)

▲27540 Open treatment of intercondylar spine(s) and/or tuberosity fracture(s) of the knee, with or without internal or external fixation

▲27550 Closed treatment of knee dislocation; without anesthesia

27552 requiring anesthesia

(27554 has been deleted. To report, see 27550, 27552, 27556, 27557, 27558)

▲27556 Open treatment of knee dislocation, with or without internal or external fixation; without primary ligamentous repair or augmentation/reconstruction

27557 with primary ligamentous repair

● 27558 with primary ligamentous repair, with augmentation/reconstruction

▲27560 Closed treatment of patellar dislocation; without anesthesia

(For recurrent dislocation, see 27420-27424)

27562 requiring anesthesia

(27564 has been deleted. To report, see 27560, 27562, 27566)

▲27566 Open treatment of patellar dislocation, with or without partial or total patellectomy

MANIPULATION

27570* Manipulation of knee joint under general anesthesia (includes application of traction or other fixation devices)

ARTHRODESIS

27580 Fusion of knee, any technique

AMPUTATION

27590 Amputation, thigh, through femur, any level;

27591 immediate fitting technique including first cast

27592 open, circular (guillotine)

27594 secondary closure or scar revision

27596 re-amputation

27598 Disarticulation at knee

MISCELLANEOUS

27599 Unlisted procedure, femur or knee

LEG (TIBIA AND FIBULA) and ANKLE JOINT

INCISION

▲**27600** Decompression fasciotomy, leg; anterior and/or lateral compartments only

▲**27601** posterior compartment(s) only

▲**27602** anterior and/or lateral, and posterior compartment(s)

(For incision and drainage procedures, superficial, see 10040-10160)

(For decompression fasciotomy with debridement, see 27892-27894)

27603 Incision and drainage, leg or ankle; deep abscess or hematoma

27604 infected bursa

27605* Tenotomy, Achilles tendon, subcutaneous (separate procedure); local anesthesia

27606 general anesthesia

27607 Incision, deep, with opening of bone cortex (eg, for osteomyelitis or bone abscess), leg or ankle

(27608 has been deleted)

27610 Arthrotomy, ankle, for infection, with exploration, drainage or removal of foreign body

(27611 has been deleted)

27612 Arthrotomy, ankle, posterior capsular release, with or without Achilles tendon lengthening

(See also 27685)

EXCISION

27613 Biopsy, soft tissue of leg or ankle area; superficial

27614 deep

(For needle biopsy of soft tissue, use 20206)

27615 Radical resection of tumor (eg, malignant neoplasm), soft tissue of leg or ankle area

27618 Excision, tumor, leg or ankle area; subcutaneous

27619 deep, subfascial or intramuscular

27620 Arthrotomy, ankle, with joint exploration, with or without biopsy, with or without removal of loose or foreign body

27625 Arthrotomy, ankle, for synovectomy;

27626 including tenosynovectomy

27630 Excision of lesion of tendon sheath or capsule (eg, cyst or ganglion), leg and/or ankle

27635 Excision or curettage of bone cyst or benign tumor, tibia or fibula;

27637 with autograft (includes obtaining graft)

27638 with allograft

27640 Partial excision (craterization, saucerization, or diaphysectomy) of bone (eg, for osteomyelitis or exostosis); tibia

27641 fibula

27645 Resection for tumor, radical; tibia

27646 fibula

27647 talus or calcaneus

INTRODUCTION OR REMOVAL

27648 Injection procedure for ankle arthrography

(For radiological supervision and interpretation, see 73615)

(For ankle arthroscopy, see 29890-29898)

REPAIR, REVISION OR RECONSTRUCTION

27650 Repair, primary, open or percutaneous, ruptured Achilles tendon;

27652 with graft (includes obtaining graft)

27654 Repair, secondary, ruptured Achilles tendon, with or without graft

27656 Repair, fascial defect of leg

27658 Repair or suture of flexor tendon of leg; primary, without graft, single, each

27659 secondary with or without graft, single tendon, each

27664 Repair or suture of extensor tendon of leg; primary, without graft, single, each

27665 secondary with or without graft, single tendon, each

27675 Repair for dislocating peroneal tendons; without fibular osteotomy

27676 with fibular osteotomy

27680 Tenolysis, including tibia, fibula and ankle flexor; single

27681 multiple (through same incision), each

27685 Lengthening or shortening of tendon, leg or ankle; single (separate procedure)

27686 multiple (through same incision), each

27687 Gastrocnemius recession (eg, Strayer procedure)

(Toe extensors are considered as a group to be a single tendon when transplanted into midfoot)

27690 Transfer or transplant of single tendon (with muscle redirection or rerouting); superficial (eg, anterior tibial extensors into midfoot)

27691 anterior tibial or posterior tibial through interosseous space

27692 each additional tendon

27695 Suture, primary, torn, ruptured or severed ligament, ankle; collateral

27696 both collateral ligaments

27698 Suture, secondary repair, torn, ruptured or severed ligament, ankle, collateral (eg, Watson-Jones procedure)

27700 Arthroplasty, ankle;

27702 with implant (''total ankle'')

27703 secondary reconstruction, total ankle

27704 Removal of ankle implant

27705 Osteotomy; tibia

27707 fibula

27709 tibia and fibula

27712 multiple, with realignment on intramedullary rod (Sofield type procedure)

(For osteotomy to correct genu varus (bowleg) or genu valgus (knock-knee), see 27455-27457)

27715 Osteoplasty, tibia and fibula, lengthening

27720 Repair of nonunion or malunion, tibia; without graft, (eg, compression technique)

27722 with sliding graft

27724 with iliac or other autograft (includes obtaining graft)

27725 by synostosis, with fibula, any method

27727 Repair of congenital pseudarthrosis, tibia

27730 Epiphyseal arrest by epiphysiodesis or stapling; distal tibia

27732 distal fibula

27734 distal tibia and fibula

27740 Epiphyseal arrest by epiphysiodesis or stapling, combined, proximal and distal tibia and fibula;

27742 and distal femur

(For epiphyseal arrest of proximal tibia and fibula, see 27477)

27745 Prophylactic treatment (nailing, pinning, plating or wiring) with or without methylmethacrylate, tibia

FRACTURES AND/OR DISLOCATIONS

▲**27750** Closed treatment of tibial shaft fracture (with or without fibular fracture); without manipulation

▲**27752** with manipulation, with or without skeletal traction

(27754 has been deleted. To report, see 27750, 27752, 27756, 27758)

▲**27756** Percutaneous skeletal fixation of tibial shaft fracture (with or without fibular fracture) (eg, pins or screws)

▲**27758** Open treatment of tibial shaft fracture, (with or without fibular fracture) with plate/screws, with or without cerclage

● **27759** Open treatment of tibial shaft fracture (with or without fibular fracture) by intramedullary implant, with or without interlocking screws and/or cerclage

▲**27760** Closed treatment of medial malleolus fracture; without manipulation

▲**27762** with manipulation, with or without skin or skeletal traction

(27764 has been deleted. To report, see 27760, 27762, 27766)

▲**27766** Open treatment of medial malleolus fracture, with or without internal or external fixation

▲**27780** Closed treatment of proximal fibula or shaft fracture; without manipulation

27781 with manipulation

(27782 has been deleted. To report, see 27780, 27781, 27784)

▲**27784** Open treatment of proximal fibula or shaft fracture, with or without internal or external fixation

▲**27786** Closed treatment of distal fibular fracture (lateral malleolus); without manipulation

27788 with manipulation

(27790 has been deleted. To report, see 27786, 27788, 27792)

▲**27792** Open treatment of distal fibular fracture (lateral malleolus), with or without internal or external fixation

(27800 has been deleted. To report, see 27750)

(27802 has been deleted. To report, see 27752)

(27804 has been deleted. To report, see 27750, 27752, 27756, 27758, 27759)

(27806 has been deleted. To report, see 27756, 27758, 27759)

▲**27808** Closed treatment of bimalleolar ankle fracture, (including Potts); without manipulation

27810 with manipulation

(27812 has been deleted. To report, see 27808, 27810, 27814)

▲**27814** Open treatment of bimalleolar ankle fracture, with or without internal or external fixation

▲**27816** Closed treatment of trimalleolar ankle fracture; without manipulation

27818 with manipulation

(27820 has been deleted. To report, see 27816, 27818, 27822, 27823)

▲**27822** Open treatment of trimalleolar ankle fracture, with or without internal or external fixation, medial and/or lateral malleolus; without fixation of posterior lip

▲**27823** with fixation of posterior lip

● **27824** Closed treatment of fracture of weight bearing articular portion of distal tibia (eg, pilon or tibial plafond), with or without anesthesia; without manipulation

● **27825** with skeletal traction and/or requiring manipulation

● **27826** Open treatment of fracture of weight bearing articular surface/portion of distal tibia (eg, pilon or tibial plafond), with internal or external fixation; of fibula only

● **27827** of tibia only

● **27828** of both tibia and fibula

● **27829** Open treatment of distal tibiofibular joint (syndesmosis) disruption, with or without internal or external fixation

▲**27830** Closed treatment of proximal tibiofibular joint dislocation; without anesthesia

27831 requiring anesthesia

▲**27832** Open treatment of proximal tibiofibular joint dislocation, with or without internal or external fixation, or with excision of proximal fibula

▲**27840** Closed treatment of ankle dislocation; without anesthesia

▲**27842** requiring anesthesia, with or without percutaneous skeletal fixation

(27844 has been deleted. To report, see 27840, 27842, 27846, 27848)

▲27846 Open treatment of ankle dislocation, with or without percutaneous skeletal fixation; without repair or internal fixation

▲27848 with repair or internal or external fixation

ARTHROSCOPY

(27850-27853 have been deleted. To report, see 29894-29898)

MANIPULATION

27860* Manipulation of ankle under general anesthesia (includes application of traction or other fixation apparatus)

ARTHRODESIS

27870 Arthrodesis, ankle, any method

27871 Arthrodesis, tibiofibular joint, proximal or distal

AMPUTATION

27880 Amputation leg, through tibia and fibula;

27881 with immediate fitting technique including application of first cast

27882 open, circular (guillotine)

27884 secondary closure or scar revision

27886 re-amputation

27888 Amputation, ankle, through malleoli of tibia and fibula (Syme, Pirogoff type procedures), with plastic closure and resection of nerves

27889 Ankle disarticulation

MISCELLANEOUS

• 27892 Decompression fasciotomy, leg; anterior and/or lateral compartments only, with debridement of nonviable muscle and/or nerve

(For decompression fasciotomy of the leg without debridement, see 27600)

• 27893 posterior compartment(s) only, with debridement of nonviable muscle and/or nerve

(For decompression fasciotomy of the leg without debridement, see 27601)

● **27894** anterior and/or lateral, and posterior compartment(s), with debridement of nonviable muscle and/or nerve

(For decompression fasciotomy of the leg without debridement, see 27602)

27899 Unlisted procedure, leg or ankle

FOOT

INCISION

(For incision and drainage procedures, superficial, see 10040-10160)

28001* Incision and drainage, infected bursa, foot

28002* Deep dissection below fascia, for deep infection of foot, with or without tendon sheath involvement; single bursal space, specify

28003 multiple areas

(28004 has been deleted)

28005 Incision, deep, with opening of bone cortex (eg, for osteomyelitis or bone abscess), foot

(28006 has been deleted)

28008 Fasciotomy, foot and/or toe

(See also 28060, 28062, 28250)

28010 Tenotomy, subcutaneous, toe; single

28011 multiple

(For open tenotomy, see 28230-28234)

28020 Arthrotomy, with exploration, drainage or removal of loose or foreign body; intertarsal or tarsometatarsal joint

28022 metatarsophalangeal joint

28024 interphalangeal joint

28030 Neurectomy of intrinsic musculature of foot

28035 Tarsal tunnel release (posterior tibial nerve decompression)

(For other nerve entrapments, see 64704, 64722)

EXCISION

28043 Excision, tumor, foot; subcutaneous

28045 deep, subfascial, intramuscular

28046 Radical resection of tumor (eg, malignant neoplasm), soft tissue of foot

28050 Arthrotomy for synovial biopsy; intertarsal or tarsometatarsal joint

28052 metatarsophalangeal joint

28054 interphalangeal joint

28060 Fasciectomy, excision of plantar fascia; partial (separate procedure)

28062 radical (separate procedure)

(For plantar fasciotomy, see 28008, 28250)

28070 Synovectomy; intertarsal or tarsometatarsal joint, each

28072 metatarsophalangeal joint, each

28080 Excision of interdigital (Morton) neuroma, single, each

28086 Synovectomy, tendon sheath, foot; flexor

28088 extensor

28090 Excision of lesion of tendon or fibrous sheath or capsule (including synovectomy) (cyst or ganglion); foot

28092 toes

28100 Excision or curettage of bone cyst or benign tumor, talus or calcaneus;

28102 with iliac or other autograft (includes obtaining graft)

28103 with allograft

28104 Excision or curettage of bone cyst or benign tumor, tarsal or metatarsal bones, except talus or calcaneus;

28106 with iliac or other autograft (includes obtaining graft)

28107 with allograft

28108 Excision or curettage of bone cyst or benign tumor, phalanges of foot

(For ostectomy, partial (eg, hallux valgus, Silver type procedure), see 28290)

(28109 has been deleted. To report, use 28899)

28110 Ostectomy, partial excision, fifth metatarsal head (bunionette) (separate procedure)

28111 Ostectomy, complete excision; first metatarsal head

28112 other metatarsal head (second, third or fourth)

28113 fifth metatarsal head

28114 all metatarsal heads, with partial proximal phalangectomy, excluding first metatarsal (Clayton type procedure)

28116 Ostectomy, excision of tarsal coalition

28118 Ostectomy, calcaneus;

28119 for spur, with or without plantar fascial release

28120 Partial excision (craterization, saucerization, sequestrectomy, or diaphysectomy) of bone (eg, for osteomyelitis or talar bossing), talus or calcaneus

(28121 has been deleted)

28122 Partial excision (craterization, saucerization, or diaphysectomy) of bone (eg, for osteomyelitis or tarsal bossing), tarsal or metatarsal bone, except talus or calcaneus

(28123 has been deleted)

28124 Partial excision (craterization, saucerization, or diaphysectomy) of bone (eg, for osteomyelitis or dorsal bossing), phalanx of toe

28126 Condylectomy, phalangeal base, single toe, each

28130 Talectomy (astragalectomy)

(28135 has been deleted. To report, use 28118)

28140 Metatarsectomy

28150 Phalangectomy of toe, single, each

28153 Resection, head of phalanx, toe

28160 Hemiphalangectomy or interphalangeal joint excision, toe, single, each

28171 Radical resection for tumor; tarsal (except talus or calcaneus)

28173 metatarsal

28175 phalanx of toe

(For talus or calcaneus, see 27647)

INTRODUCTION AND/OR REMOVAL

28190* Removal of foreign body, foot; subcutaneous

28192 deep

28193 complicated

REPAIR, REVISION OR RECONSTRUCTION

28200 Repair or suture of tendon, foot, flexor, single; primary or secondary, without free graft, each tendon

28202 secondary with free graft, each tendon (includes obtaining graft)

28208 Repair or suture of tendon, foot, extensor, single; primary or secondary, each tendon

28210 secondary with free graft, each tendon (includes obtaining graft)

28220 Tenolysis, flexor, foot; single

28222 multiple (through same incision)

28225 Tenolysis, extensor, foot; single

28226 multiple (through same incision)

28230 Tenotomy, open, flexor; foot, single or multiple (separate procedure)

28232 toe, single (separate procedure)

28234 Tenotomy, open, extensor, foot or toe

28236 Transfer of tendon, anterior tibial into tarsal bone

28238 Advancement of posterior tibial tendon with excision of accessory navicular bone (Kidner type procedure)

(For subcutaneous tenotomy, see 28010, 28011)

(For transfer or transplant of tendon with muscle redirection or rerouting, see 27690-27692)

(For extensor hallucis longus transfer with great toe IP fusion (Jones procedure), see 28760)

28240 Tenotomy, lengthening, or release, abductor hallucis muscle

28250 Division of plantar fascia and muscle ("Steindler stripping") (separate procedure)

28260 Capsulotomy, midfoot; medial release only (separate procedure)

28261 with tendon lengthening

28262 extensive, including posterior talotibial capsulotomy and tendon(s) lengthening as for resistant clubfoot deformity

28264 Capsulotomy, midtarsal (Heyman type procedure)

28270 Capsulotomy for contracture; metatarsophalangeal joint, with or without tenorrhaphy, single, each joint (separate procedure)

28272 interphalangeal joint, single, each joint (separate procedure)

28280 Webbing operation (create syndactylism of toes) for soft corn (Kelikian type procedure)

28285 Hammertoe operation; one toe (eg, interphalangeal fusion, filleting, phalangectomy)

28286 for cock-up fifth toe with plastic skin closure, (Ruiz-Mora type procedure)

28288 Ostectomy, partial, exostectomy or condylectomy, single, metatarsal head, first through fifth, each metatarsal head

28290 Hallux valgus (bunion) correction, with or without sesamoidectomy; simple exostectomy (Silver type procedure)

28292 Keller, McBride or Mayo type procedure

28293 resection of joint with implant

28294 with tendon transplants (Joplin type procedure)

28296 with metatarsal osteotomy (eg, Mitchell, Chevron, or concentric type procedures)

28297 Lapidus type procedure

28298 by phalanx osteotomy

28299 by other methods (eg, double osteotomy)

28300 Osteotomy; calcaneus (Dwyer or Chambers type procedure), with or without internal fixation

28302 talus

28304 Osteotomy, midtarsal bones, other than calcaneus or talus;

28305 with autograft (includes obtaining graft) (Fowler type)

28306 Osteotomy, metatarsal, base or shaft, single, with or without lengthening, for shortening or angular correction; first metatarsal

28307 first metatarsal with autograft

28308 other than first metatarsal

28309 Osteotomy, metatarsals, multiple, for cavus foot (Swanson type procedure)

28310 Osteotomy for shortening, angular or rotational correction; proximal phalanx, first toe (separate procedure)

28312 other phalanges, any toe

28313 Reconstruction, angular deformity of toe (overlapping second toe, fifth toe, curly toes), soft tissue procedures only

28315 Sesamoidectomy, first toe (separate procedure)

28320 Repair of nonunion or malunion; tarsal bones (eg, calcaneus, talus)

28322 metatarsal, with or without bone graft (includes obtaining graft)

28340 Reconstruction, toe, macrodactyly; soft tissue resection

28341 requiring bone resection

28344 Reconstruction, toe(s); polydactyly

28345 syndactyly, with or without skin graft(s), each web

28360 Reconstruction, cleft foot

FRACTURE AND/OR DISLOCATION

▲**28400** Closed treatment of calcaneal fracture; without manipulation

▲**28405** with manipulation

▲**28406** Percutaneous skeletal fixation of calcaneal fracture, with manipulation

(28410 has been deleted. To report, see 28400, 28405, 28406, 28415, 28420)

▲**28415** Open treatment of calcaneal fracture, with or without internal or external fixation;

28420 with primary iliac or other autogenous bone graft (includes obtaining graft)

▲**28430** Closed treatment of talus fracture; without manipulation

28435 with manipulation

▲**28436** Percutaneous skeletal fixation of talus fracture, with manipulation

(28440 has been deleted. To report, see 28430, 28435, 28436, 28445)

▲**28445** Open treatment of talus fracture, with or without internal or external fixation

▲**28450** Treatment of tarsal bone fracture (except talus and calcaneus); without manipulation, each

28455 with manipulation, each

▲**28456** Percutaneous skeletal fixation of tarsal bone fracture (except talus and calcaneus), with manipulation, each

(28460 has been deleted. To report, see 28450, 28455, 28456, 28465)

▲**28465** Open treatment of tarsal bone fracture (except talus and calcaneus), with or without internal or external fixation, each

▲**28470** Closed treatment of metatarsal fracture; without manipulation, each

28475 with manipulation, each

▲**28476** Percutaneous skeletal fixation of metatarsal fracture, with manipulation, each

(28480 has been deleted. To report, see 28470, 28475, 28476, 28485)

▲**28485** Open treatment of metatarsal fracture, with or without internal or external fixation, each

▲**28490** Closed treatment of fracture great toe, phalanx or phalanges; without manipulation

28495 with manipulation

▲**28496** Percutaneous skeletal fixation of fracture great toe, phalanx or phalanges, with manipulation

(28500 has been deleted. To report, see 28490, 28495, 28496, 28505)

▲**28505** Open treatment of fracture great toe, phalanx or phalanges, with or without internal or external fixation

▲**28510** Closed treatment of fracture, phalanx or phalanges, other than great toe; without manipulation, each

28515 with manipulation, each

(28520 has been deleted. To report, see 28510, 28515, 28525)

▲**28525** Open treatment of fracture, phalanx or phalanges, other than great toe, with or without internal or external fixation, each

▲**28530** Closed treatment of sesamoid fracture

• **28531** Open treatment of sesamoid fracture, with or without internal fixation

▲**28540** Closed treatment of tarsal bone dislocation, other than talotarsal; without anesthesia

28545 requiring anesthesia

▲**28546** Percutaneous skeletal fixation of tarsal bone dislocation, other than talotarsal, with manipulation

(28550 has been deleted. To report, see 28540, 28545, 28546, 28555)

▲28555 Open treatment of tarsal bone dislocation, with or without internal or external fixation

▲28570 Closed treatment of talotarsal joint dislocation; without anesthesia

28575 requiring anesthesia

• 28576 Percutaneous skeletal fixation of talotarsal joint dislocation, with manipulation

(28580 has been deleted. To report, see 28570, 28575, 28576, 28585)

▲28585 Open treatment of talotarsal joint dislocation, with or without internal or external fixation

▲28600 Closed treatment of tarsometatarsal joint dislocation; without anesthesia

28605 requiring anesthesia

▲28606 Percutaneous skeletal fixation of tarsometatarsal joint dislocation, with manipulation

(28610 has been deleted. To report, see 28600, 28605, 28606, 28615)

▲28615 Open treatment of tarsometatarsal joint dislocation, with or without internal or external fixation

▲28630* Closed treatment of metatarsophalangeal joint dislocation; without anesthesia

28635* requiring anesthesia

• 28636 Percutaneous skeletal fixation of metatarsophalangeal joint dislocation, with manipulation

(28640 has been deleted. To report, see 28630, 28635, 28636, 28645)

▲28645 Open treatment of metatarsophalangeal joint dislocation, with or without internal or external fixation

▲28660* Closed treatment of interphalangeal joint dislocation; without anesthesia

28665* requiring anesthesia

● **28666** Percutaneous skeletal fixation of interphalangeal joint dislocation, with manipulation

(28670 has been deleted. To report, see 28660, 28665, 28666, 28675)

▲ **28675** Open treatment of interphalangeal joint dislocation, with or without internal or external fixation

ARTHRODESIS

28705 Pantalar arthrodesis

28715 Triple arthrodesis

28725 Subtalar arthrodesis

28730 Arthrodesis, midtarsal or tarsometatarsal, multiple or transverse;

28735 with osteotomy as for flatfoot correction

28737 Arthrodesis, midtarsal navicular-cuneiform, with tendon lengthening and advancement (Miller type procedure)

28740 Arthrodesis, midtarsal or tarsometatarsal, single joint

28750 Arthrodesis, great toe; metatarsophalangeal joint

28755 interphalangeal joint

28760 Arthrodesis, great toe, interphalangeal joint, with extensor hallucis longus transfer to first metatarsal neck (Jones type procedure)

(For hammertoe operation or interphalangeal fusion, see 28285)

AMPUTATION

28800 Amputation, foot; midtarsal (Chopart type procedure)

28805 transmetatarsal

28810 Amputation, metatarsal, with toe, single

28820 Amputation, toe; metatarsophalangeal joint

28825 interphalangeal joint

(For amputation of tuft of distal phalanx, use 11752)

MISCELLANEOUS

28899 Unlisted procedure, foot or toes

APPLICATION OF CASTS AND STRAPPING

The listed procedures apply when the cast application or strapping is a replacement procedure used during or after the period of follow-up care. Additional visits are reportable only if significant identifiable further services are provided at the time of the cast application or strapping.

If cast application or strapping is provided as an initial procedure in which no surgery is performed (eg, casting of a sprained ankle or knee), use the appropriate level of office visit in addition to 99070 for supplies.

Listed procedures include removal of cast or strapping.

BODY AND UPPER EXTREMITY CASTS

29000 Application of halo type body cast (see 20661-20663 for insertion)

29010 Application of Risser jacket, localizer, body; only

29015 including head

29020 Application of turnbuckle jacket, body; only

29025 including head

29035 Application of body cast, shoulder to hips;

29040 including head, Minerva type

29044 including one thigh

29046 including both thighs

29049 Application; plaster figure-of-eight

29055 shoulder spica

29058 plaster Velpeau

29065 shoulder to hand (long arm)

29075 elbow to finger (short arm)

29085 hand and lower forearm (gauntlet)

SPLINTS

29105 Application of long arm splint (shoulder to hand)

29125 Application of short arm splint (forearm to hand); static

29126 dynamic

29130 Application of finger splint; static

29131 dynamic

STRAPPING - ANY AGE

29200 Strapping; thorax

29220 low back

29240 shoulder (eg, Velpeau)

29260 elbow or wrist

29280 hand or finger

LOWER EXTREMITY CASTS

29305 Application of hip spica cast; one leg

29325 one and one-half spica or both legs

(For hip spica (body) cast, including thighs only, see 29046)

29345 Application of long leg cast (thigh to toes);

29355 walker or ambulatory type

29358 Application of long leg cast brace

29365 Application of cylinder cast (thigh to ankle)

29405 Application of short leg cast (below knee to toes);

29425 walking or ambulatory type

29435 Application of patellar tendon bearing (PTB) cast

29440 Adding walker to previously applied cast

29450 Application of clubfoot cast with molding or manipulation, long or short leg

(29455 has been deleted. To report, use 29450 with modifier -50 or 09950)

SPLINTS

29505 Application of long leg splint (thigh to ankle or toes)

29515 Application of short leg splint (calf to foot)

STRAPPING - ANY AGE

29520 Strapping; hip

29530 knee

29540 ankle

29550 toes

29580 Unna boot

29590 Denis-Browne splint strapping

REMOVAL OR REPAIR

(Codes for cast removals should be employed only for casts applied by another physician)

29700 Removal or bivalving; gauntlet, boot or body cast

29705 full arm or full leg cast

29710 shoulder or hip spica, Minerva, or Risser jacket, etc.

29715 turnbuckle jacket

29720 Repair of spica, body cast or jacket

29730 Windowing of cast

29740 Wedging of cast (except clubfoot casts)

29750 Wedging of clubfoot cast

(29751 has been deleted. To report, use 29750 with modifier -50 or 09950)

MISCELLANEOUS

29799 Unlisted procedure, casting or strapping

ARTHROSCOPY

(Surgical arthroscopy always includes a diagnostic arthroscopy)

(When arthroscopy is performed in conjunction with arthrotomy, add modifier -51 or 09951)

29800 Arthroscopy, temporomandibular joint, diagnostic, with or without synovial biopsy (separate procedure)

29804 Arthroscopy, temporomandibular joint, surgical

29815 Arthroscopy, shoulder, diagnostic, with or without synovial biopsy (separate procedure)

29819 Arthroscopy, shoulder, surgical; with removal of loose body or foreign body

29820 synovectomy, partial

29821 synovectomy, complete

29822 debridement, limited

29823 debridement, extensive

29825 with lysis and resection of adhesions, with or without manipulation

29826 decompression of subacromial space with partial acromioplasty, with or without coracoacromial release

29830 Arthroscopy, elbow, diagnostic, with or without synovial biopsy (separate procedure)

29834 Arthroscopy, elbow, surgical; with removal of loose body or foreign body

29835 synovectomy, partial

29836 synovectomy, complete

29837 debridement, limited

29838 debridement, extensive

29840 Arthroscopy, wrist, diagnostic, with or without synovial biopsy (separate procedure)

29843 Arthroscopy, wrist, surgical; for infection, lavage and drainage

29844 synovectomy, partial

29845 synovectomy, complete

29846 excision of triangular fibrocartilage and/or joint debridement

29847 internal fixation for fracture or instability

29848 with release of transverse carpal ligament

(For open procedure, see 64721)

• **29850** Arthroscopically aided treatment of intercondylar spine(s) and/or tuberosity fracture(s) of the knee, with or without manipulation; without internal or external fixation (includes arthroscopy)

• **29851** with internal or external fixation (includes arthroscopy)

(For bone graft, use 20900, 20902)

• **29855** Arthroscopically aided treatment of tibial fracture, proximal (plateau); unicondylar, with or without internal or external fixation (includes arthroscopy)

• **29856** bicondylar, with or without internal or external fixation (includes arthroscopy)

(For bone graft, use 20900, 20902)

29870 Arthroscopy, knee, diagnostic, with or without synovial biopsy (separate procedure)

29871 Arthroscopy, knee, surgical; for infection, lavage and drainage

(29872 has been deleted)

29874 for removal of loose body or foreign body (eg, osteochondritis dissecans fragmentation, chondral fragmentation)

29875 synovectomy, limited (eg, plica or shelf resection) (separate procedure)

29876 synovectomy, major, two or more compartments (eg, medial or lateral)

29877 debridement/shaving of articular cartilage (chondroplasty)

29879 abrasion arthroplasty (includes chondroplasty where necessary) or multiple drilling

29880 with meniscectomy (medial AND lateral, including any meniscal shaving)

29881 with meniscectomy (medial OR lateral including any meniscal shaving)

29882 with meniscus repair (medial OR lateral)

29883 with meniscus repair (medial AND lateral)

29884 with lysis of adhesions, with or without manipulation (separate procedure)

29885 drilling for osteochondritis dissecans with bone grafting, with or without internal fixation (including debridement of base of lesion)

29886 drilling for intact osteochondritis dissecans lesion

29887 drilling for intact osteochondritis dissecans lesion with internal fixation

29888 Arthroscopically aided anterior cruciate ligament repair/augmentation or reconstruction

29889 Arthroscopically aided posterior cruciate ligament repair/augmentation or reconstruction

(Procedures 29888 and 29889 should not be used with reconstruction procedures 27427-27429)

(29890 has been deleted)

29894 Arthroscopy, ankle (tibiotalar and fibulotalar joints), surgical; with removal of loose body or foreign body

29895 synovectomy, partial

(29896 has been deleted)

29897 debridement, limited

29898 debridement, extensive

29909 Unlisted procedure, arthroscopy

Respiratory System

NOSE

INCISION

30000* Drainage abscess or hematoma, nasal, internal approach

(For external approach, see 10060, 10140)

30020* Drainage abscess or hematoma, nasal septum

(For lateral rhinotomy, see specific application (eg, 30118, 30320))

EXCISION

30100 Biopsy, intranasal

(For biopsy skin of nose, see 11100, 11101)

30110 Excision, nasal polyp(s), simple

(30110 would normally be completed in an office setting)

(30111 has been deleted. To report, use 30110 with modifier -50 or 09950)

30115 Excision, nasal polyp(s), extensive

(30115 would normally require the facilities available in a hospital setting)

(30116 has been deleted. To report, use 30115 with modifier -50 or 09950)

30117 Excision or destruction, any method (including laser), intranasal lesion; internal approach

30118 external approach (lateral rhinotomy)

30120 Excision or surgical planing of skin of nose for rhinophyma

30124 Excision dermoid cyst, nose; simple, skin, subcutaneous

30125 complex, under bone or cartilage

30130 Excision turbinate, partial or complete

30140 Submucous resection turbinate, partial or complete

(For submucous resection of nasal septum, use 30520)

30150 Rhinectomy; partial

30160 total

(For closure and/or reconstruction, primary or delayed, see Integumentary System, 13150-13152, 14060-14300, 15120, 15121, 15260, 15261, 15760, 20900-20912)

INTRODUCTION

30200* Injection into turbinate(s), therapeutic

30210* Displacement therapy (Proetz type)

30220 Insertion, nasal septal prosthesis (button)

ENDOSCOPY

(For nasal endoscopy, see 31250-31258)

REMOVAL FOREIGN BODY

30300* Removal foreign body, intranasal; office type procedure

30310 requiring general anesthesia

30320 by lateral rhinotomy

REPAIR

(For obtaining tissues for graft, see 20900-20926, 21210)

30400 Rhinoplasty, primary; lateral and alar cartilages and/or elevation of nasal tip

(For columellar reconstruction, see 13150 et seq)

30410 complete, external parts including bony pyramid, lateral and alar cartilages, and/or elevation of nasal tip

30420 including major septal repair

30430 Rhinoplasty, secondary; minor revision (small amount of nasal tip work)

30435 intermediate revision (bony work with osteotomies)

30450 major revision (nasal tip work and osteotomies)

● **30460** Rhinoplasty for nasal deformity secondary to congenital cleft lip and/or palate, including columellar lengthening; tip only

● **30462** tip, septum, osteotomies

(30500 has been deleted. To report, use 30520)

30520 Septoplasty or submucous resection, with or without cartilage scoring, contouring or replacement with graft

(For submucous resection of turbinates, use 30140)

30540 Repair choanal atresia; intranasal

30545 transpalatine

30560* Lysis intranasal synechia

30580 Repair fistula; oromaxillary (combine with 31030 if antrotomy is included)

30600 oronasal

▲**30620** Septal or other intranasal dermatoplasty (does not include obtaining graft)

30630 Repair nasal septal perforations

DESTRUCTION

(30800 has been deleted. To report, see 30801, 30802)

30801* Cauterization and/or ablation, mucosa of turbinates, unilateral or bilateral, any method, (separate procedure); superficial

30802 intramural

(30805, 30820 have been deleted. To report, see 30801, 30802)

OTHER PROCEDURES

(30900 has been deleted. To report, see 30901, 30903)

30901* Control nasal hemorrhage, anterior, simple (limited cautery and/or packing) any method

(30902 has been deleted. To report, use 30901 with modifier -50 or 09950)

30903* Control nasal hemorrhage, anterior, complex (extensive cautery and/or packing) any method

(30904 has been deleted. To report, use 30903 with modifier -50 or 09950)

30905* Control nasal hemorrhage, posterior, with posterior nasal packs and/or cauterization, any method; initial

30906* subsequent

30915 Ligation arteries; ethmoidal

30920 internal maxillary artery, transantral

(For ligation external carotid artery, see 37600)

30930 Fracture nasal turbinate(s), therapeutic

30999 Unlisted procedure, nose

ACCESSORY SINUSES

INCISION

31000* Lavage by cannulation; maxillary sinus (antrum puncture or natural ostium)

(31001 has been deleted. To report, use 31000 with modifier -50 or 09950)

31002* sphenoid sinus

31020 Sinusotomy, maxillary (antrotomy); intranasal

(31021 has been deleted. To report, use 31020 with modifier -50 or 09950)

31030 radical (Caldwell-Luc) without removal of antrochoanal polyps

(31031 has been deleted. To report, use 31030 with modifier -50 or 09950)

31032 radical (Caldwell-Luc) with removal of antrochoanal polyps

(31033 has been deleted. To report, use 31032 with modifier -50 or 09950)

31040 Pterygomaxillary fossa surgery, any approach

(For transantral ligation of internal maxillary artery, see 30920)

31050 Sinusotomy, sphenoid, with or without biopsy;

31051 with mucosal stripping or removal of polyp(s)

31070 Sinusotomy frontal; external, simple (trephine operation)

31071 intranasal

31075 transorbital, unilateral (for mucocele or osteoma, Lynch type)

31080 obliterative without osteoplastic flap, brow incision (includes ablation)

31081 obliterative, without osteoplastic flap, coronal incision (includes ablation)

31084 obliterative, with osteoplastic flap, brow incision

31085 obliterative, with osteoplastic flap, coronal incision

31086 nonobliterative, with osteoplastic flap, brow incision

31087 nonobliterative, with osteoplastic flap, coronal incision

31090 Sinusotomy combined, three or more sinuses

EXCISION

31200 Ethmoidectomy; intranasal, anterior

31201 intranasal, total

31205 extranasal, total

31225 Maxillectomy; without orbital exenteration

31230 with orbital exenteration (en bloc)

(For orbital exenteration only, see 65110 et seq)

(For skin grafts, see 15120 et seq)

ENDOSCOPY

(For endoscopic procedures, code appropriate endoscopy of each anatomic site examined)

(A surgical sinus endoscopy always includes a sinusotomy and diagnostic endoscopy)

31250 Nasal endoscopy, diagnostic, with or without biopsy (includes examination of the medial meatus, infundibulum and sinus ostia) (separate procedure)

31252 Nasal endoscopy, surgical; with nasal polypectomy

31254 with ethmoidectomy, partial

31255 with ethmoidectomy, anterior and posterior (total)

31256 with maxillary antrostomy

31258 with removal of foreign body(s)

31260 Maxillary sinus endoscopy, diagnostic, with or without biopsy (separate procedure)

31263 Maxillary sinus endoscopy, surgical; with removal of foreign body(s)

31265 with removal of cyst

31267 with removal of mucous membrane and/or polyps

31268 with removal of fungus ball

31270 Sphenoid endoscopy, diagnostic, with or without biopsy (separate procedure)

31275 Sphenoid endoscopy, surgical;

31277 with removal of mucous membrane

31285 Sinus endoscopy, two or more sinuses, unilateral

OTHER PROCEDURES

(For hypophysectomy, transantral or transeptal approach, see 61548)

(For transcranial hypophysectomy, see 61546)

(31245 has been deleted. To report, use 61548)

31299 Unlisted procedure, accessory sinuses

LARYNX

EXCISION

31300 Laryngotomy (thyrotomy, laryngofissure); with removal of tumor or laryngocele, cordectomy

31320 diagnostic

31360 Laryngectomy; total, without radical neck dissection

31365 total, with radical neck dissection

31367 subtotal supraglottic, without radical neck dissection

31368 subtotal supraglottic, with radical neck dissection

31370 Partial laryngectomy (hemilaryngectomy); horizontal

31375 laterovertical

31380 anterovertical

31382 antero-latero-vertical

31390 Pharyngolaryngectomy, with radical neck dissection; without reconstruction

31395 with reconstruction

31400 Arytenoidectomy or arytenoidopexy, external approach

(For endoscopic arytenoidectomy, see 31560)

31420 Epiglottidectomy

INTRODUCTION

31500 Intubation, endotracheal, emergency procedure

(For injection procedure for bronchography, see 31656, 31708, 31710)

31502 Tracheotomy tube change prior to establishment of fistula tract

ENDOSCOPY

(For endoscopic procedures, code appropriate endoscopy of each anatomic site examined)

31505 Laryngoscopy, indirect (separate procedure); diagnostic

31510 with biopsy

31511 with removal of foreign body

31512 with removal of lesion

31513 with vocal cord injection

31515 Laryngoscopy direct, with or without tracheoscopy; for aspiration

31520 diagnostic, newborn

31525 diagnostic, except newborn

31526 diagnostic, with operating microscope

31527 with insertion of obturator

31528 with dilatation, initial

31529 with dilatation, subsequent

31530 Laryngoscopy, direct, operative, with foreign body removal;

31531 with operating microscope

31535 Laryngoscopy, direct, operative, with biopsy;

31536 with operating microscope

31540 Laryngoscopy, direct, operative, with excision of tumor and/or stripping of vocal cords or epiglottis;

31541 with operating microscope

31560 Laryngoscopy, direct, operative, with arytenoidectomy;

31561 with operating microscope

31570 Laryngoscopy, direct, with injection into vocal cord(s), therapeutic;

31571 with operating microscope

31575 Laryngoscopy, flexible fiberoptic; diagnostic

31576 with biopsy

31577 with removal of foreign body

31578 with removal of lesion

31579 with stroboscopy

REPAIR

31580 Laryngoplasty; for laryngeal web, two stage, with keel insertion and removal

31582 for laryngeal stenosis, with graft or core mold, including tracheotomy

31584 with open reduction of fracture

31585 Treatment of closed laryngeal fracture; without manipulation

31586 with closed manipulative reduction

31587 Laryngoplasty, cricoid split

31588 Laryngoplasty, not otherwise specified (eg, for burns, reconstruction after partial laryngectomy)

31590 Laryngeal reinnervation by neuromuscular pedicle

DESTRUCTION

31595 Section recurrent laryngeal nerve, therapeutic (separate procedure), unilateral

OTHER PROCEDURES

31599 Unlisted procedure, larynx

TRACHEA AND BRONCHI

INCISION

31600 Tracheostomy, planned (separate procedure);

31601 under two years

31603 Tracheostomy, emergency procedure; transtracheal

31605 cricothyroid membrane

31610 Tracheostomy, fenestration procedure with skin flaps

(For endotracheal intubation, see 31500)

(For tracheal aspiration under direct vision, see 31515)

31611 Construction of tracheoesophageal fistula and subsequent insertion of an alaryngeal speech prosthesis (eg, voice button, Blom-Singer prosthesis)

31612 Tracheal puncture, percutaneous for aspiration of mucus (transtracheal aspiration)

31613 Tracheostoma revision; simple, without flap rotation

31614 complex, with flap rotation

ENDOSCOPY

(For endoscopic procedures, code appropriate endoscopy of each anatomic site examined)

(For tracheoscopy, see laryngoscopy codes 31515-31578)

31615 Tracheobronchoscopy through established tracheostomy incision

(31620, 31621 have been deleted. To report, use 31622)

31622 Bronchoscopy; diagnostic, (flexible or rigid), with or without cell washing or brushing

31625 with biopsy

(31626 has been deleted. To report, use 31625)

(31627 has been deleted. To report, use 31622)

31628 with transbronchial lung biopsy, with or without fluoroscopic guidance

31629 with transbronchial needle aspiration biopsy

31630 with tracheal or bronchial dilation or closed reduction of fracture

31631 with tracheal dilation and placement of tracheal stent

31635 with removal of foreign body

31640 with excision of tumor

31641 with destruction of tumor or relief of stenosis by any method other than excision (eg, laser)

31645 with therapeutic aspiration of tracheobronchial tree, initial (eg, drainage of lung abscess)

31646 with therapeutic aspiration of tracheobronchial tree, subsequent

(For catheter aspiration of tracheobronchial tree at bedside, use 31725)

(31650, 31651 have been deleted. To report, see 31645, 31646)

31656 with injection of contrast material for segmental bronchography (fiberscope only)

(For radiological supervision and interpretation, see 71040, 71060)

31659 with other bronchoscopic procedures

INTRODUCTION

(For endotracheal intubation, see 31500)

(For tracheal aspiration under direct vision, see 31515)

31700 Catheterization, transglottic (separate procedure)

31708 Instillation of contrast material for laryngography or bronchography, without catheterization

(For radiological supervision and interpretation, see 70373, 71040, 71060)

31710 Catheterization for bronchography, with or without instillation of contrast material

(For bronchoscopic catheterization for bronchography, fiberscope only, see 31656)

(For radiological supervision and interpretation, see 71040, 71060)

31715 Transtracheal injection for bronchography

(For radiological supervision and interpretation, see 71040, 71060)

(For prolonged services, see 99150, 99151)

31717 Catheterization with bronchial brush biopsy

(31719 has been deleted. To report, see 31730)

31720 Catheter aspiration (separate procedure); nasotracheobronchial

31725 tracheobronchial with fiberscope, bedside

• **31730** Transtracheal (percutaneous) introduction of needle wire dilator/stent or indwelling tube for oxygen therapy

REPAIR

31750 Tracheoplasty; cervical

31755 tracheopharyngeal fistulization, each stage

31760 intrathoracic

31766 Carinal reconstruction

31770 Bronchoplasty; graft repair

31775 excision stenosis and anastomosis

(For lobectomy and bronchoplasty, see 32485)

31780 Excision tracheal stenosis and anastomosis; cervical

31781 cervicothoracic

31785 Excision of tracheal tumor or carcinoma; cervical

31786 thoracic

SUTURE

31800 Suture of external tracheal wound or injury; cervical

31805 intrathoracic

31820 Surgical closure tracheostomy or fistula; without plastic repair

31825 with plastic repair

(For repair tracheoesophageal fistula, see 43305, 43312)

31830 Revision of tracheostomy scar

31899 Unlisted procedure, trachea, bronchi

LUNGS AND PLEURA

INCISION

32000* Thoracentesis, puncture of pleural cavity for aspiration, initial or subsequent

(For radiological supervision and interpretation, see 76003, 76360, 76934)

32002 Thoracentesis with insertion of tube with or without water seal (eg, for pneumothorax) (separate procedure)

32005 Chemical pleurodesis (eg, for recurrent or persistent pneumothorax)

32020 Tube thoracostomy with or without water seal (eg, for abscess, hemothorax, empyema) (separate procedure)

32035 Thoracostomy; with rib resection for empyema

32036 with open flap drainage for empyema

32095 Thoracotomy limited, for biopsy of lung or pleura

32100 Thoracotomy, major; with exploration and biopsy

32110 with control of traumatic hemorrhage and/or repair of lung tear

32120 for postoperative complications

32124 with open intrapleural pneumonolysis

32140 with cyst(s) removal, with or without a pleural procedure

32141 with excision-plication of bullae, with or without any pleural procedure

32150 with removal of intrapleural foreign body or fibrin deposit

32151 with removal of intrapulmonary foreign body

32160 with cardiac massage

(For segmental or other resections of lung, see 32480-32525)

32200 Pneumonostomy, with open drainage of abscess or cyst

32215 Pleural scarification for repeat pneumothorax

32220 Decortication, pulmonary, (separate procedure); total

32225 partial

EXCISION

32310 Pleurectomy; parietal (separate procedure)

32315 partial

32320 Decortication and parietal pleurectomy

32400* Biopsy, pleura; percutaneous needle

(For radiological supervision and interpretation, see 71036, 76360, 76942)

(For fine needle aspiration, preparation, and interpretation of smears, see 88170-88173)

32402 open

32405 Biopsy, lung or mediastinum, percutaneous needle

(For radiological supervision and interpretation, see 71036, 76360, 76942)

(For fine needle aspiration, preparation, and interpretation of smears, see 88170-88173)

32420* Pneumonocentesis, puncture of lung for aspiration

32440 Pneumonectomy, total

32445 Pneumonectomy, extrapleural; without empyemectomy

32450 with empyemectomy

32480 Lobectomy, total or segmental;

32485 with bronchoplasty

32490 with concomitant decortication

32500 Wedge resection of lung, single or multiple

32520 Resection of lung; with resection of chest wall

32522 with reconstruction of chest wall, without prosthesis

32525 with major reconstruction of chest wall, with prosthesis

32540 Extrapleural enucleation of empyema (empyemectomy);

32545 with lobectomy

ENDOSCOPY

(For endoscopic procedures, code appropriate endoscopy of each anatomic site examined)

32700 Thoracoscopy, exploratory (separate procedure);

32705 with biopsy

REPAIR

32800 Repair lung hernia through chest wall

32810 Closure of chest wall following open flap drainage for empyema (Clagett type procedure)

32815 Open closure of major bronchial fistula

32820 Major reconstruction, chest wall (post-traumatic)

SURGICAL COLLAPSE THERAPY; THORACOPLASTY

(See also 32520-32525)

32900 Resection of ribs, extrapleural, all stages

32905 Thoracoplasty, Schede type or extrapleural (all stages);

32906 with closure of bronchopleural fistula

(For open closure of major bronchial fistula, see 32815)

(For resection of first rib for thoracic outlet compression, see 21615, 21616)

32940 Pneumonolysis, extraperiosteal, including filling or packing procedures

32960* Pneumothorax, therapeutic, intrapleural injection of air

32999 Unlisted procedure, lungs and pleura

Cardiovascular System

Selective vascular catheterizations should be coded to include introduction and all lesser order selective catheterizations used in the approach (eg, the description for a selective right middle cerebral artery catheterization includes the introduction and placement catheterization of the right common and internal carotid arteries).

Additional second and/or third order arterial catheterizations within the same family of arteries supplied by a single first order artery should be expressed by 36218 or 36248. Additional first order or higher catheterizations in vascular families supplied by a first order vessel different from a previously selected and coded family should be separately coded using the conventions described above.

(For monitoring, operation of pump and other nonsurgical services, see 99150, 99151, 99291, 99292, 99190-99192)

(For other medical or laboratory related services, see appropriate section)

(For radiological supervision and interpretation, see 75600-75978)

HEART AND PERICARDIUM

PERICARDIUM

33010* Pericardiocentesis; initial

(For radiological supervision and interpretation, see 76930)

33011* subsequent

(For radiological supervision and interpretation, see 76930)

33015 Tube pericardiostomy

33020 Pericardiotomy for removal of clot or foreign body (primary procedure)

33025 Creation of pericardial window or partial resection for drainage

33030 Pericardiectomy, subtotal or complete; without cardiopulmonary bypass

33031 with cardiopulmonary bypass

(33035 has been deleted. To report, use 33031)

33050 Excision of pericardial cyst or tumor

33100 Pericardiectomy (separate procedure)

CARDIAC TUMOR

33120 Excision of intracardiac tumor, resection with cardiopulmonary bypass

33130 Resection of external cardiac tumor

PACEMAKER OR DEFIBRILLATOR

(For electronic, telephonic analysis of internal pacemaker system, see 93731-93736)

(Procedures include repositioning or replacement in first 14 days)

(For radiological supervision and interpretation with insertion of pacemaker, see 71090)

33200 Insertion of permanent pacemaker with epicardial electrode; by thoracotomy

33201 by xiphoid approach

(33205 has been deleted. To report, use 33206-33208)

33206 Insertion of permanent pacemaker with transvenous electrode(s); atrial

33207 ventricular

33208 AV sequential

33210 Insertion of temporary transvenous cardiac electrode, or pacemaker catheter (separate procedure)

33212 Insertion or replacement of pacemaker pulse generator or automatic implantable cardioverter-defibrillator pulse generator only

33216 Insertion, replacement, or repositioning of permanent transvenous electrodes only (15 days or more after initial insertion)

33218 Repair of pacemaker; electrodes only

33219 with replacement of pulse generator

33222 Revision or relocation of skin pocket for pacemaker or automatic implantable cardioverter-defibrillator

33232 Removal of permanent pacemaker

33245 Implantation of automatic implantable cardioverter-defibrillator pads, with or without sensing electrodes;

33246 with insertion of automatic implantable cardioverter-defibrillator pulse generator

33248 Revision or removal of automatic implantable cardioverter-defibrillator pads and electrodes

33250 Operative ablation of supraventricular arrhythmogenic focus or pathway (eg, Wolff-Parkinson-White, A-V node re-entry), tract(s) and/or focus (foci); without cardiopulmonary bypass

33251 with cardiopulmonary bypass

33260 Operative ablation of arrhythmogenic focus or pathway; without cardiopulmonary bypass

33261 with cardiopulmonary bypass

WOUNDS OF THE HEART AND GREAT VESSELS

33300 Repair of cardiac wound; without bypass

33305 with cardiopulmonary bypass

33310 Cardiotomy, exploratory (includes removal of foreign body); without bypass

33315 with cardiopulmonary bypass

33320 Suture repair of aorta or great vessels; without bypass

33322 with cardiopulmonary bypass

33330 Insertion of graft, aorta or great vessels; without bypass

33335 with cardiopulmonary bypass

33350 Great vessel repair with other major procedure

CARDIAC VALVES

AORTIC VALVES

33400 Valvuloplasty, aortic valve, open, with cardiopulmonary bypass

33404 Construction of apical-aortic conduit

33405 Replacement, aortic valve, with cardiopulmonary bypass

33407 Valvotomy, aortic valve (commissurotomy); with cardiopulmonary bypass

33408 with inflow occlusion

33411 Replacement, aortic valve; with aortic annulus enlargement, noncoronary cusp

33412 with transventricular aortic annulus enlargement (Konno procedure)

33415 Resection or incision of subvalvular tissue for discrete subvalvular aortic stenosis

33416 Ventriculomyotomy (-myectomy) for idiopathic hypertrophic subaortic stenosis (eg, asymmetric septal hypertrophy)

33417 Aortoplasty (gusset) for supravalvular stenosis

MITRAL VALVE

33420 Valvotomy, mitral valve (commissurotomy); closed

33422 open, with cardiopulmonary bypass

33425 Valvuloplasty, mitral valve, with cardiopulmonary bypass;

33426 with prosthetic ring

33427 radical reconstruction with or without ring

33430 Replacement, mitral valve, with cardiopulmonary bypass

TRICUSPID VALVE

(33450 has been deleted. To report, use 33452)

33452 Valvotomy, tricuspid valve, with cardiopulmonary bypass

33460 Valvuloplasty or valvectomy, tricuspid valve, with cardiopulmonary bypass;

33465 replacement

33468 Tricuspid valve repositioning and plication for Ebstein anomaly

PULMONARY VALVE

33470 Valvotomy, pulmonary valve (commissurotomy); closed (transventricular)

(33471 has been deleted. To report, see 92990)

33472 open, with inflow occlusion

33474 open, with cardiopulmonary bypass

33476 Right ventricular resection for infundibular stenosis, with or without commissurotomy

33478 Outflow tract augmentation (gusset), with or without commissurotomy or infundibular resection

(33480-33492 have been deleted. To report, see 33400-33478 and add modifier -51 to the secondary valve procedure code when multiple valve procedures are performed.)

CORONARY ARTERY AND RELATED PROCEDURES

(Basic procedures include endarterectomy or angioplasty)

▲**33500** Repair of coronary arteriovenous or arteriocardiac chamber fistula; with cardio-pulmonary bypass

● **33501** without cardio-pulmonary bypass

33502 Anomalous coronary artery; ligation

33503 graft, without cardiopulmonary bypass

33504 graft, with cardiopulmonary bypass

VENOUS GRAFTING ONLY FOR CORONARY ARTERY BYPASS

The following codes are used to report coronary artery bypass procedures using venous grafts only. These codes should NOT be used to report the performance of coronary artery bypass procedures using arterial grafts and venous grafts during the same procedure. See 33517-33523 and 33533-33536 for reporting combined arterial-venous grafts.

▲**33510** Coronary artery bypass, vein only; single coronary venous graft

▲**33511** two coronary venous grafts

▲**33512** three coronary venous grafts

▲**33513** four coronary venous grafts

▲**33514** five coronary venous grafts

▲**33516** six or more coronary venous grafts

(For separate procurement of graft, add modifier -62, Services rendered by two surgeons, or use 09962)

COMBINED ARTERIAL-VENOUS GRAFTING FOR CORONARY BYPASS

The following codes are used to report coronary artery bypass procedures using venous grafts and arterial grafts during the same procedure. These codes may NOT be used alone. To report combined arterial-venous grafts it is necessary to report two codes: 1) the appropriate combined arterial-venous graft code (33517-33523); and, 2) the appropriate arterial graft code (33533-33536).

● **33517** Coronary artery bypass, using venous graft(s) and arterial graft(s); single vein graft (list separately in addition to code for arterial graft)

● **33518** two venous grafts (list separately in addition to code for arterial graft)

● **33519** three venous grafts (list separately in addition to code for arterial graft)

(33520 has been deleted)

● **33521** four venous grafts (list separately in addition to code for arterial graft)

● **33522** five venous grafts (list separately in addition to code for arterial graft)

● **33523** six or more venous grafts (list separately in addition to code for arterial graft)

(33525 and 33528 have been deleted)

▲**33530** Reoperation, coronary artery bypass procedure or valve procedure, more than one month after original operation (list separately in addition to code for primary procedure)

(Use 33530 only for codes 33400-33478; 33510-33516)

(33532 has been deleted. To report, use 33999)

ARTERIAL GRAFTING FOR CORONARY ARTERY BYPASS

The following codes are used to report coronary artery bypass procedures using either arterial grafts only or a combination of arterial-venous grafts. The codes include the use of the internal mammary artery, gastroepiploic artery, epigastric artery, radial artery, and arterial conduits procured from other sites.

To report combined arterial-venous grafts it is necessary to report two codes: 1) the appropriate arterial graft code (33533-33536); and, 2) the appropriate combined arterial-venous graft code (33517-33523).

• **33533** Coronary artery bypass, using arterial graft(s); single arterial graft

• **33534** two coronary arterial grafts

• **33535** three coronary arterial grafts

• **33536** four or more coronary arterial grafts

33542 Myocardial resection (eg, ventricular aneurysmectomy)

33545 Repair of postinfarction ventricular septal defect, with or without myocardial resection

(33560 has been deleted)

33570 Coronary angioplasty (endarterectomy with or without gas, arterial implantation or anastomosis), with bypass;

33575 combined with vascularization

SEPTAL DEFECT

(33640 has been deleted. To report, see 33641)

33641 Repair atrial septal defect, secundum, with cardiopulmonary bypass, with or without patch

(33643 has been deleted. To report, see 33641)

33645 Direct or patch closure, sinus venosus, with or without anomalous pulmonary venous drainage

33647 Repair of atrial septal defect and ventricular septal defect, with direct or patch closure

33649 Repair of tricuspid atresia (eg, Fontan, Gago procedures)

33660 Patch closure, endocardial cushion defect, with or without repair of mitral and/or tricuspid cleft;

33665 with repair of separate ventricular septal defect

33670 Repair of complete atrioventricular canal, with or without prosthetic valve

33681 Closure of ventricular septal defect, with or without patch

(33682 has been deleted. To report, use 33681)

33684 with pulmonary valvotomy or infundibular resection (acyanotic)

33688 with removal of pulmonary artery band, with or without gusset

33690 Banding of pulmonary artery

33692 Complete repair tetralogy of Fallot;

33694 with transannular patch

33696 with closure of previous shunt

SINUS OF VALSALVA

33702 Repair sinus of Valsalva fistula, with cardiopulmonary bypass;

33710 with repair of ventricular septal defect

33720 Repair sinus of Valsalva aneurysm, with cardiopulmonary bypass

TOTAL ANOMALOUS PULMONARY VENOUS DRAINAGE

33730 Complete repair of anomalous venous return (supracardiac, intracardiac, or infracardiac types)

(For partial anomalous return, see atrial septal defect)

SHUNTING PROCEDURES

33735 Atrial septectomy or septostomy; closed (Blalock-Hanlon type operation)

33737 open, with inflow occlusion

33738 transvenous method, balloon, Rashkind type (includes cardiac catheterization)

33739 blade method (Sang-Park septostomy) (includes cardiac catheterization)

33750 Shunt; subclavian to pulmonary artery (Blalock-Taussig type operation)

33755 ascending aorta to pulmonary artery (Waterston type operation)

33762 descending aorta to pulmonary artery (Potts-Smith type operation)

33764 central, with prosthetic graft

33766 vena cava to pulmonary artery (Glenn type operation)

TRANSPOSITION OF THE GREAT VESSELS

33774 Repair of transposition of the great arteries, atrial baffle procedure (eg, Mustard or Senning type) with cardiopulmonary bypass;

33775 with removal of pulmonary band

33776 with closure of ventricular septal defect

33777 with repair of subpulmonic obstruction

33778 Repair of transposition of the great arteries, aortic pulmonary artery reconstruction (eg, Jatene type);

33779 with removal of pulmonary band

33780 with closure of ventricular septal defect

33781 with repair of subpulmonic obstruction

(33782, 33783, 33784, 33785 have been deleted. To report, see 33774-33781)

TRUNCUS ARTERIOSUS

33786 Total repair, truncus arteriosus (Rastelli type operation)

33788 Reimplantation of an anomalous pulmonary artery

(For pulmonary artery band, see 33690)

AORTIC ANOMALIES

● **33800** Aortic suspension (aortopexy) for tracheal decompression (eg, for tracheomalacia) (separate procedure)

33802 Division of aberrant vessel (vascular ring);

33803 with reanastomosis

(33810, 33812 have been deleted)

33813 Obliteration of aortopulmonary septal defect; without cardiopulmonary bypass

33814 with cardiopulmonary bypass

33820 Patent ductus arteriosus; ligation (primary procedure)

33822 division, under 18 years

33824 division, 18 years and older

33830 ligation or division when performed with another procedure

33840 Excision of coarctation of aorta, with or without associated patent ductus arteriosus; with direct anastomosis

33845 with graft

(33850 has been deleted. To report, use 33999)

33851 repair using either left subclavian artery or prosthetic material as gusset for enlargement

33852 repair of hypoplastic or interrupted aortic arch using autogenous or prosthetic material

33855 repair of hypoplastic left heart syndrome (eg, Norwood type)

THORACIC AORTIC ANEURYSM

33860 Ascending aorta graft, with cardiopulmonary bypass, with or without coronary implant, with or without valve suspension; without valve replacement

33865 with valve replacement

33870 Transverse arch graft, with cardiopulmonary bypass

33875 Descending thoracic aorta graft, with or without bypass

33877 Repair of thoracoabdominal aortic aneurysm with graft, with or without cardiopulmonary bypass

PULMONARY ARTERY

33910 Pulmonary artery embolectomy; with cardiopulmonary bypass

33915 without bypass

33916 Pulmonary endarterectomy, with or without embolectomy, with cardiopulmonary bypass

MISCELLANEOUS

33930 Donor cardiectomy-pneumonectomy, with preparation and maintenance of homograft

33935 Heart-lung transplant with recipient cardiectomy-pneumonectomy

33940 Donor cardiectomy, with preparation and maintenance of homograft

33945 Heart transplant, with or without recipient cardiectomy

(33950 has been deleted. To report, see 33940, 33945)

33960 Prolonged extracorporeal circulation for cardiopulmonary insufficiency

(For insertion of cannula for prolonged extracorporeal circulation, use 36822)

33970 Intra-aortic balloon counterpulsation; insertion only

(For percutaneous insertion, use 93536)

33971 removal of balloon including repair of artery, with or without graft

33972 monitoring only

(For sternal debridement, use 21627)

33999 Unlisted procedure, cardiac surgery

ARTERIES AND VEINS

Primary vascular procedure listings include establishing both inflow and outflow by whatever procedures necessary. Also included is that portion of the operative arteriogram performed by the surgeon, as indicated. Sympathectomy, when done, is included in the listed aortic procedures. For unlisted vascular procedure, use 37799.

ARTERIAL EMBOLECTOMY OR THROMBECTOMY, WITH OR WITHOUT CATHETER

34001 Embolectomy or thrombectomy, with or without catheter; carotid, subclavian or innominate artery, by neck incision

34051 innominate, subclavian artery, by thoracic incision

34101 axillary, brachial, innominate, subclavian artery, by arm incision

34111 radial or ulnar artery, by arm incision

34151 renal, celiac, mesentery, aortoiliac artery, by abdominal incision

34201 femoropopliteal, aortoiliac artery, by leg incision

34203 popliteal-tibio-peroneal artery, by leg incision

VENOUS THROMBECTOMY, DIRECT OR WITH CATHETER

34401 Thrombectomy, direct or with catheter; vena cava, iliac vein, by abdominal incision

34421 vena cava, iliac, femoropopliteal vein, by leg incision

34451 vena cava, iliac, femoropopliteal vein, by abdominal and leg incision

34471 subclavian vein, by neck incision

34490 axillary and subclavian vein, by arm incision

VENOUS RECONSTRUCTION

34501 Valvuloplasty, femoral vein

34510 Venous valve transposition, any vein donor

34520 Cross-over vein graft to venous system

34530 Saphenopopliteal vein anastomosis

DIRECT REPAIR OF ANEURYSM OR EXCISION (PARTIAL OR TOTAL) AND GRAFT INSERTION FOR ANEURYSM, FALSE ANEURYSM, RUPTURED ANEURYSM, OR OCCLUSIVE DISEASE

Procedures 35001-35162 include preparation of artery for anastomosis including endarterectomy

(For intracranial aneurysm, see 61700 et seq)

(For thoracic aortic aneurysm, see 33860-33875)

35001 Direct repair of aneurysm, false aneurysm, or excision (partial or total) and graft insertion, with or without patch graft; for aneurysm or occlusive disease, carotid, subclavian artery, by neck incision

35002 for ruptured aneurysm, carotid, subclavian artery, by neck incision

35005 for aneurysm, false aneurysm, or occlusive disease, vertebral artery

35011 for aneurysm or occlusive disease, axillary-brachial artery, by arm incision

35013 for ruptured aneurysm, axillary-brachial artery, by arm incision

35021 for aneurysm, false aneurysm, or occlusive disease, innominate, subclavian artery, by thoracic incision

35022 for ruptured aneurysm, innominate, subclavian artery, by thoracic incision

35045 for aneurysm, false aneurysm, or occlusive disease, radial or ulnar artery

35081 for aneurysm, false aneurysm, or occlusive disease, abdominal aorta

35082 for ruptured aneurysm, abdominal aorta

35091 for aneurysm, false aneurysm, or occlusive disease, abdominal aorta involving visceral vessels (mesenteric, celiac, renal)

35092 for ruptured aneurysm, abdominal aorta involving visceral vessels (mesenteric, celiac, renal)

35102 for aneurysm, false aneurysm, or occlusive disease, abdominal aorta involving iliac vessels (common, hypogastric, external)

35103 for ruptured aneurysm, abdominal aorta involving iliac vessels (common, hypogastric, external)

35111 for aneurysm, false aneurysm, or occlusive disease, splenic artery

35112 for ruptured aneurysm, splenic artery

35121 for aneurysm, false aneurysm, or occlusive disease, hepatic, celiac, renal, or mesenteric artery

35122 for ruptured aneurysm, hepatic, celiac, renal, or mesenteric artery

35131 for aneurysm, false aneurysm, or occlusive disease, iliac artery (common, hypogastric, external)

35132 for ruptured aneurysm, iliac artery (common, hypogastric, external)

35141 for aneurysm, false aneurysm, or occlusive disease, common femoral artery (profunda femoris, superficial femoral)

35142 for ruptured aneurysm, common femoral artery (profunda femoris, superficial femoral)

35151 for aneurysm, false aneurysm, or occlusive disease, popliteal artery

35152 for ruptured aneurysm, popliteal artery

35161 for aneurysm, false aneurysm, or occlusive disease, other arteries

35162 for ruptured aneurysm, other arteries

REPAIR ARTERIOVENOUS FISTULA

35180 Repair, congenital arteriovenous fistula; head and neck

35182 thorax and abdomen

35184 extremities

35188 Repair, acquired or traumatic arteriovenous fistula; head and neck

35189 thorax and abdomen

35190 extremities

REPAIR BLOOD VESSEL OTHER THAN FOR FISTULA, WITH OR WITHOUT PATCH GRAFT

(For AV fistula repair, see 35180-35190)

35201 Repair blood vessel, direct; neck

35206 upper extremity

35207 hand, finger

35211 intrathoracic, with bypass

35216 intrathoracic, without bypass

35221 intra-abdominal

35226 lower extremity

35231 Repair blood vessel with vein graft; neck

35236 upper extremity

35241 intrathoracic, with bypass

35246 intrathoracic, without bypass

35251 intra-abdominal

35256 lower extremity

35261 Repair blood vessel with graft other than vein; neck

35266 upper extremity

35271 intrathoracic, with bypass

35276 intrathoracic, without bypass

35281 intra-abdominal

35286 lower extremity

THROMBOENDARTERECTOMY

(For coronary artery, see 33570, 33575)

35301 Thromboendarterectomy, with or without patch graft; carotid, vertebral, subclavian, by neck incision

35311 subclavian, innominate, by thoracic incision

35321 axillary-brachial

35331 abdominal aorta

35341 mesenteric, celiac, or renal

35351 iliac

35355 iliofemoral

35361 combined aortoiliac

35363 combined aortoiliofemoral

35371 common femoral

35372 deep (profunda) femoral

35381 femoral and/or popliteal, and/or tibioperoneal

TRANSLUMINAL ANGIOPLASTY

(If done as part of another operation, use modifier -51 or 09951 or use modifier -52 or 09952)

(For radiological supervision and interpretation, see 75962-75968 and 75978)

TRANSLUMINAL ANGIOPLASTY, OPEN

▲**35450** Transluminal balloon angioplasty, open; renal or other visceral artery

35452 aortic

35454 iliac

35456 femoral-popliteal

35458 brachiocephalic

35459 tibioperoneal trunk and branches

35460 venous

TRANSLUMINAL ANGIOPLASTY, PERCUTANEOUS

▲**35470** Transluminal balloon angioplasty, percutaneous; tibioperoneal trunk and branches

35471 renal or visceral artery

35472 aortic

35473 iliac

35474 femoral-popliteal

35475 brachiocephalic

35476 venous

(For radiological supervision and interpretation, see 75978)

TRANSLUMINAL ATHERECTOMY

(If done as part of another operation, use modifier -51 or 09951 or use modifier -52 or 09952)

(For radiological supervision and interpretation, see 75992-75996)

TRANSLUMINAL ATHERECTOMY, OPEN

• **35480** Transluminal peripheral atherectomy, open; renal or other visceral artery

• **35481** aortic

• **35482** iliac

• **35483** femoral-popliteal

• **35484** brachiocephalic

• 35485 tibioperoneal trunk and branches

TRANSLUMINAL ATHERECTOMY, PERCUTANEOUS

• 35490 Transluminal peripheral atherectomy, percutaneous; renal or other visceral artery

• 35491 aortic

• 35492 iliac

• 35493 femoral-popliteal

• 35494 brachiocephalic

• 35495 tibioperoneal trunk and branches

BYPASS GRAFT—VEIN

35501 Bypass graft, with vein; carotid

35506 carotid-subclavian

35507 subclavian-carotid

35508 carotid-vertebral

35509 carotid-carotid

35511 subclavian-subclavian

35515 subclavian-vertebral

35516 subclavian-axillary

35518 axillary-axillary

35521 axillary-femoral

35526 aortosubclavian or carotid

35531 aortoceliac or aortomesenteric

35533 axillary-femoral-femoral

35536 splenorenal

35541 aortoiliac

35546 aortofemoral or bifemoral

35548 aortoiliofemoral, unilateral

35549 aortoiliofemoral, bilateral

35551 aortofemoral-popliteal

35556 femoral-popliteal

35558 femoral-femoral

35560 aortorenal

35563 ilioiliac

35565 iliofemoral

35566 femoral-anterior tibial, posterior tibial, peroneal artery or other distal vessels

35571 popliteal-tibial, -peroneal artery or other distal vessels

IN-SITU VEIN BYPASS

35582 In-situ vein bypass; aortofemoral-popliteal (only femoral-popliteal portion in-situ)

35583 femoral-popliteal

35585 femoral-anterior tibial, posterior tibial, or peroneal artery

35587 popliteal-tibial, peroneal

BYPASS GRAFT, WITH OTHER THAN VEIN

35601 Bypass graft, with other than vein; carotid

35606 carotid-subclavian

35612 subclavian-subclavian

35616 subclavian-axillary

35621 axillary-femoral

35626 aortosubclavian or carotid

35631 aortoceliac, aortomesenteric, aortorenal

35636 splenorenal

35637 vertebral-carotid transposition

35638 vertebral-subclavian transposition

35641 aortoiliac

35642 carotid-vertebral

35645 subclavian-vertebral

35646 aortofemoral or bifemoral

35650 axillary-axillary

35651 aortofemoral-popliteal

35654 axillary-femoral-femoral

35656 femoral-popliteal

35661 femoral-femoral

35663 ilioiliac

35665 iliofemoral

35666 femoral-anterior tibial, posterior tibial, or peroneal artery

35671 popliteal-tibial or -peroneal artery

35681 Bypass graft, composite

(List procedure 35681 separately in addition to code for primary procedure)

EXPLORATION

35701 Exploration (not followed by surgical repair), with or without lysis of artery; carotid artery

35721 femoral artery

35741 popliteal artery

35761 other vessels

EXPLORATION FOR POSTOPERATIVE HEMORRHAGE, THROMBOSIS OR INFECTION

35800 Exploration for postoperative hemorrhage, thrombosis or infection; neck

35820 chest

35840 abdomen

35860 extremity

35870 Repair of graft-enteric fistula

35875 Thrombectomy and/or repair of arterial or venous graft

(35880 has been deleted. To report, use 35875)

35900 Excision of infected graft;

35910 with revascularization

VASCULAR INJECTION PROCEDURES

Listed services for injection procedures include necessary local anesthesia, introduction of needles or catheter, injection of contrast media with or without automatic power injection, and/or necessary pre- and postinjection care specifically related to the injection procedure.

Catheters, drugs, and contrast media are not included in the listed service for the injection procedures.

(For injection procedures in conjunction with cardiac catheterization, see 93541-93545)

(For chemotherapy of malignant disease, see 96400-96549)

INTRAVENOUS

(An intracatheter is a sheathed combination of needle and short catheter)

36000* Introduction of needle or intracatheter, vein

(36001 has been deleted. To report, use 36000 with modifier -50 or 09950)

● **36005** Injection procedure for contrast venography (including introduction of needle or intracatheter)

36010 Introduction of catheter, superior or inferior vena cava

36011 Selective catheter placement, venous system; first order branch (eg, renal vein, jugular vein)

36012 second order, or more selective, branch (eg, left adrenal vein, petrosal sinus)

36013 Introduction of catheter, right heart or main pulmonary artery

36014 Selective catheter placement, left or right pulmonary artery

36015 Selective catheter placement, segmental or subsegmental pulmonary artery

(For insertion of flow directed catheter (eg, Swan-Ganz), see 93503)

(For venous catheterization for selective organ blood sampling, see 36500)

INTRA-ARTERIAL—INTRA-AORTIC

(For radiological supervision and interpretation, see Radiology)

36100 Introduction of needle or intracatheter, carotid or vertebral artery

(36101 has been deleted. To report, use 36100 with modifier -50 or 09950)

36120 Introduction of needle or intracatheter; retrograde brachial artery

36140 extremity artery

36145 arteriovenous shunt created for dialysis (cannula, fistula, or graft)

(For insertion of arteriovenous cannula, see 36810-36820)

36160 Introduction of needle or intracatheter, aortic, translumbar

36200 Introduction of catheter, aorta

(36210 has been deleted. To report, see 36215-36218)

36215 Selective catheter placement, arterial system; each first order thoracic or brachiocephalic branch, within a vascular family

36216 initial second order thoracic or brachiocephalic branch, within a vascular family

36217 initial third order or more selective thoracic or brachiocephalic branch, within a vascular family

36218 additional second order, third order, and beyond, thoracic or braciocephalic branch, within a vascular family (use in addition to 36216 or 36217 as appropriate)

(36220 has been deleted. To report, see 36215-36218)

36230 Selective catheter placement, coronary artery, single or multiple

(36240 has been deleted. To report, use 36248)

36245 Selective catheter placement, arterial system; each first order abdominal, pelvic or lower extremity artery branch, within a vascular family

36246 initial second order abdominal, pelvic or lower extremity branch, within a vascular family

36247 initial third order or more selective abdominal, pelvic or lower extremity branch, within a vascular family

36248 additional second order, third order, and beyond, abdominal, pelvic or lower extremity artery branch within a vascular family (use in addition to 36246 or 36247 as appropriate)

(36250 has been deleted. To report, use 36248)

36260 Insertion of implantable intra-arterial infusion pump (eg, for chemotherapy of liver)

36261 Revision of implanted intra-arterial infusion pump

36262 Removal of implanted intra-arterial infusion pump

36299 Unlisted procedure, vascular injection

VENOUS

Venipuncture, needle or catheter for diagnostic study or intravenous therapy, percutaneous.

36400 Venipuncture, under age 3 years; femoral, jugular or sagittal sinus

36405* scalp vein

36406 other vein

36410* Venipuncture, child over age 3 years or adult, necessitating physician's skill (separate procedure), for diagnostic or therapeutic purposes. Not to be used for routine venipuncture.

▲**36415*** Routine venipuncture or finger/heel/ear stick for collection of specimen(s)

36420 Venipuncture, cutdown; under age 1 year

36425 age 1 or over

36430 Transfusion, blood or blood components

(36431 has been deleted)

36440* Push transfusion, blood, 2 years or under

36450 Exchange transfusion, blood; newborn

36455 other than newborn

36460 Transfusion, intrauterine, fetal

36468 Single or multiple injections of sclerosing solutions, spider veins (telangiectasia); limb or trunk

36469 face

36470* Injection of sclerosing solution; single vein

36471* multiple veins, same leg

(36480 has been deleted. To report, use 36488 or 36489)

36481 Percutaneous portal vein catheterization by any method

(36485 has been deleted. To report, use 36490 or 36491)

36488* Placement of central venous catheter (subclavian, jugular, or other vein) (eg, for central venous pressure, hyperalimentation, hemodialysis, or chemotherapy); percutaneous, age 2 years or under

36489* percutaneous, over age 2

36490* cutdown, age 2 years or under

36491* cutdown, over age 2

(For examination of patient and instruction to patient, review of prescription of fluids for long-term or permanent hyperalimentation, use levels of care listed in office or hospital visits category or consultative follow-up codes as appropriate)

36493 Repositioning of previously placed central venous catheter under fluoroscopic guidance

(For radiological supervision and interpretation, see Radiology)

(36495-36497 have been deleted. To report, see 36530-36535)

36500 Venous catheterization for selective organ blood sampling

(For catheterization in superior or inferior vena cava, see 36010)

(For radiological supervision and interpretation, see 75893)

36510* Catheterization of umbilical vein for diagnosis or therapy, newborn

36520 Therapeutic apheresis (plasma and/or cell exchange)

36522 Photopheresis, extracorporeal

36530 Insertion of implantable intravenous infusion pump

36531 Revision of implantable intravenous infusion pump

36532 Removal of implantable intravenous infusion pump

36533 Insertion of implantable venous access port, with or without subcutaneous reservoir

36534 Revision of implantable venous access port and/or subcutaneous reservoir

36535 Removal of implantable venous access port and/or subcutaneous reservoir

ARTERIAL

36600* Arterial puncture, withdrawal of blood for diagnosis

36620 Arterial catheterization or cannulation for sampling, monitoring or transfusion (separate procedure); percutaneous

36625 cutdown

36640 Arterial catheterization for prolonged infusion therapy (chemotherapy), cutdown

(See also 96526)

(For arterial catheterization for occlusion therapy, see 75894)

36660* Catheterization, umbilical artery, newborn, for diagnosis or therapy

INTRAOSSEOUS

36680 Placement of needle for intraosseous infusion

INTERVASCULAR CANNULIZATION OR SHUNT (SEPARATE PROCEDURE)

36800 Insertion of cannula for hemodialysis, other purpose; vein to vein

36810 arteriovenous, external (Scribner type)

36815 arteriovenous, external revision or closure

36820 arteriovenous, internal (Cimino type)

36821 Arteriovenous anastomosis, direct, any site

36822 Insertion of cannula(s) for prolonged extracorporeal circulation for cardiopulmonary insufficiency (ECMO)

(For maintenance of prolonged extracorporal circulation, use 33960)

36825 Creation of arteriovenous fistula; autogenous graft

36830 nonautogenous graft

36832 Revision of an arteriovenous fistula, with or without thrombectomy, autogenous or non-autogenous graft

36835 Insertion of Thomas shunt

36840 Insertion mandril

36845 Anastomosis mandril

36860 Cannula declotting; without balloon catheter

36861 with balloon catheter

37140 Anastomosis; portocaval

(For peritoneal-venous shunt, see 49425)

37145 renoportal

37160 caval-mesenteric

37180 splenorenal, proximal

37181 splenorenal, distal (selective decompression of esophagogastric varices, any technique)

37190 Plastic repair of arteriovenous aneurysm

TRANSCATHETER THERAPY AND BIOPSY

(For radiological supervision and interpretation, see Radiology)

37200 Transcatheter biopsy

(For radiological supervision and interpretation, see 75970)

37201 Transcatheter therapy, infusion for thrombolysis other than coronary

37202 Transcatheter therapy, infusion other than for thrombolysis, any type (eg, spasmolytic, vasoconstrictive)

(For thrombolysis of coronary vessels, see 92975, 92977)

37203 Transcatheter retrieval, percutaneous, of intravascular foreign body (eg, fractured venous or arterial catheter)

(For radiological supervision and interpretation, see 75961)

37204 Transcatheter occlusion or embolization (eg, for tumor destruction, to achieve hemostasis, to occlude a vascular malformation), percutaneous, any method, each location, non-central nervous system, non-head or neck

(See also 61624, 61626)

(For radiological supervision and interpretation, see 75894)

TRANSCATHETER THERAPY AND BIOPSY

(For radiological supervision and interpretation, see Radiology)

• **37205** Transcatheter placement of an intravascular stent(s), (non-coronary vessel), percutaneous; initial vessel

• **37206** each additional vessel

• **37207** Transcatheter placement of an intravascular stent(s), (non-coronary vessel), open; initial vessel

• **37208** each additional vessel

LIGATION AND OTHER PROCEDURES

(37400-37560 have been deleted. To report, see 35201-35286)

37565 Ligation of internal jugular vein

37600 Ligation; external carotid artery

37605 internal or common carotid artery

37606 internal or common carotid artery, with gradual occlusion, as with Selverstone or Crutchfield clamp

(For ligation treatment of intracranial aneurysm, see 61703)

37609 Ligation or biopsy, temporal artery

37615 Ligation, major artery (eg, post-traumatic, rupture); neck

37616 chest

37617 abdomen

37618 extremity

37620 Interruption, partial or complete, of inferior vena cava by suture, ligation, plication, clip, extravascular, intravascular (umbrella device)

(For radiological supervision and interpretation, see 75940)

37650 Interruption, partial or complete, of femoral vein, by ligature, intravascular device

(37651 has been deleted. To report, use 37650 with modifier -50 or 09950)

37660 Interruption, partial or complete, of common iliac vein by ligature, intravascular device

37700 Ligation and division of long saphenous vein at saphenofemoral junction, or distal interruptions

(37701 has been deleted. To report, use 37700 with modifier -50 or 09950)

37720 Ligation and division and complete stripping of long or short saphenous veins

(37721 has been deleted. To report, use 37720 with modifier -50 or 09950)

37730 Ligation and division and complete stripping of long and short saphenous veins

(37731 has been deleted. To report, use 37730 with modifier -50 or 09950)

37735 Ligation and division and complete stripping of long or short saphenous veins with radical excision of ulcer and skin graft and/or interruption of communicating veins of lower leg, with excision of deep fascia

(37737 has been deleted. To report, use 37735 with modifier -50 or 09950)

37760 Ligation of perforators, subfascial, radical (Linton type), with or without skin graft

37780 Ligation and division of short saphenous vein at saphenopopliteal junction (separate procedure)

(37781 has been deleted. To report, use 37780 with modifier -50 or 09950)

37785 Ligation, division, and/or excision of recurrent or secondary varicose veins (clusters), one leg

(37787 has been deleted. To report, use 37785 with modifier -50 or 09950)

37788 Penile revascularization, artery, with or without vein graft

37799 Unlisted procedure, vascular surgery

Hemic and Lymphatic Systems

SPLEEN

EXCISION

(38090 has been deleted. To report, use 38999)

38100 Splenectomy (separate procedure); total

38101 partial

REPAIR

38115 Repair of ruptured spleen (splenorrhaphy) with or without partial splenectomy

INTRODUCTION

38200 Injection procedure for splenoportography

(For radiological supervision and interpretation, see 75810)

BONE MARROW TRANSPLANTATION SERVICES

38230 Bone marrow harvesting for transplantation

38240 Bone marrow transplantation; allogenic

38241 autologous

(For compatibility studies, see 86810-86822)

LYMPH NODES AND LYMPHATIC CHANNELS

INCISION

38300* Drainage of lymph node abscess or lymphadenitis; simple

38305 extensive

38308 Lymphangiotomy or other operations on lymphatic channels

38380 Suture and/or ligation of thoracic duct; cervical approach

38381 thoracic approach

38382 abdominal approach

EXCISION

38500 Biopsy or excision of lymph node(s); superficial (separate procedure)

38505 by needle, superficial (eg, cervical, inguinal, axillary)

(For fine needle aspiration, use 88170)

38510 deep cervical node(s)

38520 deep cervical node(s) with excision scalene fat pad

38525 deep axillary node(s)

38530 internal mammary node(s) (separate procedure)

(For percutaneous needle biopsy, retroperitoneal lymph node or mass, see 49180; for fine needle aspiration, use 88171)

(38540 has been deleted. To report, see 38510, 38520)

38542 Dissection, deep jugular node(s)

(For radical cervical neck dissection, see 38720)

38550 Excision of cystic hygroma, axillary or cervical, without deep neurovascular dissection; simple

38555 complex

LIMITED LYMPHADENECTOMY FOR STAGING (SEPARATE PROCEDURE)

38562 Limited lymphadenectomy for staging (separate procedure); pelvic and para-aortic

(When combined with prostatectomy, use 55812 or 55842)

(When combined with insertion of radioactive substance into prostate, use 55862)

38564 retroperitoneal (aortic and/or splenic)

RADICAL LYMPHADENECTOMY (RADICAL RESECTION OF LYMPH NODES)

(For limited pelvic and retroperitoneal lymphadenectomies, see 38562, 38564)

38700 Suprahyoid lymphadenectomy

(38701 has been deleted. To report, use 38700 with modifier -50 or 09950)

38720 Cervical lymphadenectomy (complete)

(38721 has been deleted. To report, use 38720 with modifier -50 or 09950)

38724 Cervical lymphadenectomy (modified radical neck dissection)

38740 Axillary lymphadenectomy; superficial

38745 complete

38760 Inguinofemoral lymphadenectomy, superficial, including Cloquet's node (separate procedure)

(38761 has been deleted. To report, use 38760 with modifier -50 or 09950)

38765 Inguinofemoral lymphadenectomy, superficial, in continuity with pelvic lymphadenectomy, including external iliac, hypogastric, and obturator nodes (separate procedure)

(38766 has been deleted. To report, use 38765 with modifier -50 or 09950)

38770 Pelvic lymphadenectomy, including external iliac, hypogastric, and obturator nodes (separate procedure)

(38771 has been deleted. To report, use 38770 with modifier -50 or 09950)

38780 Retroperitoneal transabdominal lymphadenectomy, extensive, including pelvic, aortic, and renal nodes (separate procedure)

(For excision and repair of lymphedematous skin and subcutaneous tissue, see 15000, 15570-15650)

INTRODUCTION

38790 Injection procedure for lymphangiography

(For radiological supervision and interpretation, see 75801-75807)

(38791 has been deleted. To report, use 38790 with modifier -50 or 09950)

38794 Cannulation, thoracic duct

38999 Unlisted procedure, hemic or lymphatic system

Mediastinum and Diaphragm

MEDIASTINUM

INCISION

39000 Mediastinotomy with exploration, drainage, or removal of foreign body; cervical approach

39010 transthoracic

39020 sternal split

(39050-39070 have been deleted. To report, see 39000-39020)

EXCISION

39200 Excision of mediastinal cyst

39220 Excision of mediastinal tumor

(For substernal thyroidectomy, see 60270)

(For thymectomy, see 60520)

ENDOSCOPY

39400 Mediastinoscopy, with or without biopsy

REPAIR

39499 Unlisted procedure, mediastinum

DIAPHRAGM

REPAIR

(39500 has been deleted. To report, see 43324, 43325)

39501 Repair, laceration of diaphragm

39502 Repair, paraesophageal hiatus hernia, transabdominal, with or without fundoplasty, vagotomy, and/or pyloroplasty, except neonatal

39503 Repair, neonatal diaphragmatic hernia, with or without chest tube insertion and with or without creation of ventral hernia

(39510 has been deleted. To report, see 43324, 43325)

39520 Repair, diaphragmatic hernia (esophageal hiatal); transthoracic

39530 combined, thoracoabdominal

39531 combined, thoracoabdominal, with dilation of stricture (with or without gastroplasty)

39540 Repair, diaphragmatic hernia (other than neonatal), traumatic; acute

39541 chronic

39545 Imbrication of diaphragm for eventration; paralytic

39547 nonparalytic

39599 Unlisted procedure, diaphragm

Digestive System

MOUTH

INCISION

(For drainage of abscess, see appropriate anatomic areas)

LIPS

(For procedures on skin of lips, see 10040 et seq)

EXCISION

40490 Biopsy of lip

40500 Vermilionectomy (lip shave), with mucosal advancement

40510 Excision of lip; transverse wedge excision with primary closure

40520 V-excision with primary direct linear closure

(For excision of mucous lesions, see 40810-40816)

40525 full thickness, reconstruction with local flap (eg, Estlander or fan)

40527 full thickness, reconstruction with cross lip flap (Abbe-Estlander)

40530 Resection of lip, more than one-fourth, without reconstruction

(For reconstruction, see 13131 et seq)

REPAIR (CHEILOPLASTY)

40650 Repair lip, full thickness; vermilion only

40652 up to half vertical height

40654 over one-half vertical height, or complex

40700 Plastic repair of cleft lip/nasal deformity; primary, partial or complete, unilateral

40701 primary bilateral, one stage procedure

40702 primary bilateral, one of two stages

40720 secondary, by recreation of defect and reclosure

(To report rhinoplasty only for nasal deformity secondary to congenital cleft lip, see 30460, 30462)

(40740 has been deleted. To report, use 40720 with modifier -50 or 09950)

(40760 has been deleted. To report, use 40527)

40761 with cross lip pedicle flap (Abbe-Estlander type), including sectioning and inserting of pedicle

(For repair cleft palate, see 42200 et seq)

(For other reconstructive procedures, see 14060, 14061, 15120-15261, 15574, 15576, 15630)

OTHER PROCEDURES

40799 Unlisted procedure, lips

VESTIBULE OF MOUTH

The vestibule is the part of the oral cavity outside the dentoalveolar structures; it includes the mucosal and submucosal tissue of lips and cheeks.

INCISION

40800* Drainage of abscess, cyst, hematoma, vestibule of mouth; simple

40801 complicated

40804* Removal of embedded foreign body, vestibule of mouth; simple

40805 complicated

40806 Incision of labial frenum (frenotomy)

EXCISION, DESTRUCTION

40808 Biopsy, vestibule of mouth

40810 Excision of lesion of mucosa and submucosa, vestibule of mouth; without repair

40812 with simple repair

40814 with complex repair

40816 complex, with excision of underlying muscle

40818 Excision of mucosa of vestibule of mouth as donor graft

40819 Excision of frenum, labial or buccal (frenumectomy, frenulectomy, frenectomy)

40820 Destruction of lesion or scar of vestibule of mouth by physical methods (eg, laser, thermal, cryo, chemical)

REPAIR

40830 Closure of laceration, vestibule of mouth; 2.5 cm or less

40831 over 2.5 cm or complex

40840 Vestibuloplasty; anterior

40842 posterior, unilateral

40843 posterior, bilateral

40844 entire arch

40845 complex (including ridge extension, muscle repositioning)

(For skin grafts, see 15000 et seq)

OTHER PROCEDURES

40899 Unlisted procedure, vestibule of mouth

TONGUE, FLOOR OF MOUTH

INCISION

41000* Intraoral incision and drainage of abscess, cyst, or hematoma of tongue or floor of mouth; lingual

41005* sublingual, superficial

41006 sublingual, deep, supramylohyoid

41007 submental space

41008 submandibular space

41009 masticator space

41010 Incision of lingual frenum (frenotomy)

41015 Extraoral incision and drainage of abscess, cyst, or hematoma of floor of mouth; sublingual

41016 submental

41017 submandibular

41018 masticator space

(For frenoplasty, see 41520)

EXCISION

41100 Biopsy of tongue; anterior two-thirds

41105 posterior one-third

41108 Biopsy of floor of mouth

41110 Excision of lesion of tongue without closure

41112 Excision of lesion of tongue with closure; anterior two-thirds

41113 posterior one-third

41114 with local tongue flap

(List 41114 in addition to code 41112 or 41113)

41115 Excision of lingual frenum (frenectomy)

41116 Excision, lesion of floor of mouth

41120 Glossectomy; less than one-half tongue

41130 hemiglossectomy

41135 partial, with unilateral radical neck dissection

41140 complete or total, with or without tracheostomy, without radical neck dissection

41145 complete or total, with or without tracheostomy, with unilateral radical neck dissection

41150 composite procedure with resection floor of mouth and mandibular resection, without radical neck dissection

41153 composite procedure with resection floor of mouth, with suprahyoid neck dissection

41155 composite procedure with resection floor of mouth, mandibular resection, and radical neck dissection (Commando type)

REPAIR

41250* Repair of laceration 2.5 cm or less; floor of mouth and/or anterior two-thirds of tongue

41251* posterior one-third of tongue

41252* Repair of laceration of tongue, floor of mouth, over 2.6 cm or complex

OTHER PROCEDURES

41500 Fixation of tongue, mechanical, other than suture (eg, K-wire)

41510 Suture of tongue to lip for micrognathia (Douglas type procedure)

41520 Frenoplasty (surgical revision of frenum, eg, with Z-plasty)

(For frenotomy, see 40806, 41010)

41599 Unlisted procedure, tongue, floor of mouth

DENTOALVEOLAR STRUCTURES

INCISION

41800* Drainage of abscess, cyst, hematoma from dentoalveolar structures

41805 Removal of embedded foreign body from dentoalveolar structures; soft tissues

41806 bone

EXCISION, DESTRUCTION

41820 Gingivectomy, excision gingiva, each quadrant

41821 Operculectomy, excision pericoronal tissues

41822 Excision of fibrous tuberosities, dentoalveolar structures

41823 Excision of osseous tuberosities, dentoalveolar structures

41825 Excision of lesion or tumor (except listed above), dentoalveolar structures; without repair

41826 with simple repair

41827 with complex repair

(For nonexcisional destruction, see 41850)

41828 Excision of hyperplastic alveolar mucosa, each sextant or quadrant (specify)

41830 Alveolectomy, including curettage of osteitis or sequestrectomy

41850 Destruction of lesion (except excision), dentoalveolar structures

OTHER PROCEDURES

41870 Periodontal mucosal grafting

41872 Gingivoplasty

41874 Alveoplasty

(For closure of lacerations, see 40830, 40831)

(For segmental osteotomy, see 21202, 21206)

(For reduction of fractures, see 21421-21490)

41899 Unlisted procedure, dentoalveolar structures

PALATE, UVULA

INCISION

42000* Drainage of abscess of palate, uvula

EXCISION, DESTRUCTION

42100 Biopsy of palate, uvula

42104 Excision, lesion of palate, uvula; without closure

42106 with simple primary closure

42107 with local flap closure

(For skin graft, see 14040-14300)

(For mucosal graft, see 40818)

42120 Resection of palate or extensive resection of lesion

(For reconstruction of palate with extraoral tissue, see 14040-14300, 15050, 15120, 15240, 15576)

42140 Uvulectomy, excision of uvula

42145 Palatopharyngoplasty (eg, uvulopalatopharyngoplasty, uvulopharyngoplasty)

(42150 has been deleted. To report, see 21031, 21032)

42160 Destruction of lesion, palate or uvula (thermal, cryo or chemical)

REPAIR

42180 Repair, laceration of palate; up to 2 cm

42182 over 2 cm or complex

42200 Palatoplasty for cleft palate, soft and/or hard palate only

42205 Palatoplasty for cleft palate, with closure of alveolar ridge; soft tissue only

42210 with bone graft to alveolar ridge (includes obtaining graft)

42215 Palatoplasty for cleft palate; major revision

42220 secondary lengthening procedure

42225 attachment pharyngeal flap

42226 Lengthening of palate, and pharyngeal flap

42227 Lengthening of palate, with island flap

42235 Repair of anterior palate, including vomer flap

(42250 has been deleted. To report, use 30600)

42260 Repair of nasolabial fistula

(For repair of cleft lip, see 40700 et seq)

42280 Maxillary impression for palatal prosthesis

42281 Insertion of pin-retained palatal prosthesis

OTHER PROCEDURES

42299 Unlisted procedure, palate, uvula

SALIVARY GLAND AND DUCTS

INCISION

42300* Drainage of abscess; parotid, simple

42305 parotid, complicated

42310* Drainage of abscess; submaxillary or sublingual, intraoral

42320* submaxillary, external

42325 Fistulization of sublingual salivary cyst (ranula);

42326 with prosthesis

42330 Sialolithotomy; submandibular (submaxillary), sublingual or parotid, uncomplicated, intraoral

42335 submandibular (submaxillary), complicated, intraoral

42340 parotid, extraoral or complicated intraoral

EXCISION

42400* Biopsy of salivary gland; needle

42405 incisional

42408 Excision of sublingual salivary cyst (ranula)

42409 Marsupialization of sublingual salivary cyst (ranula)

(For fistulization of sublingual salivary cyst, see 42325)

42410 Excision of parotid tumor or parotid gland; lateral lobe, without nerve dissection

42415 lateral lobe, with dissection and preservation of facial nerve

42420 total, with dissection and preservation of facial nerve

42425 total, en bloc removal with sacrifice of facial nerve

42426 total, with unilateral radical neck dissection

(For suture or grafting of facial nerve, see 64864, 64865, 69740, 69745)

42440 Excision of submandibular (submaxillary) gland

42450 Excision of sublingual gland

REPAIR

42500 Plastic repair of salivary duct, sialodochoplasty; primary or simple

42505 secondary or complicated

42507 Parotid duct diversion, bilateral (Wilke type procedure);

42508 with excision of one submandibular gland

42509 with excision of both submandibular glands

42510 with ligation of both submandibular (Wharton's) ducts

OTHER PROCEDURES

42550 Injection procedure for sialography

(For radiological supervision and interpretation, see 70390)

42600 Closure salivary fistula

42650* Dilation salivary duct

42660* Dilation and catheterization of salivary duct, with or without injection

42665 Ligation salivary duct, intraoral

42699 Unlisted procedure, salivary glands or ducts

PHARYNX, ADENOIDS, AND TONSILS

INCISION

42700* Incision and drainage abscess; peritonsillar

42720 retropharyngeal or parapharyngeal, intraoral approach

42725 retropharyngeal or parapharyngeal, external approach

EXCISION, DESTRUCTION

42800 Biopsy; oropharynx

42802 hypopharynx

42804 nasopharynx, visible lesion, simple

42806 nasopharynx, survey for unknown primary lesion

(For laryngoscopic biopsy, see 31510, 31535, 31536)

42808 Excision or destruction of lesion of pharynx, any method

42809 Removal of foreign body from pharynx

42810 Excision branchial cleft cyst or vestige, confined to skin and subcutaneous tissues

42815 Excision branchial cleft cyst, vestige, or fistula, extending beneath subcutaneous tissues and/or into pharynx

42820 Tonsillectomy and adenoidectomy; under age 12

42821 age 12 or over

42825 Tonsillectomy, primary or secondary; under age 12

42826 age 12 or over

42830 Adenoidectomy, primary; under age 12

42831 age 12 or over

42835 Adenoidectomy, secondary; under age 12

42836 age 12 or over

42842 Radical resection of tonsil, tonsillar pillars, and/or retromolar trigone; without closure

42844 closure with local flap (eg, tongue, buccal)

42845 closure with other flap

(For closure with other flap(s), use appropriate number for flap(s))

(When combined with radical neck dissection, use also 38720)

42860 Excision of tonsil tags

42870 Excision or destruction lingual tonsil, any method (separate procedure)

42880 Excision nasopharyngeal lesion (eg, fibroma)

(For excision and repair of hypopharyngeal diverticulum, cervical approach, see 43130)

42890 Limited pharyngectomy

42892 Resection of lateral pharyngeal wall or pyriform sinus, direct closure by advancement of lateral and posterior pharyngeal walls

(When combined with radical neck dissection, use also 38720)

42894 Resection of pharyngeal wall requiring closure with myocutaneous flap

(When combined with radical neck dissection, use also 38720)

(42895 has been deleted. To report, use 38720 with 42890)

REPAIR

42900 Suture pharynx for wound or injury

42950 Pharyngoplasty (plastic or reconstructive operation on pharynx)

(For pharyngeal flap, see 42225)

42953 Pharyngoesophageal repair

(For closure with myocutaneous or other flap, use appropriate number in addition)

OTHER PROCEDURES

42955 Pharyngostomy (fistulization of pharynx, external for feeding)

42960 Control oropharyngeal hemorrhage, primary or secondary (eg, posttonsillectomy); simple

42961 complicated, requiring hospitalization

42962 with secondary surgical intervention

42970 Control of nasopharyngeal hemorrhage, primary or secondary (eg, postadenoidectomy); simple, with posterior nasal packs, with or without anterior packs and/or cauterization

42971 complicated, requiring hospitalization

42972 with secondary surgical intervention

42999 Unlisted procedure, pharynx, adenoids, or tonsils

ESOPHAGUS

INCISION

43000 Esophagotomy, cervical approach; without removal of foreign body

43020 with removal of foreign body

43030 Cricopharyngeal myotomy

43040 Esophagotomy, thoracic approach; without removal of foreign body

43045 with removal of foreign body

EXCISION

43100 Excision of local lesion, esophagus, with primary repair; cervical approach

43101 thoracic approach

43105 Wide excision of malignant lesion of cervical esophagus, with or without laryngectomy;

43106 with radical neck dissection (Wookey type procedure)

43110 Esophagectomy (at upper two-thirds level) and gastric anastomosis with vagotomy; with or without pyloroplasty

43111 with second stage pyloroplasty

43115 Esophagectomy (at upper two-thirds level) with segment replacement, one or two stages

43119 Total esophagectomy with gastropharyngostomy, without thoracotomy

43120 Esophagogastrectomy (lower third) and vagotomy, combined thoracicoabdominal, with or without pyloroplasty

43130 Diverticulectomy of hypopharynx or esophagus, with or without myotomy; cervical approach

43135 thoracic approach

43136 Diverticulopexy of hypopharynx, with or without myotomy

ENDOSCOPY

(For endoscopic procedures, code appropriate endoscopy of each anatomic site examined)

43200 Esophagoscopy, rigid or flexible fiberoptic (specify); diagnostic procedure

43202 for biopsy and/or collection of specimen by brushing or washing

43204 for injection sclerosis of esophageal varices

43215 for removal of foreign body

(For radiological supervision and interpretation, see 74235)

43217 for removal of polypoid lesion(s)

(43218 has been deleted. To report, use 43499)

43219 for insertion of plastic tube or stent

43220 for dilation, direct, any method

(For dilation without visualization, see 43450-43456)

(43221 has been deleted. To report, use 43200 or 43235)

(43222 has been deleted. To report, use 43202 or 43239)

(43223 has been deleted. To report, use 43215 or 43247)

(43224 has been deleted. To report, use 43217 or 43251)

(43225 has been deleted. To report, use 43499)

43226 for insertion of wire to guide dilation

43227 for control of hemorrhage (eg, electrocoagulation, laser photocoagulation)

43228 for ablation of tumor or mucosal lesion (eg, electrocoagulation, laser photocoagulation)

43234 Upper gastrointestinal endoscopy, simple primary examination (eg, with small diameter flexible fiberscope)

43235 Upper gastrointestinal endoscopy including esophagus, stomach, and either the duodenum and/or jejunum as appropriate; complex diagnostic

43239 for biopsy and/or collection of specimen by brushing or washing

43241 with transendoscopic tube or catheter placement

43243 for injection sclerosis of esophageal and/or gastric varices

43245 for dilation of gastric outlet for obstruction

43246 for directed placement of percutaneous gastrostomy tube

(For radiological supervision and interpretation, see 74350)

43247 for removal of foreign body

(For radiological supervision and interpretation, see 74235)

43251 for removal of polypoid lesion(s)

43255 for control of hemorrhage (eg, electrocoagulation, laser photocoagulation)

43258 for ablation of tumor or mucosal lesion (eg, electrocoagulation, laser photocoagulation, hot biopsy/fulguration)

(For injection sclerosis of esophageal varices, use 43204 or 43243)

43260 Endoscopic retrograde cholangiopancreatography (ERCP), with or without biopsy and/or collection of specimen;

(For radiological supervision and interpretation, see 74328, 74329, 74330)

43262 for sphincterotomy/papillotomy

(For radiological supervision and interpretation, see 74328, 74329, 74330)

43263 for pressure measurement of sphincter of Oddi

(For radiological supervision and interpretation, see 74328, 74329, 74330)

43264 for removal of stone(s) from biliary and/or pancreatic ducts

(For radiological supervision and interpretation, see 74328, 74329, 74330)

43265 for destruction, lithotripsy of stone, any method

(When done with sphincterotomy, also use 43262)

(For radiological supervision and interpretation, see 74328, 74329, 74330)

43267 for insertion of nasobiliary or nasopancreatic drainage tube

(When done with sphincterotomy, also use 43262)

(For radiological supervision and interpretation, see 74328, 74329, 74330)

43268 for insertion of tube or stent into bile or pancreatic duct

(When done with sphincterotomy, also use 43262)

(For radiological supervision and interpretation, see 74328, 74329, 74330)

43269 for removal and/or change of tube, stent or foreign body

(For radiological supervision and interpretation, see 74328, 74329, 74330)

43271 for balloon dilation of ampulla, biliary or pancreatic duct

(For radiological supervision and interpretation, see 74328, 74329, 74330)

43272 for ablation of tumor or mucosal lesion (eg, laser, hot biopsy/fulguration)

(For radiological supervision and interpretation, see 74328, 74329, 74330)

REPAIR

43300 Esophagoplasty, (plastic repair or reconstruction), cervical approach; without repair of tracheoesophageal fistula

43305 with repair of tracheoesophageal fistula

43310 Esophagoplasty, (plastic repair or reconstruction), thoracic approach; without repair of tracheoesophageal fistula

43312 with repair of tracheoesophageal fistula

43320 Esophagogastrostomy (cardioplasty), with or without vagotomy and pyloroplasty; abdominal approach

43321 thoracic approach

43324 Esophagogastric fundoplasty (eg, Nissen, Belsey IV, Hill procedures)

43325 Esophagogastric fundoplasty; with fundic patch (Thal-Nissen procedure)

(For cricopharyngeal myotomy, see 43030)

43326 with gastroplasty (eg, Collis)

43330 Esophagomyotomy ((Heller type), with or without hiatal hernia repair); abdominal approach

43331 thoracic approach

43340 Esophagojejunostomy (without total gastrectomy); abdominal approach

43341 thoracic approach

43350 Esophagostomy, fistulization of esophagus, external; abdominal approach

43351 thoracic approach

43352 cervical approach

SUTURE

43400 Ligation, direct, esophageal varices

43401 Transection of esophagus with repair, for esophageal varices

43410 Suture of esophageal wound or injury; cervical approach

43415 thoracic approach

43420 Closure of esophagostomy or fistula; cervical approach

43425 thoracic approach

(For repair of esophageal hiatal hernia, see 39520 et seq)

MANIPULATION

(For associated esophagogram, use 74220)

43450* Dilation of esophagus, by unguided sound or bougie, single or multiple passes; initial session

43451* subsequent session

43453 Dilation of esophagus, over guide wire or string

(For dilation with direct visualization, see 43220)

43455 Dilation of esophagus, by balloon or dilator; under fluoroscopic guidance

(For radiological supervision and interpretation, see 74360)

43456 retrograde

(For radiological supervision and interpretation, see 74360)

43460 Esophagogastric tamponade, with balloon (Sengstaaken type)

(For removal of esophageal foreign body by balloon catheter, see 43215, 43247, 74235)

43499 Unlisted procedure, esophagus

STOMACH

INCISION

43500 Gastrotomy; with exploration or foreign body removal

43501 with suture repair of bleeding ulcer or esophagogastric laceration

43510 with esophageal dilation and insertion of plastic tubes

43520 Pyloromyotomy, cutting of pyloric muscle (Fredet-Ramstedt type operation)

EXCISION

43600 Biopsy of stomach; by capsule, tube, peroral (one or more specimens)

43605 by laparotomy

43610 Excision, local, of ulcer or tumor of stomach

43620 Gastrectomy, total; including intestinal anastomosis

43625 with repair by intestinal transplant

43630 Hemigastrectomy or distal subtotal gastrectomy including pyloroplasty, gastroduodenostomy or gastrojejunostomy; without vagotomy

43635 with vagotomy, any type

43638 Hemigastrectomy or proximal subtotal gastrectomy, thoracic or abdominal approach

43640 Vagotomy including pyloroplasty, with or without gastrostomy; truncal or selective

(For pyloroplasty, see 43800)

(For vagotomy, see 64752-64760)

43641 parietal cell (highly selective)

ENDOSCOPY

(For upper gastrointestinal endoscopy, see 43234-43258)

(43700 has been deleted. To report, use 43235)

(43702 has been deleted. To report, use 43239)

(43709 has been deleted. To report, use 43247)

(43711 has been deleted. To report, use 43251)

(43712 has been deleted. To report, use 43255)

(43714 has been deleted. To report, use 43258)

INTRODUCTION

43750 Percutaneous placement of gastrostomy tube

(For radiological supervision and interpretation, see 74350)

43760* Change of gastrostomy tube

(For radiological supervision and interpretation, see 74350)

43761 Repositioning of the gastric feeding tube through the duodenum for enteric nutrition

(43765 has been deleted. To report, use 43760)

SUTURE

43800 Pyloroplasty

(For pyloroplasty and vagotomy, see 43640)

43810 Gastroduodenostomy

43820 Gastrojejunostomy;

43825 with vagotomy, any type

43830 Gastrostomy, temporary (tube, rubber or plastic) (separate procedure);

43831 neonatal, for feeding

(For change of gastrostomy tube, see 43760)

43832 Gastrostomy, permanent, with construction of gastric tube

(43834 has been deleted. To report, use 43246)

43840 Gastrorrhaphy, suture of perforated duodenal or gastric ulcer, wound, or injury

● **43842** Gastroplasty, vertical-banded, for morbid obesity

● **43843** Gastroplasty, other than vertical-banded, for morbid obesity

▲ **43844** Gastric bypass, other than with Roux-en-Y gastroenterostomy, for morbid obesity

(43845 has been deleted. To report, see 43842, 43843)

43846 Gastric bypass with Roux-en-Y gastroenterostomy for morbid obesity

43850 Revision of gastroduodenal anastomosis (gastroduodenostomy) with reconstruction; without vagotomy

43855 with vagotomy

43860 Revision of gastrojejunal anastomosis (gastrojejunostomy) with reconstruction, with or without partial gastrectomy or bowel resection; without vagotomy

43865 with vagotomy

43870 Closure of gastrostomy, surgical

43880 Closure of gastrocolic fistula

43885 Anterior gastropexy for hiatal hernia (separate procedure)

43999 Unlisted procedure, stomach

INTESTINES (EXCEPT RECTUM)

INCISION

(44000 has been deleted)

44005 Enterolysis (freeing of intestinal adhesion) (separate procedure)

44010 Duodenotomy, for exploration, biopsy(s), or foreign body removal

44015 Tube jejunostomy for enteral alimentation, intraoperative, any method (List separately in addition to primary procedure)

44020 Enterotomy, small bowel, other than duodenum; for exploration, biopsy(s), or foreign body removal

44021 for decompression (eg, Baker tube)

44025 Colotomy, for exploration, biopsy(s), or foreign body removal

44040 Exteriorization of intestine (Mikulicz resection with crushing of spur)

44050 Reduction of volvulus, intussusception, internal hernia, by laparotomy

44055 Correction of malrotation by lysis of duodenal bands and/or reduction of midgut volvulus (eg, Ladd procedure)

(44060 has been deleted. To report, use 44799)

EXCISION

44100 Biopsy of intestine by capsule, tube, peroral (one or more specimens)

44110 Excision of one or more lesions of small or large bowel not requiring anastomosis, exteriorization, or fistulization; single enterotomy

44111 multiple enterotomies

(44115 has been deleted. To report, use 44799)

44120 Enterectomy, resection of small intestine; with anastomosis

44125 with double-barrel enterostomy

44130 Enteroenterostomy, anastomosis of intestine; (separate procedure)

44131 intestinal bypass for morbid obesity

44140 Colectomy, partial; with anastomosis

44141 with skin level cecostomy or colostomy

44143 with end colostomy and closure of distal segment (Hartmann type procedure)

44144 with resection, with colostomy or ileostomy and creation of mucofistula

44145 with coloproctostomy (low pelvic anastomosis)

44146 with coloproctostomy (low pelvic anastomosis), with colostomy

44147 abdominal and transanal approach

44150 Colectomy, total, abdominal, without proctectomy; with ileostomy or ileoproctostomy

44151 with continent ileostomy

44152 with rectal mucosectomy, ileoanal anastomosis, with or without loop ileostomy

44153 with rectal mucosectomy, ileoanal anastomosis, creation of ileal reservoir (S or J), with or without loop ileostomy

44155 Colectomy, total, abdominal, with proctectomy; with ileostomy

44156 with continent ileostomy

44160 Colectomy with removal of terminal ileum and ileocolostomy

ENTEROSTOMY—EXTERNAL FISTULIZATION OF INTESTINES

44300 Enterostomy or cecostomy, tube (eg, for decompression or feeding) (separate procedure)

(44305 has been deleted.)

(44308 has been deleted. To report, use 44799)

44310 Ileostomy or jejunostomy, non-tube (separate procedure)

44312 Revision of ileostomy; simple (release of superficial scar) (separate procedure)

44314 complicated (reconstruction in-depth) (separate procedure)

44316 Continent ileostomy (Kock procedure) (separate procedure)

(For fiberoptic evaluation, see 44385)

44320 Colostomy or skin level cecostomy; (separate procedure)

44322 with multiple biopsies (eg, for Hirschsprung disease) (separate procedure)

44340 Revision of colostomy; simple (release of superficial scar) (separate procedure)

44345 complicated (reconstruction in-depth) (separate procedure)

44346 with repair of paracolostomy hernia (separate procedure)

ENDOSCOPY, SMALL BOWEL AND STOMAL

(For upper gastrointestinal endoscopy, see 43234-43258)

44360 Small intestinal endoscopy, enteroscopy beyond second portion of duodenum; diagnostic

44361 with biopsy and/or collection of specimen by brushing or washing

44363 with removal of foreign body

44364 with removal of polypoid lesion(s)

44366 with control of hemorrhage (eg, electrocoagulation, laser photocoagulation)

44369 with ablation of tumor or mucosal lesion (eg, laser, hot biopsy/fulguration)

44372 with placement of percutaneous jejunostomy tube

44373 with conversion of percutaneous gastrostomy tube to percutaneous jejunostomy tube

(44375 has been deleted. To report, use 43235)

44380 Fiberoptic ileoscopy through stoma;

44382 with biopsy and/or collection of specimen by brushing or washing

44385 Fiberoptic evaluation of small intestinal (Kock) or pelvic pouch;

44386 with biopsy and/or collection of specimen by brushing or washing

44388 Fiberoptic colonoscopy through colostomy;

44389 with biopsy and/or collection of specimen by brushing or washing

44390 with removal of foreign body

44391 with control of hemorrhage (eg, electrocoagulation, laser photocoagulation)

44392 with removal of polypoid lesion(s)

44393 with ablation of tumor or mucosal lesion (eg, laser, hot biopsy/fulguration)

(For colonoscopy per rectum, see 45330-45385)

(44400, 44405 have been deleted. To report, use 44799)

SUTURE

44600 Suture of intestine (enterorrhaphy), large or small, for perforated ulcer, diverticulum, wound, injury or rupture; single

44605 with colostomy

44610 multiple

44620 Closure of enterostomy, large or small intestine;

44625 with resection and anastomosis

44640 Closure of intestinal cutaneous fistula

44650 Closure of enteroenteric or enterocolic fistula

44660 Closure of enterovesical fistula; without intestinal or bladder resection

44661 with bowel and/or bladder resection

(For closure of renocolic fistula, see 50525, 50526)

(For closure of gastrocolic fistula, see 43880)

(For closure of rectovesical fistula, see 45800, 45805)

44680 Intestinal plication (separate procedure)

44799 Unlisted procedure, intestine

MECKEL'S DIVERTICULUM AND THE MESENTERY

EXCISION

44800 Excision of Meckel's diverticulum (diverticulectomy) or omphalomesenteric duct

44820 Excision of lesion of mesentery (separate procedure)

(With bowel resection, see 44120 or 44140 et seq)

SUTURE

44850 Suture of mesentery (separate procedure)

(For reduction and repair of internal hernia, see 44050)

44899 Unlisted procedure, Meckel's diverticulum and the mesentery

APPENDIX

INCISION

44900 Incision and drainage of appendiceal abscess, transabdominal

EXCISION

44950 Appendectomy;

(Incidental appendectomy during intra-abdominal surgery does not usually warrant a separate identification. If necessary to report, add modifier -52 or 09952)

44955 when done for indicated purpose at time of other major procedure (not as separate procedure)

44960 for ruptured appendix with abscess or generalized peritonitis

RECTUM

INCISION

45000 Transrectal drainage of pelvic abscess

45005 Incision and drainage of submucosal abscess, rectum

45020 Incision and drainage of deep supralevator, pelvirectal, or retrorectal abscess

(See also 46050, 46060)

EXCISION

45100 Biopsy of anorectal wall, anal approach (eg, congenital megacolon)

(45105 has been deleted. To report, use 45100)

(For endoscopic biopsy, see 45305)

45108 Anorectal myomectomy

45110 Proctectomy; complete, combined abdominoperineal, with colostomy, one or two stages

45111 partial resection of rectum

45112 Proctectomy, combined abdominoperineal, pull-through procedure, one or two stages

45114 Proctectomy, partial, with anastomosis; abdominal and transacral approach, one or two stages

45116 transacral approach only (Kraske type)

45120 Proctectomy, complete; (eg, for congenital megacolon, Swenson, Duhamel, or Soave type operation)

45121 with subtotal or total colectomy, with multiple biopsies (eg, for colonic aganglionosis)

45130 Excision of rectal procidentia, with anastomosis; perineal approach

45135 abdominal and perineal approach

45150 Division of stricture of rectum

45160 Excision of rectal tumor by proctotomy, transacral or transcoccygeal approach

45170 Excision of rectal tumor, transanal approach

45180 Excision and/or electrodesiccation of malignant tumor of rectum, transanal approach

(45181 has been deleted. To report, use 45180)

ENDOSCOPY

PROCTOSIGMOIDOSCOPY is the examination of the rectum and sigmoid colon.

SIGMOIDOSCOPY is the examination of the entire rectum, sigmoid colon and may include examination of a portion of the descending colon.

COLONOSCOPY is the examination of the entire colon, from the rectum to the cecum, and may include the examination of the terminal ileum.

For an incomplete colonoscopy, with full preparation for a colonoscopy, use a colonoscopy code with the modifier -52 or 09952 and provide documentation.

45300 Proctosigmoidoscopy; diagnostic (separate procedure)

45302 with collection of specimen by brushing or washing

45303 with dilation, direct, instrumental

(For radiological supervision and interpretation, see 74360)

45305 with biopsy

45307 with removal of foreign body

45310 with removal of polyp or papilloma

45315 with removal of multiple excrescences, papillomata or polyps

45317 with control of hemorrhage (eg, electrocoagulation, laser photocoagulation)

(45319 has been deleted. To report, use 45999)

45320 with ablation of tumor (eg, electrocoagulation, photocoagulation, hot biopsy/fulguration)

45321 with decompression of volvulus

(45325 colonoscopy has been renumbered 45355 without change in terminology)

45330 Sigmoidoscopy, flexible fiberoptic; diagnostic

45331 with biopsy and/or collection of specimen by brushing or washing

45332 with removal of foreign body

45333 with removal of polypoid lesion(s)

45334 with control of hemorrhage (eg, electrocoagulation, laser photocoagulation)

45336 with ablation of tumor or mucosal lesion (eg, electrocoagulation, photocoagulation, hot biopsy/fulguration)

45337 with decompression of volvulus

45355 Colonoscopy, with standard sigmoidoscope, transabdominal via colotomy, single or multiple

(45360-45372 have been deleted. To report, see 45330-45337)

45378 Colonoscopy, fiberoptic, beyond splenic flexure; diagnostic, with or without colon decompression

45379 with removal of foreign body

45380 with biopsy and/or collection of specimen by brushing or washing

45382 with control of hemorrhage (eg, electrocoagulation, laser photocoagulation)

45383 with ablation of tumor or mucosal lesion (eg, electrocoagulation, laser photocoagulation, hot biopsy/fulguration)

45385 with removal of polypoid lesion(s)

(45386 has been deleted. To report, use 44799)

(For small bowel and stomal endoscopy, see 44360-44393)

REPAIR

45500 Proctoplasty; for stenosis

45505 for prolapse of mucous membrane

45520 Perirectal injection of sclerosing solution for prolapse

(45521 has been deleted)

45540 Proctopexy for prolapse; abdominal approach

45541 perineal approach

45550 Proctopexy combined with sigmoid resection, abdominal approach

45560 Repair of rectocele (separate procedure)

(For repair of rectocele with posterior colporrhaphy, see 57250)

SUTURE

45800 Closure of rectovesical fistula;

45805 with colostomy

45820 Closure of rectourethral fistula;

45825 with colostomy

(For rectovaginal fistula closure, see 57300-57307)

MANIPULATION

45900* Reduction of procidentia (separate procedure) under anesthesia

45905* Dilation of anal sphincter (separate procedure) under anesthesia other than local

45910 Dilation of rectal stricture (separate procedure) under anesthesia other than local

45915* Removal of fecal impaction or foreign body (separate procedure) under anesthesia

45999 Unlisted procedure, rectum

ANUS

INCISION

46000* Fistulotomy, subcutaneous

(For fistulectomy, see 46060, 46270-46285)

46030* Removal of anal seton, other marker

(46032 has been deleted. To report, use 46999)

46040 Incision and drainage of ischiorectal and/or perirectal abscess (separate procedure)

46045 Incision and drainage of intramural, intramuscular or submucosal abscess, transanal, under anesthesia

46050* Incision and drainage, perianal abscess, superficial

(See also 45020, 46060)

46060 Incision and drainage of ischiorectal or intramural abscess, with fistulectomy, submuscular

(See also 45020)

46070 Incision, anal septum (infant)

(For anoplasty, see 46700-46705)

46080* Sphincterotomy, anal, division of sphincter (separate procedure)

46083 Incision of thrombosed hemorrhoid, external

EXCISION

46200 Fissurectomy, with or without sphincterotomy

46210 Cryptectomy; single

46211 multiple (separate procedure)

46220 Papillectomy or excision of single tag, anus (separate procedure)

46221 Hemorrhoidectomy, by simple ligature (eg, rubber band)

46230 Excision of external hemorrhoid tags and/or multiple papillae

46250 Hemorrhoidectomy, external, complete

46255 Hemorrhoidectomy internal and external, simple;

46257 with fissurectomy

46258 with fistulectomy, with or without fissurectomy

46260 Hemorrhoidectomy, internal and external, complex or extensive;

46261 with fissurectomy

46262 with fistulectomy, with or without fissurectomy

46270 Fistulectomy; subcutaneous

46275 submuscular

46280 complex or multiple

46285 second stage

46320* Enucleation or excision of external thrombotic hemorrhoid

INTRODUCTION

46500* Injection of sclerosing solution, hemorrhoids

(46510, 46530 have been deleted. To report, use 46999)

ENDOSCOPY

46600 Anoscopy; diagnostic (separate procedure)

46602 for collection of specimen by brushing or washing

46604 for dilation, direct, instrumental

46606 for biopsy

46608 for removal of foreign body

46610 for removal of polyp

46612 for multiple polyp removal

46614 with coagulation for control of hemorrhage and/or fulguration of mucosal lesion

REPAIR

46700 Anoplasty, plastic operation for stricture; adult

46705 infant

(For simple incision of anal septum, see 46070)

46715 Repair of congenital anovaginal fistula (''cut-back'' type procedure)

46716 Perineal transplant of anovaginal fistula

46730 Construction of anus for congenital absence; perineal or sacrococcygeal approach

46735 combined abdominal and perineal approach

46740 Construction of anus for congenital absence, with repair of urinary fistula

46750 Sphincteroplasty, anal, for incontinence or prolapse; adult

46751 child

46753 Graft (Thiersch operation) for rectal incontinence and/or prolapse

46754 Removal of Thiersch wire or suture, anal canal

46760 Sphincteroplasty, anal, for incontinence, adult; muscle transplant

46761 levator muscle imbrication (Park posterior anal repair)

46762 implantation artificial sphincter

DESTRUCTION

46900* Destruction of lesion(s), anus (eg, condyloma, papilloma, molluscum contagiosum, herpetic vesicle), simple; chemical

46910* electrodesiccation

46916 cryosurgery

46917 laser surgery

(46920 has been deleted. To report, use 46922)

46922 surgical excision

46924 Destruction of lesion(s), anus (eg, condyloma, papilloma, molluscum contagiosum, herpetic vesicle), extensive, any method

(46930 has been deleted. To report, use 46924)

(46932 has been deleted. To report, use 46916)

(46933 has been deleted. To report, use 46924)

46934 Destruction of hemorrhoids, any method; internal

46935 external

46936 internal and external

46937 Cryosurgery of rectal tumor; benign

46938 malignant

46940 Curettage or cauterization of anal fissure, including dilation of anal sphincter (separate procedure); initial

46942 subsequent

SUTURE

46945 Ligation of internal hemorrhoids; single procedure

46946 multiple procedures

OTHER PROCEDURES

46999 Unlisted procedure, anus

LIVER

INCISION

47000* Biopsy of liver, percutaneous needle;

(For radiological supervision and interpretation, see 76003, 76360, 76942)

47001 when done for indicated purpose at time of other major procedure (not as separate procedure)

(For radiological supervision and interpretation, see 76003, 76360, 76942)

(For fine needle aspiration, preparation, and interpretation of smears, see 88170-88173)

47010 Hepatotomy for drainage of abscess or cyst, one or two stages

EXCISION

47100 Biopsy of liver, wedge (separate procedure)

47120 Hepatectomy, resection of liver; partial lobectomy

47122 trisegmentectomy

47125 total left lobectomy

47130 total right lobectomy

47133 Donor hepatectomy, with preparation and maintenance of homograft

47135 Liver transplant, with or without recipient hepatectomy

REPAIR

47300 Marsupialization of cyst or abscess of liver

SUTURE

47350 Hepatorrhaphy, suture of liver wound or injury; simple

47355 with common duct or gallbladder drainage

47360 complex, with or without hepatic artery ligation

47399 Unlisted procedure, liver

BILIARY TRACT

INCISION

47400 Hepaticotomy or hepaticostomy with exploration, drainage, or removal of calculus

47420 Choledochotomy or choledochostomy with exploration, drainage, or removal of calculus, with or without cholecystotomy;

47425 with transduodenal sphincterotomy or sphincteroplasty

47440 Duodenocholedochotomy, transduodenal choledocholithotomy

47460 Transduodenal sphincterotomy or sphincteroplasty (separate procedure)

47480 Cholecystotomy or cholecystostomy with exploration, drainage, or removal of calculus (separate procedure)

47490 Percutaneous cholecystostomy

(For radiological supervision and interpretation, see 75989)

INTRODUCTION

47500 Injection procedure for percutaneous transhepatic cholangiography

(For radiological supervision and interpretation, see 74320)

• **47505** Injection procedure for cholangiography through an existing catheter (eg, percutaneous transhepatic or T-tube)

47510 Introduction of percutaneous transhepatic catheter for biliary drainage

(For radiological supervision and interpretation, see 75980)

47511 Introduction of percutaneous transhepatic stent for internal and external biliary drainage

(For radiological supervision and interpretation, see 75982)

47525 Change of percutaneous biliary drainage catheter

(For radiological supervision and interpretation, see 75984)

47530 Revision and/or reinsertion of transhepatic T-tube

(For radiological supervision and interpretation, see 75984)

ENDOSCOPY

47550 Biliary endoscopy, intraoperative (choledochoscopy)

(Use 47550 with either 47420 or 47610)

47552 Biliary endoscopy, percutaneous via T-tube or other tract; diagnostic

47553 for biopsy and/or collection of specimen by brushing or washing

47554 for removal of stone(s)

47555 for dilation of biliary duct stricture(s) without stent

(For peroral biliary endoscopic procedure, see 43260-43272)

(For radiological supervision and interpretation, see 74363)

47556 for dilation of biliary duct stricture(s) with stent

(For radiological supervision and interpretation, see 75982)

EXCISION

47600 Cholecystectomy;

47605 with cholangiography

(For laparoscopic cholecystectomy, see 49310, 49311)

47610 Cholecystectomy with exploration of common duct;

(47611 has been deleted. To report, use 47610 with 47550)

47612 with choledochoenterostomy

47620 with transduodenal sphincterotomy or sphincteroplasty, with or without cholangiography

47630 Biliary duct stone extraction, percutaneous via T-tube tract, basket or snare (eg, Burhenne technique)

(For radiological supervision and interpretation, see 74327)

47700 Exploration for congenital atresia of bile ducts, without repair, with or without liver biopsy, with or without cholangiography

47701 Portoenterostomy (eg, Kasai procedure)

47710 Excision of bile duct tumor, with repair

47715 Excision of choledochal cyst

47716 Anastomosis, choledochal cyst, without excision

REPAIR

47720 Cholecystoenterostomy; direct

47721 with gastroenterostomy

47740 Roux-en-Y

47760 Anastomosis, direct, of extrahepatic biliary ducts and gastrointestinal tract

47765 Anastomosis, direct, of intrahepatic ducts and gastrointestinal tract

47780 Anastomosis, Roux-en-Y, of extrahepatic biliary ducts and gastrointestinal tract

47800 Reconstruction, plastic, of extrahepatic biliary ducts with end-to-end anastomosis

47801 Placement of choledochal stent

47802 U-tube hepaticoenterostomy

(47810 has been deleted. To report, use 47999)

OTHER PROCEDURES

(47850, 47855 have been deleted. To report, use 47999)

47999 Unlisted procedure, biliary tract

PANCREAS

INCISION

48000 Drainage of abdomen for pancreatitis

48020 Removal of pancreatic calculus

EXCISION

48100 Biopsy of pancreas (separate procedure)

48102* Biopsy of pancreas, percutaneous needle

(For radiological supervision and interpretation, see 76003, 76360, 76942)

(For fine needle aspiration, preparation, and interpretation of smears, see 88170-88173)

48120 Excision of lesion of pancreas (eg, cyst, adenoma)

48140 Pancreatectomy, distal subtotal, with or without splenectomy;

48145 with pancreaticojejunostomy

48148 Excision of ampulla of Vater, simple

48150 Pancreatectomy, proximal subtotal, with pancreaticoduodenectomy (Whipple type procedure), and pancreatic jejunostomy

48151 Pancreatectomy, near-total, with preservation of duodenum (Child type procedure)

48155 Pancreatectomy, total;

48160 with transplantation

48180 Pancreaticojejunostomy, side-to-side anastomosis (Puestow type operation) (separate procedure)

ENDOSCOPY

(For peroral pancreatic endoscopic procedures, see 43260-43272)

REPAIR

48500 Marsupialization of cyst of pancreas

48510 External drainage, pseudocyst of pancreas

48520 Internal anastomosis of pancreatic cyst to gastrointestinal tract; direct

48540 Roux-en-Y

48999 Unlisted procedure, pancreas

ABDOMEN, PERITONEUM, AND OMENTUM

INCISION

49000 Exploratory laparotomy, exploratory celiotomy with or without biopsy(s) (separate procedure)

49002 Reopening of recent laparotomy

49010 Exploration, retroperitoneal area with or without biopsy(s) (separate procedure)

49020 Drainage of peritoneal abscess or localized peritonitis, exclusive of appendiceal abscess, transabdominal

(For appendiceal abscess, see 44900)

49040 Drainage of subdiaphragmatic or subphrenic abscess

49060 Drainage of retroperitoneal abscess

49080* Peritoneocentesis, abdominal paracentesis, or peritoneal lavage (diagnostic or therapeutic); initial

49081* subsequent

49085 Removal of peritoneal foreign body from peritoneal cavity

(For lysis of intestinal adhesions, see 44005)

EXCISION AND DESTRUCTION

49180* Biopsy, abdominal or retroperitoneal mass, percutaneous needle

(For radiological supervision and interpretation, see 76003, 76360, 76365, 76942)

(For fine needle aspiration, preparation, and interpretation of smears, see 88170-88173)

49200 Excision or destruction by any method of intra-abdominal or retroperitoneal tumors or cysts or endometriomas;

49201 extensive

49215 Excision of presacral or sacrococcygeal tumor

49220 Staging celiotomy (laparotomy) for Hodgkin's disease or lymphoma (includes splenectomy, needle or open biopsies of both liver lobes, possibly also removal of abdominal nodes, abdominal node and/or bone marrow biopsies, ovarian repositioning)

49250 Umbilectomy, omphalectomy, excision of umbilicus (separate procedure)

49255 Omentectomy, epiploectomy, resection of omentum (separate procedure)

ENDOSCOPY

49300 Peritoneoscopy; without biopsy

49301 with biopsy

49302 Peritoneoscopy with guided transhepatic cholangiography; without biopsy

49303 with biopsy

(For sterilization by laparoscopic technique, see 58982)

49310 Laparoscopy, surgical; cholecystectomy (any method)

49311 cholecystectomy with cholangiography

• **49315** appendectomy

INTRODUCTION AND REVISION

49400* Pneumoperitoneum (separate procedure); initial

49401* subsequent

49420* Insertion of intraperitoneal cannula or catheter for drainage or dialysis; temporary

49421 permanent

49425 Peritoneal-venous shunt (eg, LeVeen shunt)

49426 Revision of peritoneal-venous shunt

(For shunt patency test, see 78291)

• **49427** Injection procedure (eg, contrast media) for evaluation of previously placed peritoneal-venous shunt

(For radiological supervision and interpretation, see 75809)

(49430, 49440 have been deleted. To report, use 49999)

REPAIR

HERNIOPLASTY, HERNIORRHAPHY, HERNIOTOMY

(For reduction and repair of intra-abdominal hernia, see 44050)

(For debridement of abdominal wall, see 11042, 11043)

(All codes for bilateral procedures in hernia repair have been deleted. To report, add modifier -50 or 09950)

49500 Repair inguinal hernia, under age 5 years, with or without hydrocelectomy

49505 Repair inguinal hernia, age 5 or over;

49510 with orchiectomy, with or without implantation of prosthesis

49515 with excision of hydrocele or spermatocele

49520 Repair inguinal hernia, any age; recurrent

49525 sliding

49530 incarcerated

49535 strangulated

49540 Repair lumbar hernia

49550 Repair femoral hernia, groin incision

49552 Repair femoral hernia, Henry approach

49555 Repair femoral hernia, recurrent, any approach

49560 Repair ventral (incisional) hernia (separate procedure);

49565 recurrent

49570 Repair epigastric hernia, properitoneal fat (separate procedure); simple

49575 complex

49580 Repair umbilical hernia; under age 5 years

49581 age 5 or over

49590 Repair spigelian hernia

49600 Repair of omphalocele; small, with primary closure

49605 large or gastroschisis, with or without prosthesis

49606 with staged closure of prosthesis, reduction in operating room, under anesthesia

49610 Repair of omphalocele (Gross type operation); first stage

49611 second stage

(For diaphragmatic or hiatal hernia repair, see 39502-39541)

(49630-49640 have been deleted. For surgical repair of omentum, use 49999)

SUTURE

49900 Suture, secondary, of abdominal wall for evisceration or dehiscence

(For suture of ruptured diaphragm, see 39540, 39541)

(For debridement of abdominal wall, see 11042, 11043)

OTHER PROCEDURES

● **49905** Omental flap (eg, for reconstruction of sternal and chest wall defects) (list separately in addition to code for primary procedure)

(49910 has been deleted. To report, use 49999)

49999 Unlisted procedure, abdomen, peritoneum and omentum

Urinary System

(For provision of chemotherapeutic agents, use 96545 in addition to primary procedure)

KIDNEY

INCISION

(For retroperitoneal exploration, abscess, tumor, or cyst, see 49010, 49060, 49200, 49201)

50010 Renal exploration, not necessitating other specific procedures

50020 Drainage of perirenal or renal abscess (separate procedure)

50040 Nephrostomy, nephrotomy with drainage

50045 Nephrotomy, with exploration

(For renal endoscopy performed in conjunction with this procedure, see 50570-50580)

50060 Nephrolithotomy; removal of calculus

50065 secondary surgical operation for calculus

50070 complicated by congenital kidney abnormality

50075 removal of large staghorn calculus filling renal pelvis and calyces (including anatrophic pyelolithotomy)

50080 Percutaneous nephrostolithotomy or pyelostolithotomy, with or without dilation, endoscopy, lithotripsy, stenting or basket extraction; up to 2 cm

50081 over 2 cm

(For establishment of nephrostomy without nephrostolithotomy, see 50040, 50395, 52334)

(For fluoroscopic guidance, see 76000, 76001)

50100 Transection or repositioning of aberrant renal vessels (separate procedure)

50120 Pyelotomy; with exploration

(For renal endoscopy performed in conjunction with this procedure, see 50570-50580)

50125 with drainage, pyelostomy

50130 with removal of calculus (pyelolithotomy, pelviolithotomy, including coagulum pyelolithotomy)

50135 complicated (eg, secondary operation, congenital kidney abnormality)

(For supply of anticarcinogenic agents, use 99070 in addition to primary procedure)

EXCISION

(For excision of retroperitoneal tumor or cyst, see 49200, 49201)

50200* Renal biopsy; percutaneous, by trocar or needle

(For radiological supervision and interpretation, see 76003, 76360, 76942)

(For fine needle aspiration, preparation, and interpretation of smears, see 88170-88173)

50205 by surgical exposure of kidney

50220 Nephrectomy, including partial ureterectomy, any approach including rib resection;

50225 complicated because of previous surgery on same kidney

50230 radical, with regional lymphadenectomy and/or vena caval thrombectomy

(When vena caval resection with reconstruction is necessary, use 37799)

50234 Nephrectomy with total ureterectomy and bladder cuff; through same incision

50236 through separate incision

50240 Nephrectomy, partial

50280 Excision or unroofing of cyst(s) of kidney

50290 Excision of perinephric cyst

RENAL TRANSPLANTATION

(For dialysis, see 90935-90999)

50300 Donor nephrectomy, with preparation and maintenance of homograft; from cadaver donor, unilateral or bilateral

50320 from living donor, unilateral

50340 Recipient nephrectomy (separate procedure)

(50341 has been deleted. To report, use 50340 with modifier -50 or 09950)

50360 Renal homotransplantation, implantation of graft; excluding donor and recipient nephrectomy

50365 with recipient nephrectomy

(50366 has been deleted. To report, use 50365 with modifier -50 or 09950)

50370 Removal of transplanted homograft (eg, infarcted or rejected kidney)

50380 Renal autotransplantation, reimplantation of kidney

(For extra-corporeal "bench" surgery, use autotransplantation as the primary procedure and add the secondary procedure (eg, partial nephrectomy, nephrolithotomy), and use the modifier -51 or 09951)

INTRODUCTION

50390* Aspiration and/or injection of renal cyst or pelvis by needle, percutaneous

(For radiological supervision and interpretation, see 74425, 74470, 76003, 76365, 76938)

(For fine needle aspiration, preparation, and interpretation of smears, see 88170-88173)

50392 Introduction of intracatheter or catheter into renal pelvis for drainage and/or injection, percutaneous

(For radiological supervision and interpretation, see 74475, 76365, 76938)

50393 Introduction of ureteral catheter or stent into ureter through renal pelvis for drainage and/or injection, percutaneous

(For radiological supervision and interpretation, see 74480, 76003, 76365, 76938)

50394 Injection procedure for pyelography (as nephrostogram, pyelostogram, antegrade pyeloureterograms) through nephrostomy or pyelostomy tube, or indwelling ureteral catheter

(For radiological supervision and interpretation, see 74425)

50395 Introduction of guide into renal pelvis and/or ureter with dilation to establish nephrostomy tract, percutaneous

(For radiological supervision and interpretation, see 74475, 74480, 74485)

(For nephrostolithotomy, see 50080, 50081)

(For retrograde percutaneous nephrostomy, use 52334)

(For endoscopic surgery, see 50551-50561)

50396 Manometric studies through nephrostomy or pyelostomy tube, or indwelling ureteral catheter

(For radiological supervision and interpretation, see 74425, 74475, 74480)

50398* Change of nephrostomy or pyelostomy tube

(For fluoroscopic guidance, use 76000)

(For radiological supervision and interpretation, see 75984)

REPAIR

50400 Pyeloplasty (Foley Y-pyeloplasty), plastic operation on renal pelvis, with or without plastic operation on ureter, nephropexy, nephrostomy, pyelostomy, or ureteral splinting; simple

50405 complicated (congenital kidney abnormality, secondary pyeloplasty, solitary kidney, calycoplasty)

(50420 has been deleted)

SUTURE

50500 Nephrorrhaphy, suture of kidney wound or injury

50520 Closure of nephrocutaneous or pyelocutaneous fistula

50525 Closure of nephrovisceral fistula (eg, renocolic), including visceral repair; abdominal approach

50526 thoracic approach

50540 Symphysiotomy for horseshoe kidney with or without pyeloplasty and/or other plastic procedure, unilateral or bilateral (one operation)

ENDOSCOPY

(For supplies and materials, use 99070)

(References to office and hospital have been deleted)

50551 Renal endoscopy through established nephrostomy or pyelostomy, with or without irrigation, instillation, or ureteropyelography, exclusive of radiologic service;

50553 with ureteral catheterization, with or without dilation of ureter

50555 with biopsy

50557 with fulguration and/or incision, with or without biopsy

50559 with insertion of radioactive substance with or without biopsy and/or fulguration

50561 with removal of foreign body or calculus

(When procedures 50570-50580 provide a significant identifiable service, they may be added to 50045 and 50120)

50570 Renal endoscopy through nephrotomy or pyelotomy, with or without irrigation, instillation, or ureteropyelography, exclusive of radiologic service;

(For nephrotomy, see 50045)

(For pyelotomy, see 50120)

50572 with ureteral catheterization, with or without dilation of ureter

50574 with biopsy

50576 with fulguration and/or incision, with or without biopsy

50578 with insertion of radioactive substance, with or without biopsy and/or fulguration

50580 with removal of foreign body or calculus

OTHER PROCEDURES

50590 Lithotripsy, extracorporeal shock wave

URETER

INCISION

50600 Ureterotomy with exploration or drainage (separate procedure)

(For ureteral endoscopy performed in conjunction with this procedure, see 50970-50980)

50605 Ureterotomy for insertion of indwelling stent, all types

50610 Ureterolithotomy; upper one-third of ureter

50620 middle one-third of ureter

50630 lower one-third of ureter

(For transvesical ureterolithotomy, see 51060)

(For cystotomy with stone basket extraction of ureteral calculus, see 51065)

(For endoscopic extraction or manipulation of ureteral calculus, see 50080, 50081, 50561, 50961, 50980, 52320-52330, 52336, 52337)

EXCISION

(For ureterocele, see 51535, 51536, 52300)

50650 Ureterectomy, with bladder cuff (separate procedure)

50660 Ureterectomy, total, ectopic ureter, combination abdominal, vaginal and/or perineal approach

INTRODUCTION

50684 Injection procedure for ureterography or ureteropyelography through ureterostomy or indwelling ureteral catheter

(For radiological supervision and interpretation, see 74425)

50686 Manometric studies through ureterostomy or indwelling ureteral catheter

50688* Change of ureterostomy tube

(For radiological supervision and interpretation, see 74425)

50690 Injection procedure for visualization of ileal conduit and/or ureteropyelography, exclusive of radiologic service

(For radiological supervision and interpretation, see 74425)

REPAIR

50700 Ureteroplasty, plastic operation on ureter (eg, stricture)

50715 Ureterolysis, with or without repositioning of ureter for retroperitoneal fibrosis

(50716 has been deleted. To report, use 50715 with modifier -50 or 09950)

50722 Ureterolysis for ovarian vein syndrome

50725 Ureterolysis for retrocaval ureter, with reanastomosis of upper urinary tract or vena cava

● **50727** Revision of urinary-cutaneous anastomosis (any type urostomy);

● **50728** with repair of fascial defect and hernia

50740 Ureteropyelostomy, anastomosis of ureter and renal pelvis

50750 Ureterocalycostomy, anastomosis of ureter to renal calyx

50760 Ureteroureterostomy

50770 Transureteroureterostomy, anastomosis of ureter to contralateral ureter

(Codes 50780-50785 include minor procedures to prevent vesicoureteral reflux)

▲**50780** Ureteroneocystostomy; anastomosis of single ureter to bladder

(50781 has been deleted. To report, use 50780 with modifier -50 or 09950)

(When combined with cystourethroplasty or vesical neck revision, see 51820)

● **50782** anastomosis of duplicated ureter to bladder

● **50783** with extensive ureteral tailoring

▲**50785** with vesico-Psoas hitch or bladder flap

(50786 has been deleted. To report, use 50785 with modifier -50 or 09950)

50800 Ureteroenterostomy, direct anastomosis of ureter to intestine

(50801 has been deleted. To report, use 50800 with modifier -50 or 09950)

50810 Ureterosigmoidostomy, with creation of sigmoid bladder and establishment of abdominal or perineal colostomy, including bowel anastomosis

50815 Ureterocolon conduit, including bowel anastomosis

(50816 has been deleted. To report, use 50815 with modifier -50 or 09950)

50820 Ureteroileal conduit (ileal bladder), including bowel anastomosis (Bricker operation)

(50821 has been deleted. To report, use 50820 with modifier -50 or 09950)

(For combination of 50800-50820 with cystectomy, see 51580-51595)

50825 Continent diversion, including bowel anastomosis using any segment of small and/or large bowel (Kock pouch or Camey enterocystoplasty)

50830 Urinary undiversion (eg, taking down of ureteroileal conduit, ureterosigmoidostomy or ureteroenterostomy with ureteroureterostomy or ureteroneocystostomy)

50840 Replacement of all or part of ureter by bowel segment, including bowel anastomosis

(50841 has been deleted. To report, use 50840 with modifier -50 or 09950)

50860 Ureterostomy, transplantation of ureter to skin

(50861 has been deleted. To report, use 50860 with modifier -50 or 09950)

SUTURE

50900 Ureterorrhaphy, suture of ureter (separate procedure)

50920 Closure of ureterocutaneous fistula

50930 Closure of ureterovisceral fistula (including visceral repair)

50940 Deligation of ureter

(For ureteroplasty, ureterolysis, see 50700-50860)

ENDOSCOPY

(References to office and hospital have been deleted)

50951 Ureteral endoscopy through established ureterostomy, with or without irrigation, instillation, or ureteropyelography, exclusive of radiologic service;

50953 with ureteral catheterization, with or without dilation of ureter

50955 with biopsy

50957 with fulguration and/or incision, with or without biopsy

50959 with insertion of radioactive substance, with or without biopsy and/or fulguration (not including provision of material)

50961 with removal of foreign body or calculus

(When procedures 50970-50980 provide a significant identifiable service, they may be added to 50600)

50970 Ureteral endoscopy through ureterotomy, with or without irrigation, instillation, or ureteropyelography, exclusive of radiologic service;

(For ureterotomy, see 50600)

50972 with ureteral catheterization, with or without dilation of ureter

50974 with biopsy

50976 with fulguration and/or incision, with or without biopsy

50978 with insertion of radioactive substance, with or without biopsy and/or fulguration (not including provision of material)

50980 with removal of foreign body or calculus

BLADDER

INCISION

51000* Aspiration of bladder by needle

51005* Aspiration of bladder; by trocar or intracatheter

51010 with insertion of suprapubic catheter

51020 Cystotomy or cystostomy; with fulguration and/or insertion of radioactive material

51030 with cryosurgical destruction of intravesical lesion

51040 Cystostomy, cystotomy with drainage

51045 Cystotomy, with insertion of ureteral catheter or stent (separate procedure)

51050 Cystolithotomy, cystotomy with removal of calculus, without vesical neck resection

51060 Transvesical ureterolithotomy

51065 Cystotomy, with stone basket extraction and/or ultrasonic or electrohydraulic fragmentation of ureteral calculus

51080 Drainage of perivesical or prevesical space abscess

EXCISION

51500 Excision of urachal cyst or sinus, with or without umbilical hernia repair

51520 Cystotomy; for simple excision of vesical neck (separate procedure)

51525 for excision of bladder diverticulum, single or multiple (separate procedure)

51530 for excision of bladder tumor

(For transurethral resection, see 52234-52240, 52305)

51535 Cystotomy for excision, incision, or repair of ureterocele

(For transurethral excision, see 52300)

(51536 has been deleted. To report, use 51535 with modifier -50 or 09950)

51550 Cystectomy, partial; simple

51555 complicated (eg, postradiation, previous surgery, difficult location)

51565 Cystectomy, partial, with reimplantation of ureter(s) into bladder (ureteroneocystostomy)

51570 Cystectomy, complete; (separate procedure)

51575 with bilateral pelvic lymphadenectomy, including external iliac, hypogastric and obturator nodes

51580 Cystectomy, complete, with ureterosigmoidostomy or ureterocutaneous transplantations;

51585 with bilateral pelvic lymphadenectomy, including external iliac, hypogastric and obturator nodes

51590 Cystectomy, complete, with ureteroileal conduit or sigmoid bladder, including bowel anastomosis;

51595 with bilateral pelvic lymphadenectomy, including external iliac, hypogastric and obturator nodes

51596 Cystectomy, complete, with continent diversion, any technique, using any segment of small and/or large bowel to construct neobladder

51597 Pelvic exenteration, complete, for vesical, prostatic or urethral malignancy, with removal of bladder and ureteral transplantations, with or without hysterectomy and/or abdominoperineal resection of rectum and colon and colostomy, or any combination thereof

(For pelvic exenteration for gynecologic malignancy, use 58240)

INTRODUCTION

(For bladder catheterization, see 53670, 53675)

51600* Injection procedure for cystography or voiding urethrocystography

(For radiological supervision and interpretation, see 74430, 74455)

51605 Injection procedure and placement of chain for contrast and/or chain urethrocystography

(For radiological supervision and interpretation, see 74430)

51610 Injection procedure for retrograde urethrocystography

(For radiological supervision and interpretation, see 74450)

51700* Bladder irrigation, simple, lavage and/or instillation

51705* Change of cystostomy tube; simple

51710* complicated

51720 Bladder instillation of anticarcinogenic agent (including detention time)

URODYNAMICS

The following section (51725-51797) lists procedures that may be used separately or in many and varied combinations. When multiple procedures are performed in the same investigative session, either modifier - 51 or code 09951 should be employed.

All procedures in this section imply that these services are performed by, or are under the direct supervision of, a physician and that all instruments, equipment, fluids, gases, probes, catheters, technician's fees, medications, gloves, trays, tubing and other sterile supplies be provided by the physician. When the physician only interprets the results and/or operates the equipment, a professional component, modifier -26 or code 09926, should be used to identify physicians' services.

51725 Simple cystometrogram (CMG) (eg, spinal manometer)

51726 Complex cystometrogram (eg, calibrated electronic equipment)

(51727-51733 have been deleted. To report, use 51726)

51736 Simple uroflowmetry (UFR) (eg, stop-watch flow rate, mechanical uroflowmeter)

(51737, 51738 have been deleted. To report, use 51736)

51739 Sound recording of external stream (eg, Lyons type, Keitzer type)

51741 Complex uroflowmetry (eg, calibrated electronic equipment)

(51742-51749 have been deleted. To report, use 51741)

(51751-51769 have been deleted. To report, use 53899)

51772 Urethral pressure profile studies (UPP) (urethral closure pressure profile), any technique

(51773-51783 have been deleted. To report, use 51772)

51785 Electromyography studies (EMG) of anal or urethral sphincter, any technique

(51786-51791 have been deleted. To report, use 51785)

51792 Stimulus evoked response (eg, measurement of bulbocavernosus reflex latency time)

51795 Voiding pressure studies (VP); bladder voiding pressure, any technique

(51796 has been deleted. To report, use 51795)

51797 intra-abdominal voiding pressure (AP) (rectal, gastric, intraperitoneal)

REPAIR

51800 Cystoplasty or cystourethroplasty, plastic operation on bladder and/or vesical neck (anterior Y-plasty, vesical fundus resection), any procedure, with or without wedge resection of posterior vesical neck

51820 Cystourethroplasty with unilateral or bilateral ureteroneocystostomy

51840 Anterior vesicourethropexy, or urethropexy (Marshall-Marchetti-Krantz type); simple

51841 complicated (eg, secondary repair)

(For urethropexy (Pereyra type), see 57289)

51845 Abdomino-vaginal vesical neck suspension, with or without endoscopic control (eg, Stamey, Raz, modified Pereyra)

51860 Cystorrhaphy, suture of bladder wound, injury or rupture; simple

51865 complicated

51880 Closure of cystostomy (separate procedure)

51900 Closure of vesicovaginal fistula, abdominal approach

(For vaginal approach, see 57320-57330)

51920 Closure of vesicouterine fistula;

51925 with hysterectomy

(For closure of vesicoenteric fistula, see 44660, 44661)

(For closure of rectovesical fistula, see 45800-45805)

51940 Closure of bladder exstrophy

(See also 54390)

51960 Enterocystoplasty, including bowel anastomosis

51980 Cutaneous vesicostomy

ENDOSCOPY—CYSTOSCOPY, URETHROSCOPY, CYSTOURETHROSCOPY

Endoscopic descriptions are listed so that the main procedure can be identified without having to list all the minor related functions performed at the same time. For example: meatotomy, urethral calibration and/or dilation, urethroscopy, and cystoscopy prior to a transurethral resection of prostate; ureteral catheterization following extraction of ureteral calculus; internal urethrotomy and bladder neck fulguration when performing a cystourethroscopy for the female urethral syndrome. When the secondary procedure requires significant additional time and effort, it may be identified by the addition of either modifier -22 or 09922. For example: urethrotomy performed for a documented pre-existing stricture or bladder neck contracture.

(References to office and hospital have been deleted)

52000 Cystourethroscopy (separate procedure)

52005 Cystourethroscopy, with ureteral catheterization, with or without irrigation, instillation, or ureteropyelography, exclusive of radiologic service;

52007 with brush biopsy of ureter and/or renal pelvis

52010 Cystourethroscopy, with ejaculatory duct catheterization, with or without irrigation, instillation, or duct radiography, exclusive of radiologic service

(For radiological supervision and interpretation, see 74440)

(52190 has been deleted)

TRANSURETHRAL SURGERY (URETHRA AND BLADDER)

(References to office and hospital have been deleted)

52204 Cystourethroscopy, with biopsy

52214 Cystourethroscopy, with fulguration (including cryosurgery or laser surgery) of trigone, bladder neck, prostatic fossa, urethra, or periurethral glands

52224 Cystourethroscopy, with fulguration (including cryosurgery or laser surgery) or treatment of MINOR (less than 0.5 cm) lesion(s) with or without biopsy

52234 Cystourethroscopy, with fulguration (including cryosurgery or laser surgery) and/or resection of; SMALL bladder tumor(s) (0.5 to 2.0 cm)

52235 MEDIUM bladder tumor(s) (2.0 to 5.0 cm)

52240 LARGE bladder tumor(s)

52250 Cystourethroscopy with insertion of radioactive substance, with or without biopsy or fulguration

52260 Cystourethroscopy, with dilation of bladder for interstitial cystitis; general or conduction (spinal) anesthesia

52265 local anesthesia

52270 Cystourethroscopy, with internal urethrotomy; female

52275 male

52276 Cystourethroscopy with direct vision internal urethrotomy

52277 Cystourethroscopy, with resection of external sphincter (sphincterotomy)

52281 Cystourethroscopy, with calibration and/or dilation of urethral stricture or stenosis, with or without meatotomy and injection procedure for cystography, male or female

52283 Cystourethroscopy, with steroid injection into stricture

52285 Cystourethroscopy for treatment of the female urethral syndrome with any or all of the following: urethral meatotomy, urethral dilation, internal urethrotomy, lysis of urethrovaginal septal fibrosis, lateral incisions of the bladder neck, and fulguration of polyp(s) of urethra, bladder neck, and/or trigone

52290 Cystourethroscopy; with ureteral meatotomy, unilateral or bilateral

52300 with resection or fulguration of ureterocele(s), unilateral or bilateral

52305 with incision or resection of orifice of bladder diverticulum, single or multiple

52310 Cystourethroscopy, with removal of foreign body, calculus, or ureteral stent from urethra or bladder (separate procedure); simple

52315 complicated

52317 Litholapaxy: crushing or fragmentation of calculus by any means in bladder and removal of fragments, simple; small (less than 2.5 cm)

52318 complicated or large (over 2.5 cm)

TRANSURETHRAL SURGERY (URETER AND PELVIS)

(The insertion of a stent is included in 52320-52339 when done and should not be reported separately)

52320 Cystourethroscopy (including ureteral catheterization); with removal of ureteral calculus

52325 with fragmentation of ureteral calculus (eg, ultrasonic or electro-hydraulic technique)

52330 with manipulation, without removal of ureteral calculus

52332 Cystourethroscopy, with insertion of indwelling ureteral stent (eg, Gibbons or double-J type)

52334 Cystourethroscopy with insertion of ureteral guide wire through kidney to establish a percutaneous nephrostomy, retrograde

(For percutaneous nephrostolithotomy, see 50080, 50081; for establishment of nephrostomy tract only, see 50395)

▲**52335** Cystourethroscopy, with ureteroscopy and/or pyeloscopy (includes dilation of the ureter and/or pyeloureteral junction by any method);

(For radiological supervision and interpretation, see 74485)

52336 with removal or manipulation of calculus (ureteral catheterization is included)

52337 with lithotripsy (ureteral catheterization is included)

52338 with biopsy and/or fulguration of lesion

● **52339** with resection of tumor

TRANSURETHRAL SURGERY (VESICAL NECK AND PROSTATE)

52340 Cystourethroscopy with incision, fulguration, or resection of bladder neck and/or posterior urethra (congenital valves, obstructive hypertrophic mucosal folds)

52450 Transurethral incision of prostate

52500 Transurethral resection of bladder neck (separate procedure)

52510 Transurethral balloon dilation of the prostatic urethra, any method

52601 Transurethral resection of prostate, including control of postoperative bleeding, complete (vasectomy, meatotomy, cystourethroscopy, urethral calibration and/or dilation, and internal urethrotomy are included)

(For other approaches, see 55801-55845)

52606 Transurethral fulguration for postoperative bleeding occurring after the usual follow-up time

(52605 has been deleted. To report, use 52606)

52612 Transurethral resection of prostate; first stage of two-stage resection (partial resection)

52614 second stage of two-stage resection (resection completed)

52620 Transurethral resection; of residual obstructive tissue after 90 days postoperative

52630 of regrowth of obstructive tissue longer than one year postoperative

52640 of postoperative bladder neck contracture

52650 Transurethral cryosurgical removal of prostate (postoperative irrigations and aspiration of sloughing tissue included)

52700 Transurethral drainage of prostatic abscess

(52800, 52805 have been deleted. To report, use 52317, 52318)

URETHRA

(For endoscopy, see cystoscopy, urethroscopy, cystourethroscopy, 52000-52700)

(For injection procedure for urethrocystography, see 51600-51610)

INCISION

53000 Urethrotomy or urethrostomy, external (separate procedure); pendulous urethra

53010 perineal urethra, external

53020 Meatotomy, cutting of meatus (separate procedure); except infant

(53021 has been deleted. To report, use 53020)

53025 infant

53040 Drainage of deep periurethral abscess

(For subcutaneous abscess, see 10060, 10061)

53060 Drainage of Skene's gland abscess or cyst

53080 Drainage of perineal urinary extravasation; uncomplicated (separate procedure)

53085 complicated

EXCISION

53200 Biopsy of urethra

53210 Urethrectomy, total, including cystostomy; female

53215 male

53220 Excision or fulguration of carcinoma of urethra

53230 Excision of urethral diverticulum (separate procedure); female

53235 male

53240 Marsupialization of urethral diverticulum, male or female

53250 Excision of bulbourethral gland (Cowper's gland)

53260 Excision or fulguration; urethral polyp(s), distal urethra

(For endoscopic approach, see 52214, 52224)

53265 urethral caruncle

53270 Skene's glands

53275 urethral prolapse

REPAIR

(For hypospadias, see 54300-54352)

53400 Urethroplasty; first stage, for fistula, diverticulum, or stricture (eg, Johannsen type)

53405 second stage (formation of urethra), including urinary diversion

53410 Urethroplasty, one-stage reconstruction of male anterior urethra

53415 Urethroplasty, transpubic or perineal, one stage, for reconstruction or repair of prostatic or membranous urethra

53420 Urethroplasty, two-stage reconstruction or repair of prostatic or membranous urethra; first stage

53425 second stage

53430 Urethroplasty, reconstruction of female urethra

53440 Operation for correction of male urinary incontinence, with or without introduction of prosthesis

53442 Removal of perineal prosthesis introduced for continence

53443 Urethroplasty with tubularization of posterior urethra and/or lower bladder for incontinence (eg, Tenago, Leadbetter procedure)

53445 Operation for correction of urinary incontinence with placement of inflatable urethral or bladder neck sphincter, including placement of pump and/or reservoir

53447 Removal, repair or replacement of inflatable sphincter including pump and/or reservoir and/or cuff

53449 Surgical correction of hydraulic abnormality of inflatable sphincter device

53450 Urethromeatoplasty, with mucosal advancement

(For meatotomy, see 53020, 53025)

53460 Urethromeatoplasty, with partial excision of distal urethral segment (Richardson type procedure)

SUTURE

53502 Urethrorrhaphy, suture of urethral wound or injury, female

53505 Urethrorrhaphy, suture of urethral wound or injury; penile

53510 perineal

53515 prostatomembranous

53520 Closure of urethrostomy or urethrocutaneous fistula, male (separate procedure)

(For closure of urethrovaginal fistula, see 57310)

(For closure of urethrorectal fistula, see 45820, 45825)

MANIPULATION

(For radiological supervision and interpretation, see 74485)

53600* Dilation of urethral stricture by passage of sound or urethral dilator, male; initial

53601* subsequent

53605 Dilation of urethral stricture or vesical neck by passage of sound or urethral dilator, male, general or conduction (spinal) anesthesia

53620* Dilation of urethral stricture by passage of filiform and follower, male; initial

53621* subsequent

53640* Passage of filiform and follower for acute vesical retention, male

53660* Dilation of female urethra including suppository and/or instillation; initial

53661* subsequent

53665 Dilation of female urethra, general or conduction (spinal) anesthesia

53670* Catheterization, urethra; simple

53675* complicated (may include difficult removal of balloon catheter)

OTHER PROCEDURES

53800 Two or three glass test including examination of urine specimen(s), any method

53899 Unlisted procedure, urinary system

Male Genital System

PENIS

INCISION

54000 Slitting of prepuce, dorsal or lateral (separate procedure); newborn

54001 except newborn

54015 Incision and drainage of penis, deep

(For skin and subcutaneous abscess, see 10040-10160)

DESTRUCTION

54050* Destruction of lesion(s), penis (eg, condyloma, papilloma, molluscum contagiosum, herpetic vesicle), simple; chemical

54055* electrodesiccation

54056 cryosurgery

54057 laser surgery

54060 surgical excision

54065 Destruction of lesion(s), penis (eg, condyloma, papilloma, molluscum contagiosum, herpetic vesicle), extensive, any method

(For destruction or excision of other lesions, see Integumentary System)

EXCISION

54100 Biopsy of penis; cutaneous (separate procedure)

54105 deep structures

54110 Excision of penile plaque (Peyronie disease);

54111 with graft to 5 cm in length

54112 with graft greater than 5 cm in length

54115 Removal foreign body from deep penile tissue (eg, plastic implant)

54120 Amputation of penis; partial

54125 complete

54130 Amputation of penis, radical; with bilateral inguinofemoral lymphadenectomy

54135 in continuity with bilateral pelvic lymphadenectomy, including external iliac, hypogastric and obturator nodes

(For lymphadenectomy (separate procedure), see 38760-38770)

54150 Circumcision, using clamp or other device; newborn

54152 except newborn

(54154 has been deleted. To report, use 54152)

54160 Circumcision, surgical excision other than clamp, device or dorsal slit; newborn

54161 except newborn

INTRODUCTION

54200* Injection procedure for Peyronie disease;

54205 with surgical exposure of plaque

54220 Irrigation of corpora cavernosa for priapism

54230 Injection procedure for corpora cavernosography

(For radiological supervision and interpretation, see 74445)

54235 Injection of corpora cavernosa with pharmacologic agent(s) (eg, papaverine, phentolamine)

54240 Penile plethysmography

54250 Nocturnal penile tumescence and/or rigidity test

REPAIR

(For other urethroplasties, see 53400-53430)

(For penile revascularization, see 37788)

54300 Plastic operation of penis for straightening of chordee (eg, hypospadias), with or without mobilization of urethra

54304 Plastic operation on penis for correction of chordee or for first stage hypospadias repair with or without transplantation of prepuce and/or skin flaps

(54305 has been deleted. To report, see 54304 et seq)

54308 Urethroplasty for second stage hypospadias repair (including urinary diversion); less than 3 cm

54312 greater than 3 cm

54316 Urethroplasty for second stage hypospadias repair (including urinary diversion) with free skin graft obtained from site other than genitalia

54318 Urethroplasty for third stage hypospadias repair to release penis from scrotum (eg, third stage Cecil repair)

(54320, 54325, 54330 have been deleted. To report, see 54308 et seq)

54322 One stage distal hypospadias repair (with or without chordee or circumcision); with simple meatal advancement (eg, Magpi, V-flap)

54324 with urethroplasty by local skin flaps (eg, flip-flap, prepucial flap)

54326 with urethroplasty by local skin flaps and mobilization of urethra

54328 with extensive dissection to correct chordee and urethroplasty with local skin flaps, skin graft patch, and/or island flap

54332 One stage proximal penile or penoscrotal hypospadias repair requiring extensive dissection to correct chordee and urethroplasty by use of skin graft tube and/or island flap

54336 One stage perineal hypospadias repair requiring extensive dissection to correct chordee and urethroplasty by use of skin graft tube and/or island flap

54340 Repair of hypospadias complications (ie, fistula, stricture, diverticula); by closure, incision, or excision, simple

54344 requiring mobilization of skin flaps and urethroplasty with flap or patch graft

54348 requiring extensive dissection and urethroplasty with flap, patch or tubed graft (includes urinary diversion)

54352 Repair of hypospadias cripple requiring extensive dissection and excision of previously constructed structures including re-release of chordee and reconstruction of urethra and penis by use of local skin as grafts and island flaps and skin brought in as flaps or grafts

54360 Plastic operation on penis to correct angulation

54380 Plastic operation on penis for epispadias distal to external sphincter;

54385 with incontinence

54390 with exstrophy of bladder

54400 Insertion of penile prosthesis; non-inflatable (semi-rigid)

54401 inflatable (self-contained)

54402 Removal or replacement of non-inflatable (semi-rigid) or inflatable (self-contained) penile prosthesis

54405 Insertion of inflatable (multi-component) penile prosthesis, including placement of pump, cylinders, and/or reservoir

54407 Removal, repair, or replacement of inflatable (multi-component) penile prosthesis, including pump and/or reservoir and/or cylinders

54409 Surgical correction of hydraulic abnormality of inflatable (multi-component) prosthesis including pump and/or reservoir and/or cylinders

54420 Corpora cavernosa-saphenous vein shunt (priapism operation), unilateral or bilateral

54430 Corpora cavernosa-corpus spongiosum shunt (priapism operation), unilateral or bilateral

54435 Corpora cavernosa-glans penis fistulization (eg, biopsy needle, Winter procedure, rongeur, or punch) for priapism

54440 Plastic operation of penis for injury

MANIPULATION

54450 Foreskin manipulation including lysis of preputial adhesions and stretching

TESTIS

EXCISION

54500 Biopsy of testis, needle (separate procedure)

(For fine needle aspiration, preparation, and interpretation of smears, see 88170-88173)

54505 Biopsy of testis, incisional (separate procedure)

(When combined with vasogram, seminal vesiculogram, or epididymogram, see 55300)

(54506 has been deleted. To report, use 54505 with modifier -50 or 09950)

54510 Excision of local lesion of testis

54520 Orchiectomy, simple (including subcapsular), with or without testicular prosthesis, scrotal or inguinal approach

(54521 has been deleted. To report, use 54520 with modifier -50 or 09950)

54530 Orchiectomy, radical, for tumor; inguinal approach

54535 with abdominal exploration

(For orchiectomy with repair of hernia, see 49510)

(For radical retroperitoneal lymphadenectomy, see 38780)

54550 Exploration for undescended testis (inguinal or scrotal area)

(54555 has been deleted. To report, use 54550 with modifier -50 or 09950)

54560 Exploration for undescended testis with abdominal exploration

(54565 has been deleted. To report, use 54560 with modifier -50 or 09950)

REPAIR

54600 Reduction of torsion of testis, surgical, with or without fixation of contralateral testis

54620 Fixation of contralateral testis (separate procedure)

54640 Orchiopexy, any type, with or without hernia repair

(54641 has been deleted. To report, use 54640 with modifier -50 or 09950)

54645 second stage (Torek type)

54660 Insertion of testicular prosthesis (separate procedure)

(54661 has been deleted. To report, use 54660 with modifier -50 or 09950)

54670 Suture or repair of testicular injury

54680 Transplantation of testis(es) to thigh (because of scrotal destruction)

EPIDIDYMIS

INCISION

54700 Incision and drainage of epididymis, testis and/or scrotal space (eg, abscess or hematoma)

EXCISION

54800 Biopsy of epididymis, needle

(For fine needle aspiration, preparation, and interpretation of smears, see 88170-88173)

54820 Exploration of epididymis, with or without biopsy

54830 Excision of local lesion of epididymis

54840 Excision of spermatocele, with or without epididymectomy

(With hernia repair, see 49515)

54860 Epididymectomy; unilateral

54861 bilateral

REPAIR

54900 Epididymovasostomy, anastomosis of epididymis to vas deferens; unilateral

54901 bilateral

(For microsurgical repair with use of operating microscope, add modifier -20 or 09920)

TUNICA VAGINALIS

INCISION

55000* Puncture aspiration of hydrocele, tunica vaginalis, with or without injection of medication

EXCISION

55040 Excision of hydrocele; unilateral

55041 bilateral

(With hernia repair, see 49500, 49515)

REPAIR

55060 Repair of tunica vaginalis hydrocele (Bottle type)

SCROTUM

INCISION

55100* Drainage of scrotal wall abscess

(See also 54700)

55110 Scrotal exploration

55120 Removal of foreign body in scrotum

EXCISION

(For excision of local lesion of skin of scrotum, see Integumentary System)

55150 Resection of scrotum

REPAIR

(55170 has been deleted. To report, see 55175, 55180)

55175 Scrotoplasty; simple

55180 complicated

VAS DEFERENS

INCISION

55200 Vasotomy, cannulization with or without incision of vas, unilateral or bilateral (separate procedure)

EXCISION

55250 Vasectomy, unilateral or bilateral (separate procedure), including postoperative semen examination(s)

INTRODUCTION

55300 Vasotomy for vasograms, seminal vesiculograms, or epididymograms, unilateral or bilateral

(For radiological supervision and interpretation, see 74440)

(When combined with biopsy of testis, see 54505 and use modifier -51 or 09951)

REPAIR

55400 Vasovasostomy, vasovasorrhaphy

(55401 has been deleted. To report, use 55400 with modifier -50 or 09950)

(For microsurgical repair with use of operating microscope, add modifier -20 or 09920)

SUTURE

55450 Ligation (percutaneous) of vas deferens, unilateral or bilateral (separate procedure)

SPERMATIC CORD

EXCISION

55500 Excision of hydrocele of spermatic cord, unilateral (separate procedure)

55520 Excision of lesion of spermatic cord (separate procedure)

55530 Excision of varicocele or ligation of spermatic veins for varicocele; (separate procedure)

55535 abdominal approach

55540 with hernia repair

SEMINAL VESICLES

INCISION

55600 Vesiculotomy;

(55601 has been deleted. To report, use 55600 with modifier -50 or 09950)

55605 complicated

EXCISION

55650 Vesiculectomy, any approach

(55651 has been deleted. To report, use 55650 with modifier -50 or 09950)

55680 Excision of Mullerian duct cyst

(For injection procedure, see 52010, 55300)

PROSTATE

INCISION

55700 Biopsy, prostate; needle or punch, single or multiple, any approach

(For fine needle aspiration, preparation, and interpretation of smears, see 88170-88173)

55705 incisional, any approach

55720 Prostatotomy, external drainage of prostatic abscess, any approach; simple

55725 complicated

(For transurethral drainage, see 52700)

(55740 has been deleted. To report, use 55899)

EXCISION

(For transurethral removal of prostate, see 52601-52650)

(For limited pelvic lymphadenectomy for staging (separate procedure), use 38562)

(For independent node dissection, see 38770-38780)

55801 Prostatectomy, perineal, subtotal (including control of postoperative bleeding, vasectomy, meatotomy, urethral calibration and/or dilation, and internal urethrotomy)

55810 Prostatectomy, perineal radical;

55812 with lymph node biopsy(s) (limited pelvic lymphadenectomy)

55815 with bilateral pelvic lymphadenectomy, including external iliac, hypogastric and obturator nodes

(If 55815 is carried out on separate days, use 38770 with modifier -50 and 55810)

55821 Prostatectomy (including control of postoperative bleeding, vasectomy, meatotomy, urethral calibration and/or dilation, and internal urethrotomy); suprapubic, subtotal, one or two stages

55831 retropubic, subtotal

55840 Prostatectomy, retropubic radical;

55842 with lymph node biopsy(s) (limited pelvic lymphadenectomy)

55845 with bilateral pelvic lymphadenectomy, including external iliac, hypogastric and obturator nodes

(If 55845 is carried out on separate days, use 38770 with modifier -50 and 55840)

55860 Exposure of prostate, any approach, for insertion of radioactive substance;

(For application of interstital radioelement, see 77776-77778)

55862 with lymph node biopsy(s) (limited pelvic lymphadenectomy)

55865 with bilateral pelvic lymphadenectomy, including external iliac, hypogastric and obturator nodes

OTHER PROCEDURES

(For artificial insemination, see 58310, 58311)

55870 Electroejaculation

55899 Unlisted procedure, male genital system

Intersex Surgery

55970 Intersex surgery; male to female

55980 female to male

Female Genital System

(For pelvic laparotomy, see 49000)

(For excision or destruction of endometriomas, open method, see 49200, 49201)

(For paracentesis, see 49080, 49081)

(For secondary closure of abdominal wall evisceration or disruption, see 49900)

(For fulguration or excision of lesions, laparoscopic approach, see 58984)

(For chemotherapy, see 96400-96549)

(56000 has been deleted. To report, see 56405)

(56100 has been deleted. To report, see 56605)

(56200 has been deleted. To report, see 56810)

ENDOSCOPY-LAPAROSCOPY-HYSTEROSCOPY

The endoscopic descriptors in this publication are listed so that the main procedure can easily be identified without having to list all the minor related procedures that may be performed at the same time (such as lysis of adhesions and fulguration of bleeding points during laparoscopy with fulguration transection of the oviducts). When the laparoscopy requires mini-laparotomy (Hasson technique) or when secondary procedures involve significant additional time and effort, they may be reported by using either modifier -22 or code 09922.

Operative laparoscopy and hysteroscopy may utilize many methods to accomplish the same result (eg, hot cautery, CO_2 laser, ND-YAG laser, pelvioscopy). The CPT code is the same regardless which technique is employed to achieve the desired result.

(For peritoneoscopy, see 49300-49303)

- **56300** Laparoscopy, diagnostic (separate procedure)
- **56301** Laparoscopy, surgical; with fulguration of oviducts (with or without transection)
- **56302** with occlusion of oviducts by device (eg, band, clip, or Falope ring)
- **56303** with fulguration or excision of lesions of the ovary, pelvic viscera, or peritoneal surface by any method
- **56304** with lysis of adhesions
- **56305** with biopsy (single or multiple)
- **56306** with aspiration (single or multiple)
- **56307** with removal of adnexal structures (partial or total oophorectomy and/or salpingectomy)
- **56308** with vaginal hysterectomy with or without removal of tube(s), with or without removal of ovary(s) (laparoscopic assisted vaginal hysterectomy)
- **56309** with removal of leiomyomata, subserosal (single or multiple)
- **56350** Hysteroscopy, diagnostic (separate procedure)
- **56351** Hysteroscopy, surgical; with sampling (biopsy) of endometrium and/or polypectomy, with or without D & C

● **56352** with lysis of intrauterine adhesions (any method)

● **56353** with division or resection of intrauterine septum (any method)

● **56354** with removal of leiomyomata

● **56355** with removal of impacted foreign body

● **56356** with endometrial ablation (any method)

VULVA, PERINEUM AND INTROITUS

The following definitions apply to the vulvectomy codes (56620-56640).

Simple: The removal of skin and superficial subcutaneous tissue.

Radical: The removal of skin and deep subcutaneous tissue.

Partial: Removal of less than 80% of the vulvar area.

Complete: The removal of greater than 80% of the vulvar area.

INCISION

(For incision and drainage of sebaceous cyst, furuncle, or abscess, see 10040, 10060, 10061)

(56400 has been deleted. To report, see 56405)

● **56405*** Incision and drainage of vulva or perineal abscess

56420* Incision and drainage of Bartholin's gland abscess

(For incision and drainage of Skene's gland abscess or cyst, see 53060)

56440 Marsupialization of Bartholin's gland cyst

56441 Lysis of labial adhesions

DESTRUCTION

(56500 has been deleted. To report, use 56501)

56501 Destruction of lesion(s), vulva; simple, any method

(56505-56507, 56510 have been deleted. To report, use 56501)

56515 extensive, any method

(56520, 56521 have been deleted. To report, use 56501 or 56515)

(For destruction of Skene's gland cyst or abscess, see 53270)

(For cautery destruction of urethral caruncle, see 53265)

EXCISION

(56600 has been deleted. To report, see 56605)

● **56605*** Biopsy of vulva or perineum (separate procedure); one lesion

● **56606*** each separate additional lesion

(For excision of local lesion, see 11420-11426, 11620-11626)

▲ **56620** Vulvectomy simple; partial

▲ **56625** complete

(For skin graft, see 15000 et seq)

▲ **56630** Vulvectomy, radical, partial;

(For skin graft, if used, see 15000, 15120, 15121, 15240, 15241)

● **56631** with unilateral inguinofemoral lymphadenectomy

● **56633** Vulvectomy, radical, complete;

● **56634** with unilateral inguinofemoral lymphadenectomy

(56635 has been deleted. To report, see 56634, 56637)

(56636 has been deleted. To report, see 56634, 56637)

● **56637** with bilateral inguinofemoral lymphadenectomy

▲ **56640** Vulvectomy, radical, complete, with inguinofemoral, iliac, and pelvic lymphadenectomy

(56641 has been deleted. To report, use 56640 with modifier -50 or 09950)

(For lymphadenectomy, see 38760-38780)

(56680, 56685 have been deleted)

56700 Partial hymenectomy or revision of hymenal ring

(56710 has been deleted. To report, see 56700)

56720* Hymenotomy, simple incision

56740 Excision of Bartholin's gland or cyst

(For excision of Skene's gland, see 53270)

(For excision of urethral caruncle, see 53265)

(For excision or fulguration of urethral carcinoma, see 53220)

(For excision or marsupialization of urethral diverticulum, see 53230, 53240)

REPAIR

(For repair of urethra for mucosal prolapse, see 53275)

56800 Plastic repair of introitus

56805 Clitoroplasty for adrenogenital syndrome

REPAIR

• **56810** Perineoplasty, repair of perineum, non-obstetrical (separate procedure)

(See also 56800)

(For repair of wounds to genitalia, see 12001-12007, 12041-12047, 13131, 13132)

(For repair of recent injury of vagina and perineum, nonobstetrical, see 57210)

(For anal sphincteroplasty, see 46750, 46751)

SUTURE

(For episiorrhaphy, episioperineorrhaphy for recent injury of vulva and/or perineum, nonobstetrical, see 57210)

VAGINA

INCISION

57000 Colpotomy; with exploration

57010 with drainage of pelvic abscess

57020* Colpocentesis (separate procedure)

DESTRUCTION

(57050, 57057, 57060 have been deleted. To report, use 57061 or 57065)

57061 Destruction of vaginal lesion(s); simple, any method

(57063 has been deleted. To report, use 57061 or 57065)

57065 extensive, any method

EXCISION

57100* Biopsy of vaginal mucosa; simple (separate procedure)

57105 extensive, requiring suture (including cysts)

57108 Colpectomy, obliteration of vagina; partial

57110 complete

57120 Colpocleisis (Le Fort type)

57130 Excision of vaginal septum

57135 Excision of vaginal cyst or tumor

INTRODUCTION

57150* Irrigation of vagina and/or application of medicament for treatment of bacterial, parasitic, or fungoid disease

57160* Insertion of pessary

57170 Diaphragm or cervical cap fitting with instructions

57180 Introduction of any hemostatic agent or pack for spontaneous or traumatic nonobstetrical vaginal hemorrhage (separate procedure)

REPAIR

(For urethral suspension, Marshall-Marchetti-Krantz type, abdominal approach, see 51840, 51841)

57200 Colporrhaphy, suture of injury of vagina (nonobstetrical)

57210 Colpoperineorrhaphy, suture of injury of vagina and/or perineum (nonobstetrical)

57220 Plastic operation on urethral sphincter, vaginal approach (eg, Kelly urethral plication)

57230 Plastic repair of urethrocele

57240 Anterior colporrhaphy, repair of cystocele with or without repair of urethrocele

57250 Posterior colporrhaphy, repair of rectocele with or without perineorrhaphy

(For repair of rectocele (separate procedure) without posterior colporrhaphy, see 45560)

57260 Combined anteroposterior colporrhaphy;

57265 with enterocele repair

57268 Repair of enterocele, vaginal approach (separate procedure)

57270 Repair of enterocele, abdominal approach (separate procedure)

57280 Colpopexy, abdominal approach

▲**57282** Sacrospinous ligament fixation for prolapse of vagina

57288 Sling operation for stress incontinence (eg, fascia or synthetic)

57289 Pereyra procedure, including anterior colporrhaphy

(57290 has been deleted. To report, use 57291, 57292)

57291 Construction of artificial vagina; without graft

57292 with graft

57300 Closure of rectovaginal fistula; vaginal or transanal approach

57305 abdominal approach

57307 abdominal approach, with concomitant colostomy

57310 Closure of urethrovaginal fistula;

57311 with bulbocavernosus transplant

57320 Closure of vesicovaginal fistula; vaginal approach

(For concomitant cystostomy, see 51005-51040)

57330 transvesical and vaginal approach

(For abdominal approach, see 51900)

57335 Vaginoplasty for adrenogenital syndrome

MANIPULATION

57400* Dilation of vagina under anesthesia

57410* Pelvic examination under anesthesia

● **57415** Removal of impacted vaginal foreign body (separate procedure) under anesthesia

(For removal without anesthesia of an impacted vaginal foreign body, use the appropriate evaluation and management code)

ENDOSCOPY

(57450, 57451 have been deleted)

57452* Colposcopy (vaginoscopy); (separate procedure)

57454* with biopsies, or biopsy of the cervix

• **57460** with loop electrosurgical excision(s) of the cervix (LEEP)

CERVIX UTERI

EXCISION

(For radical surgical procedures, see 58200-58240)

57500* Biopsy, single or multiple, or local excision of lesion, with or without fulguration (separate procedure)

57505 Endocervical curettage (not done as part of a dilation and curettage)

57510 Cauterization of cervix; electro or thermal

57511* cryocautery, initial or repeat

57513 laser ablation

57520 Conization of cervix, with or without fulguration, with or without dilation and curettage, with or without repair (any method)

(See also 58120)

57530 Trachelectomy (cervicectomy), amputation of cervix (separate procedure)

57540 Excision of cervical stump, abdominal approach;

57545 with pelvic floor repair

57550 Excision of cervical stump, vaginal approach;

57555 with anterior and/or posterior repair

57556 with repair of enterocele

INTRODUCTION

(For insertion of intrauterine device, see 58300)

(57600-57620 have been deleted. For insertion of any hemostatic agent or pack for control of spontaneous non-obstetrical hemorrhage, see 57180)

REPAIR

57700 Cerclage of uterine cervix, nonobstetrical

57720 Trachelorrhaphy, plastic repair of uterine cervix, vaginal approach

MANIPULATION

57800* Dilation of cervical canal, instrumental (separate procedure)

57820 Dilation and curettage of cervical stump

CORPUS UTERI

EXCISION

▲**58100*** Endometrial and/or endocervical sampling (biopsy), without cervical dilation, any method (separate procedure)

(58101, 58102, 58103 have been deleted)

58120 Dilation and curettage, diagnostic and/or therapeutic (nonobstetrical)

(For postpartum hemorrhage, see 59160)

58140 Myomectomy, excision of fibroid tumor of uterus, single or multiple (separate procedure); abdominal approach

58145 vaginal approach

58150 Total abdominal hysterectomy (corpus and cervix), with or without removal of tube(s), with or without removal of ovary(s);

58152 with colpo-urethrocystopexy (Marshall-Marchetti-Krantz type)

(For urethrocystopexy without hysterectomy, see 51840, 51841)

58180 Supracervical abdominal hysterectomy (subtotal hysterectomy), with or without removal of tube(s), with or without removal of ovary(s)

▲**58200** Total abdominal hysterectomy, including partial vaginectomy, with para-aortic and pelvic lymph node sampling, with or without removal of tube(s), with or without removal of ovary(s)

(58205 has been deleted. For hysterectomy with pelvic lymphadenectomy, use 58210)

▲**58210** Radical abdominal hysterectomy, with bilateral total pelvic lymphadenectomy and para-aortic lymph node sampling (biopsy), with or without removal of tube(s), with or without removal of ovary(s)

(For radical hysterectomy with ovarian transposition, use also 58825)

▲**58240** Pelvic exenteration for gynecologic malignancy, with total abdominal hysterectomy or cervicectomy, with or without removal of tube(s), with or without removal of ovary(s), with removal of bladder and ureteral transplantations, and/or abdominoperineal resection of rectum and colon and colostomy, or any combination thereof

(For pelvic exenteration for lower urinary tract or male genital malignancy, use 51597)

▲**58260** Vaginal hysterectomy;

• **58262** with removal of tube(s), and/or ovary(s)

• **58263** with removal of tube(s), and/or ovary(s), with repair of enterocele

(58265 has been deleted. To report, see 57240, 57250, 57260, 57265)

58267 with colpo-urethrocystopexy (Marshall-Marchetti-Krantz type, Pereyra type, with or without endoscopic control)

58270 with repair of enterocele

(For repair of enterocele with removal of tubes and/or ovaries, see 58263)

58275 Vaginal hysterectomy, with total or partial colpectomy;

58280 with repair of enterocele

58285 Vaginal hysterectomy, radical (Schauta type operation)

INTRODUCTION

(For insertion/removal of implantable contraceptive capsules, see 11975, 11976, 11977)

58300* Insertion of intrauterine device (IUD)

58301 Removal of intrauterine device (IUD)

58310 Artificial insemination;

58311 with sperm washing and capacitation

(58320 has been deleted)

58340* Injection procedure for hysterosalpingography

(For radiological supervision and interpretation, see 74740)

• **58345** Transcervical introduction of fallopian tube catheter for diagnosis and/or re-establishing patency (any method), with or without hysterosalpingography

(For radiological supervision and interpretation, see 74742)

58350* Hydrotubation of oviduct, including materials

(For materials supplied by physician, see 99070)

REPAIR

58400 Uterine suspension, with or without shortening of round ligaments, with or without shortening of sacrouterine ligaments; (separate procedure)

58410 with presacral sympathectomy

(58430 has been deleted. To report, use 58999)

(58500 has been deleted. To report, use 58752)

58520 Hysterorrhaphy, repair of ruptured uterus (nonobstetrical)

58540 Hysteroplasty, repair of uterine anomaly (Strassman type)

SUTURE

(For closure of vesicouterine fistula, see 51920)

OVIDUCT

INCISION

58600 Ligation or transection of fallopian tube(s), abdominal or vaginal approach, unilateral or bilateral

58605 Ligation or transection of fallopian tube(s), abdominal or vaginal approach, postpartum, unilateral or bilateral, during same hospitalization (separate procedure)

(For laparoscopic procedures, see 56301, 56302)

(58610 has been deleted. To report, see 58600-58611)

58611 Ligation or transection of fallopian tube(s) when done at the time of cesarean section or intra-abdominal surgery (not a separate procedure)

58615 Occlusion of fallopian tube(s) by device (eg, band, clip, Falope ring) vaginal or suprapubic approach

(For laparoscopic approach, see 56302)

(58618 has been deleted. To report, use 58740)

EXCISION

58700 Salpingectomy, complete or partial, unilateral or bilateral (separate procedure)

58720 Salpingo-oophorectomy, complete or partial, unilateral or bilateral (separate procedure)

REPAIR

58740 Lysis of adhesions (salpingolysis, ovariolysis)

(For laparascopic approach, see 56304)

(For excision or destruction of endometriomas, open method, see 49200, 49201)

(For fulguration or excision of lesions, laparoscopic approach, see 56303)

58750 Tubotubal anastomosis

58752 Tubouterine implantation

58760 Fimbrioplasty

58770 Salpingostomy (salpingoneostomy)

OVARY

INCISION

58800 Drainage of ovarian cyst(s), unilateral or bilateral, (separate procedure); vaginal approach

58805 abdominal approach

58820 Drainage of ovarian abscess; vaginal approach

58822 abdominal approach

58825 Transposition, ovary(s)

EXCISION

58900 Biopsy of ovary, unilateral or bilateral (separate procedure)

58920 Wedge resection or bisection of ovary, unilateral or bilateral

58925 Ovarian cystectomy, unilateral or bilateral

58940 Oophorectomy, partial or total, unilateral or bilateral;

(58942 has been deleted. To report, use 58952)

58943 for ovarian malignancy, with para-aortic and pelvic lymph node biopsies, peritoneal washings, peritoneal biopsies, diaphragmatic assessments, with or without salpingectomy(s), with or without omentectomy

(58945 has been deleted. To report, use 58950)

58950 Resection of ovarian malignancy with bilateral salpingo-oophorectomy and omentectomy;

58951 with total abdominal hysterectomy, pelvic and limited para-aortic lymphadenectomy

58952 with radical dissection for debulking

58960 Laparotomy, for staging or restaging of ovarian malignancy ("second look"), with or without omentectomy, peritoneal washing, biopsy of abdominal and pelvic peritoneum, diaphragmatic assessment with pelvic and limited para-aortic lymphadenectomy

IN VITRO FERTILIZATION

58970 Follicle puncture for oocyte retrieval, any method

(For radiological supervision and interpretation, see 76948)

58972 Culture and fertilization of oocyte(s)

58974 Embryo transfer, any method (separate procedure)

58976 Gamete or zygote intrafallopian transfer, any method

(58980 has been deleted. To report, see 56300)

(58982 has been deleted. To report, see 56301)

(58983 has been deleted. To report, see 56302)

(58984 has been deleted. To report, see 56303)

Maternity
59000 - 59899

(58985 has been deleted. To report, see 56304)

(58986 has been deleted. To report, see 56305)

(58987 has been deleted. To report, see 56306)

(58988 has been deleted. To report, see 56307)

(58990 has been deleted. To report, see 56350)

(58992 has been deleted. To report, see 56352)

(58994 has been deleted. To report, see 56354)

(58995 has been deleted. To report, see 56352, 56354, 56356)

(58996 has been deleted. To report, see 56356)

OTHER PROCEDURES

58999 Unlisted procedure, female genital system (nonobstetrical)

Maternity Care and Delivery

The services normally provided in uncomplicated maternity cases include antepartum care, delivery, and postpartum care.

Antepartum care includes the initial and subsequent history, physical examinations, recording of weight, blood pressures, fetal heart tones, routine chemical urinalysis, and monthly visits up to 28 weeks gestation, biweekly visits to 36 weeks gestation, and weekly visits until delivery. Any other visits or services within this time period should be coded separately.

Delivery services include admission to the hospital, the admission history and physical examination, management of uncomplicated labor, vaginal delivery (with or without episiotomy, with or without forceps), or cesarean delivery. Medical problems complicating labor and and delivery management may require additional resources and should be identified by utilizing the codes in the MEDICINE section in addition to codes for maternity care.

Postpartum care includes hospital and office visits following vaginal or cesarean section delivery.

For medical complications of pregnancy (eg, cardiac problems, neurological problems, diabetes, hypertension, toxemia, hyperemesis, pre-term labor, premature rupture of membranes), see services in the

MEDICINE section. For surgical complications of pregnancy (eg, appendectomy, hernia, ovarian cyst, Bartholin cyst), see services in the SURGERY section.

If a physician provides all or part of the antepartum and/or postpartum patient care but does not perform delivery due to termination of pregnancy by abortion or referral to another physician for delivery, see appropriate evaluation and management codes.

(For circumcision of newborn, see 54150, 54160)

INCISION

59000* Amniocentesis, any method

(For radiological supervision and interpretation, see 76946)

(59010, 59011 have been deleted)

59012 Cordocentesis (intrauterine), any method

59015 Chorionic villus sampling, any method

59020* Fetal contraction stress test

59025 Fetal non-stress test

59030* Fetal scalp blood sampling

(59031 has been deleted. To report, use 59030 and see modifiers -76 and -77)

59050 Initiation and/or supervision of internal fetal monitoring during labor by consultant with report (separate procedure)

59100 Hysterotomy, abdominal (eg, for hydatidiform mole, abortion)

(When tubal ligation is performed at the same time as hysterotomy, use 58611 in addition to 59100)

(59101, 59105, 59106 have been deleted. To report, see 59100, 58611)

EXCISION

59120 Surgical treatment of ectopic pregnancy; tubal or ovarian, requiring salpingectomy and/or oophorectomy, abdominal or vaginal approach

59121 tubal or ovarian, without salpingectomy and/or oophorectomy

(59125, 59126 have been deleted. To report, see 59120, 59121)

59130 abdominal pregnancy

59135 interstitial, uterine pregnancy requiring total hysterectomy

59136 interstitial, uterine pregnancy with partial resection of uterus

59140 cervical, with evacuation

59150 Laparoscopic treatment of ectopic pregnancy; without salpingectomy and/or oophorectomy

59151 with salpingectomy and/or oophorectomy

59160 Curettage, postpartum (separate procedure)

INTRODUCTION

(For intrauterine fetal transfusion, see 36460)

(For introduction of hypertonic solution and/or prostaglandins to initiate labor, see 59850)

59200 Insertion of cervical dilator (eg, laminaria, prostaglandin) (separate procedure)

REPAIR

(For tracheloplasty, see 57700)

59300 Episiotomy or vaginal repair, by other than attending physician

(59305 has been deleted)

59320 Cerclage of cervix, during pregnancy; vaginal

59325 abdominal

59350 Hysterorrhaphy of ruptured uterus

(59351 has been deleted)

DELIVERY, ANTEPARTUM AND POSTPARTUM CARE

59400 Routine obstetric care including antepartum care, vaginal delivery (with or without episiotomy, and/or forceps) and postpartum care

59410 Vaginal delivery only (with or without episiotomy and/or forceps) including postpartum care

59412 External cephalic version, with or without tocolysis (list in addition to code(s) for delivery)

59414 Delivery of placenta (separate procedure)

(59420 has been deleted. To report, see appropriate evaluation and management codes)

59430 Postpartum care only (separate procedure)

CESAREAN DELIVERY

(For standby attendance for infant, see 99150, 99151)

(59500, 59501 have been deleted. To report, see 59510, 59515, 59525)

59510 Routine obstetric care including antepartum care, cesarean delivery, and postpartum care

59515 Cesarean delivery only including postpartum care

(59520, 59521 have been deleted. To report, see 59510, 59515, 59525)

59525 Subtotal or total hysterectomy after cesarean delivery (list in addition to 59510 or 59515)

(59540, 59541, 59560, 59561, 59580, 59581 have been deleted. To report, see 59510, 59515, 59525)

ABORTION

(For medical treatment of spontaneous complete abortion, any trimester, use evaluation and management codes 99201-99233)

(59800, 59810 have been deleted. To report, see 99201-99233)

(59801, 59811 have been deleted. To report, see 59812)

▲**59812** Treatment of incomplete abortion, any trimester, completed surgically

59820 Treatment of missed abortion, completed surgically; first trimester

59821 second trimester

59830 Treatment of septic abortion, completed surgically

59840 Induced abortion, by dilation and curettage

59841 Induced abortion, by dilation and evacuation

59850 Induced abortion, by one or more intra-amniotic injections (amniocentesis-injections), including hospital admission and visits, delivery of fetus and secundines);

59851 with dilation and curettage and/or evacuation

59852 with hysterotomy (failed intra-amniotic injection)

(For insertion of cervical dilator, see 59200)

OTHER PROCEDURES

59870 Uterine evacuation and curettage for hydatidiform mole

59899 Unlisted procedure, maternity care and delivery

Endocrine System

(For pituitary and pineal surgery, see Nervous System)

THYROID GLAND

INCISION

60000* Incision and drainage of thyroglossal cyst, infected

EXCISION

60100* Biopsy thyroid, percutaneous needle

(For radiological supervision and interpretation, see 76360, 76942)

(For fine needle aspiration, preparation, and interpretation of smears, see 88170-88173)

60200 Excision of cyst or adenoma of thyroid, or transection of isthmus

60220 Total thyroid lobectomy, unilateral;

60225 with contralateral subtotal lobectomy, including isthmus

60240 Thyroidectomy, total or complete

(60242 has been deleted. To report, use 60245)

60245 Thyroidectomy, subtotal or partial;

60246 with removal of substernal thyroid gland, cervical approach

60252 Thyroidectomy, total or subtotal for malignancy; with limited neck dissection

60254 with radical neck dissection

60260 Thyroidectomy, secondary

(60261 has been deleted. To report, use 60260 with modifier -50 or 09950)

60270 Thyroidectomy, including substernal thyroid gland, sternal split or transthoracic approach

60280 Excision of thyroglossal duct cyst or sinus;

60281 recurrent

PARATHYROID, THYMUS, ADRENAL GLANDS, AND CAROTID BODY

EXCISION

(For pituitary and pineal surgery, see Nervous System)

60500 Parathyroidectomy or exploration of parathyroid(s);

60502 re-exploration

60505 with mediastinal exploration, sternal split or transthoracic approach

(60510 has been deleted)

60520 Thymectomy, partial or total (separate procedure)

60540 Adrenalectomy, partial or complete, or exploration of adrenal gland with or without biopsy, transabdominal, lumbar or dorsal (separate procedure);

60545 with excision of adjacent retroperitoneal tumor

(For excision of remote or disseminated pheochromocytoma, see 49200, 49201)

(60550, 60555 have been deleted. To report, use 60540 with modifier -50 or 09950)

60600 Excision of carotid body tumor; without excision of carotid artery

60605 with excision of carotid artery

60699 Unlisted procedure, endocrine system

Nervous System

SKULL, MENINGES, AND BRAIN

(For injection procedure for cerebral angiography, see 36100-36218)

(For injection procedure for ventriculography, see 61026, 61120, 61130)

(For injection procedure for pneumoencephalography, see 61055)

PUNCTURE FOR INJECTION, DRAINAGE OR ASPIRATION

61000* Subdural tap through fontanelle, or suture, infant, unilateral or bilateral; initial

61001* subsequent taps

61020* Ventricular puncture through previous burr hole, fontanelle, suture, or implanted ventricular catheter/reservoir; without injection

(61025 has been deleted. To report, use 61026)

61026* with injection of drug or other substance for diagnosis or treatment

(61030, 61045 have been deleted. To report, use 61026)

61050* Cisternal or lateral cervical (C1-C2) puncture; without injection (separate procedure)

(61051, 61052, 61053 have been deleted. To report, use 61055)

61055* with injection of drug or other substance for diagnosis or treatment (eg, C1-C2)

(For radiological supervision and interpretation, see Radiology)

61070* Puncture of shunt tubing or reservoir for aspiration or injection procedure

(For radiological supervision and interpretation, see 75809)

TWIST DRILL, BURR HOLE(S) OR TREPHINE

61105* Twist drill hole for subdural or ventricular puncture; not followed by other surgery

61106 followed by other surgery

61107* for implanting ventricular catheter or pressure recording device

61108 for evacuation and/or drainage of subdural hematoma

61120 Burr hole(s) for ventricular puncture (including injection of gas, contrast media, dye, or radioactive material); not followed by other surgery

61130 followed by other surgery

61140 Burr hole(s) or trephine; with biopsy of brain or intracranial lesion

61150 with drainage of brain abscess or cyst

61151 with subsequent tapping (aspiration) of intracranial abscess or cyst

61154 Burr hole(s) with evacuation and/or drainage of hematoma, extradural or subdural

(61155 has been deleted. To report, use 61154 with modifier -50 or 09950)

61156 Burr hole(s); with aspiration of hematoma or cyst, intracerebral

61210* for implanting ventricular catheter, reservoir, EEG electrode(s) or pressure recording device (separate procedure)

61215 Insertion of subcutaneous reservoir, pump or continuous infusion system for connection to ventricular catheter

(For chemotherapy, see 96450)

61250 Burr hole(s) or trephine, supratentorial, exploratory, not followed by other surgery

(61251 has been deleted. To report, use 61250 with modifier -50 or 09950)

61253 Burr hole(s) or trephine, infratentorial, unilateral or bilateral

(If burr hole(s) or trephine are followed by craniotomy at same operative session, use 61304-61321; do not use 61250 or 61253)

CRANIECTOMY OR CRANIOTOMY

61304 Craniectomy or craniotomy, exploratory; supratentorial

61305 infratentorial (posterior fossa)

(61310, 61311 have been deleted. To report, see 61312-61315)

61312 Craniectomy or craniotomy for evacuation of hematoma, supratentorial; extradural or subdural

61313 intracerebral

61314 Craniectomy or craniotomy for evacuation of hematoma, infratentorial; extradural or subdural

61315 intracerebellar

61320 Craniectomy or craniotomy, drainage of intracranial abscess; supratentorial

61321 infratentorial

61330 Decompression of orbit only, transcranial approach

(61331 has been deleted. To report, use 61330 with modifier -50 or 09950)

61332 Exploration of orbit (transcranial approach); with biopsy

61333 with removal of lesion

61334 with removal of foreign body

61340 Other cranial decompression (eg, subtemporal), supratentorial

(61341 has been deleted. To report, use 61340 with modifier -50 or 09950)

61343 Craniectomy, suboccipital with cervical laminectomy for decompression of medulla and spinal cord, with or without dural graft (eg, Arnold-Chiari malformation)

61345 Other cranial decompression, posterior fossa

(For orbital decompression by lateral wall approach, Kroenlein type, see 67445)

61440 Craniotomy for section of tentorium cerebelli (separate procedure)

61450 Craniectomy, subtemporal, for section, compression, or decompression of sensory root of gasserian ganglion

61458 Craniectomy, suboccipital; for exploration or decompression of cranial nerves

61460 for section of one or more cranial nerves

61470 for medullary tractotomy

61480 for mesencephalic tractotomy or pedunculotomy

61490 Craniotomy for lobotomy, including cingulotomy

(61491 has been deleted. To report, use 61490 with modifier -50 or 09950)

61500 Craniectomy; with excision of tumor or other bone lesion of skull

61501 for osteomyelitis

61510 Craniectomy, trephination, bone flap craniotomy; for excision of brain tumor, supratentorial, except meningioma

61512 for excision of meningioma, supratentorial

61514 for excision of brain abscess, supratentorial

61516 for excision or fenestration of cyst, supratentorial

(For excision of pituitary tumor or craniopharyngioma, see 61545, 61546, 61548)

61518 Craniectomy for excision of brain tumor, infratentorial or posterior fossa; except meningioma, cerebellopontine angle tumor, or midline tumor at base of skull

61519 meningioma

61520 cerebellopontine angle tumor

61521 midline tumor at base of skull

61522 Craniectomy, infratentorial or posterior fossa; for excision of brain abscess

61524 for excision or fenestration of cyst

61526 Craniectomy, bone flap craniotomy, transtemporal (mastoid) for excision of cerebellopontine angle tumor;

61530 combined with middle/posterior fossa craniotomy/craniectomy

● **61531** Subdural implantation of strip electrodes through one or more burr or trephine hole(s) for long term seizure monitoring

(For stereotactic implantation of electrodes, see 61760)

(61532 has been deleted. To report, see 61680-61692)

▲ **61533** Craniotomy with elevation of bone flap for subdural implantation of an electrode array; for long term seizure monitoring

(For continuous EEG monitoring, see 95950-95954)

61534 for excision of epileptogenic focus without electrocorticography during surgery

61535 for removal of epidural or subdural electrode array, without excision of cerebral tissue (separate procedure)

61536 for excision of cerebral epileptogenic focus, with electrocorticography during surgery (includes removal of electrode array)

61538 for lobectomy with electrocorticography during surgery, temporal lobe

61539 for lobectomy with electrocorticography during surgery, other than temporal lobe, partial or total

61541 for transection of corpus callosum

61542 for total hemispherectomy

61543 for partial or subtotal hemispherectomy

61544 for excision or coagulation of choroid plexus

61545 for excision of craniopharyngioma

61546 Craniotomy for hypophysectomy or excision of pituitary tumor, intracranial approach

61548 Hypophysectomy or excision of pituitary tumor, transnasal or transseptal approach, nonstereotactic

61550 Craniectomy for craniosynostosis; single cranial suture

61552 multiple cranial sutures

(61553 has been deleted. To report, see 61552, 61558, 61559)

(61555 has been deleted. To report, see 21172-21180, 61552, 61558, 61559)

(For cranial reconstruction for orbital hypertelorism, see 21260-21263)

61556 Craniotomy for craniosynostosis; frontal or parietal bone flap

61557 bifrontal bone flap

61558 Extensive craniectomy for multiple cranial suture craniosynostosis (eg, cloverleaf skull); not requiring bone grafts

61559 recontouring with multiple osteotomies and bone autografts (eg, barrel-stave procedure) (includes obtaining grafts)

(61561 has been deleted. To report, see 21172-21180)

61563 Excision, intra and extracranial, benign tumor of cranial bone (eg, fibrous dysplasia); without optic nerve decompression

61564 with optic nerve decompression

(For reconstruction, see 21181-21183)

61570 Craniectomy or craniotomy; with excision of foreign body from brain

61571 with treatment of penetrating wound of brain

(For sequestrectomy for osteomyelitis, see 61501)

61575 Transoral approach to skull base, brain stem or upper spinal cord for biopsy, decompression or excision of lesion;

61576 requiring splitting of tongue and/or mandible (including tracheostomy)

(For arthrodesis, use 22548)

ENDOVASCULAR SURGERY

61624 Transcatheter occlusion or embolization (eg, for tumor destruction, to achieve hemostasis, to occlude a vascular malformation), percutaneous, any method; central nervous system (intracranial, spinal cord)

61626 non-central nervous system, head or neck (extracranial, brachiocephalic branch)

(See also 37204)

(For radiological supervision and interpretation, see 75894)

SURGERY FOR ANEURYSM, ARTERIOVENOUS MALFORMATION OR VASCULAR DISEASE

(Includes craniotomy when appropriate for procedure)

61680 Surgery of intracranial arteriovenous malformation; supratentorial, simple

61682 supratentorial, complex

61684 infratentorial, simple

61686 infratentorial, complex

61690 dural, simple

61692 dural, complex

61700 Surgery of intracranial aneurysm, intracranial approach; carotid circulation

61702 vertebral-basilar circulation

61703 Surgery of intracranial aneurysm, cervical approach by application of occluding clamp to cervical carotid artery (Selverstone-Crutchfield type)

(For cervical approach for direct ligation of carotid artery, see 37600-37606)

61705 Surgery of aneurysm, vascular malformation or carotid-cavernous fistula; by intracranial and cervical occlusion of carotid artery

61708 by intracranial electrothrombosis

(For ligation or gradual occlusion of internal/common carotid artery, see 37605, 37606)

61710 by intra-arterial embolization, injection procedure, or balloon catheter

61711 Anastomosis, arterial, extracranial-intracranial (eg, middle cerebral/cortical) arteries

(For carotid or vertebral thromboendarterectomy, see 35301)

61712 Microdissection, intracranial or spinal procedure (list separately in addition to code for primary procedure)

STEREOTAXIS

61720 Creation of lesion by stereotactic method, including burr hole(s) and localizing and recording techniques, single or multiple stages; globus pallidus or thalamus

61735 subcortical structure(s) other than globus pallidus or thalamus

61750 Stereotactic biopsy, aspiration, or excision, including burr hole(s), for intracranial lesion;

61751 with computerized axial tomography

● **61760** Stereotactic implantation of depth electrodes into the cerebrum for long term seizure monitoring

61770 Stereotactic localization, any method, including burr hole(s); with insertion of catheter(s) for brachytherapy

(61780 has been deleted. To report, see 61760)

61790 Creation of lesion by stereotactic method, percutaneous, by neurolytic agent (eg, alcohol, thermal, electrical, radiofrequency); gasserian ganglion

61791 trigeminal medullary tract

61793 Stereotactic focused proton beam or gamma radiosurgery

61795 Stereotactic computer assisted volumetric intracranial procedure (list separately in addition to code for primary procedure)

NEUROSTIMULATORS, INTRACRANIAL

61850 Twist drill or burr hole(s) for implantation of neurostimulator electrodes; cortical

61855 subcortical

61860 Craniectomy or craniotomy for implantation of neurostimulator electrodes, cerebral; cortical

61865 subcortical

61870 Craniectomy for implantation of neurostimulator electrodes, cerebellar; cortical

61875 subcortical

61880 Revision or removal of intracranial neurostimulator electrodes

61885 Incision and subcutaneous placement of cranial neurostimulator pulse generator or receiver, direct or inductive coupling

61888 Revision or removal of cranial neurostimulator pulse generator or receiver

REPAIR

62000 Elevation of depressed skull fracture; simple, extradural

62005 compound or comminuted, extradural

62010 with repair of dura and/or debridement of brain

62100 Craniotomy for repair of dural/CSF leak, including surgery for rhinorrhea/otorrhea

(For repair of spinal dural/CSF leak, see 63707, 63709)

62115 Reduction of craniomegalic skull (eg, treated hydrocephalus); not requiring bone grafts or cranioplasty

62116 with simple cranioplasty

62117 requiring craniotomy and reconstruction with or without bone graft (includes obtaining grafts)

62120 Repair of encephalocele, skull vault, including cranioplasty

62121 Craniotomy for repair of encephalocele, skull base

62140 Cranioplasty for skull defect; up to 5 cm diameter

62141 larger than 5 cm diameter

62142 Removal of bone flap or prosthetic plate of skull

62143 Replacement of bone flap or prosthetic plate of skull

62145 Cranioplasty for skull defect with reparative brain surgery

62146 Cranioplasty with autograft (includes obtaining bone grafts); up to 5 cm diameter

62147 larger than 5 cm diameter

CSF SHUNT

62180 Ventriculocisternostomy (Torkildsen type operation)

62190 Creation of shunt; subarachnoid/subdural-atrial, -jugular, -auricular

62192 subarachnoid/subdural-peritoneal, -pleural, other terminus

62194 Replacement or irrigation, subarachnoid/subdural catheter

62200 Ventriculocisternostomy, third ventricle;

62201 stereotactic method

62220 Creation of shunt; ventriculo-atrial, -jugular, -auricular

62223 ventriculo-peritoneal, -pleural, other terminus

62225 Replacement or irrigation, ventricular catheter

62230 Replacement or revision of CSF shunt, obstructed valve, or distal catheter in shunt system

62256 Removal of complete CSF shunt system; without replacement

62258 with replacement by similar or other shunt at same operation

(For percutaneous irrigation or aspiration of shunt reservoir, see 61070)

SPINE AND SPINAL CORD

(For application of caliper or tongs, see 20660)

(For treatment of fracture or dislocation of spine, see 22305-22327)

PUNCTURE FOR INJECTION, DRAINAGE, OR ASPIRATION

62268* Percutaneous aspiration, spinal cord cyst or syrinx

(For radiological supervision and interpretation, see 76003, 76365, 76938)

62269* Biopsy of spinal cord, percutaneous needle

(For radiological supervision and interpretation, see 76003, 76360, 76942)

62270* Spinal puncture, lumbar, diagnostic

62272* Spinal puncture, therapeutic, for drainage of spinal fluid (by needle or catheter)

62273* Injection, lumbar epidural, of blood or clot patch

62274* Injection of anesthetic substance (including narcotics), diagnostic or therapeutic; subarachnoid or subdural, single

62275 epidural, cervical or thoracic, single

62276* subarachnoid or subdural, differential

62277* subarachnoid or subdural, continuous

▲**62278*** epidural, lumbar or caudal, single

▲**62279*** epidural, lumbar or caudal, continuous

62280* Injection of neurolytic substance (eg, alcohol, phenol, iced saline solutions); subarachnoid

62281* epidural, cervical or thoracic

▲**62282*** epidural, lumbar or caudal

62284* Injection procedure for myelography and/or computerized axial tomography, spinal (other than C1-C2 and posterior fossa)

(For injection procedure at C1-C2, see 61055)

(For radiological supervision and interpretation, see Radiology)

(62286 has been deleted. To report, use 64999)

62287 Aspiration procedure, percutaneous, of nucleus pulposus of intervertebral disk, any method, single or multiple levels, lumbar

62288* Injection of substance other than anesthetic, contrast, or neurolytic solutions; subarachnoid (separate procedure)

62289* lumbar or caudal epidural (separate procedure)

62290* Injection procedure for diskography, each level; lumbar

▲**62291*** cervical

(For radiological supervision and interpretation, see 72285, 72295)

62292 Injection procedure for chemonucleolysis, including diskography, intervertebral disk, single or multiple levels, lumbar

(62293 has been deleted)

62294 Injection procedure, arterial, for occlusion of arteriovenous malformation, spinal

62298* Injection of substance other than anesthetic, contrast, or neurolytic solutions, epidural, cervical or thoracic (separate procedure)

POSTERIOR EXTRADURAL LAMINOTOMY OR LAMINECTOMY FOR EXPLORATION/DECOMPRESSION OF NEURAL ELEMENTS OR EXCISION OF HERNIATED INTERVERTEBRAL DISKS

(62295-62303 have been deleted. To report, see 63001-63017)

63001 Laminectomy with exploration and/or decompression of spinal cord and/or cauda equina, without facetectomy, foraminotomy or diskectomy, (eg, spinal stenosis), one or two vertebral segments; cervical

63003 thoracic

63005 lumbar, except for spondylolisthesis

(63010 has been deleted. To report, use 63012)

63011 sacral

63012 Laminectomy with removal of abnormal facets and/or pars inter-articularis with decompression of cauda equina and nerve roots for spondylolisthesis, lumbar (Gill type procedure)

63015 Laminectomy with exploration and/or decompression of spinal cord and/or cauda equina, without facetectomy, foraminotomy or diskectomy, (eg, spinal stenosis), more than 2 vertebral segments; cervical

63016 thoracic

63017 lumbar

63020 Laminotomy (hemilaminectomy), with decompression of nerve root(s), including partial facetectomy, foraminotomy and/or excision of herniated intervertebral disk; one interspace, cervical

(63021 has been deleted. To report, use 63020 with modifier -50 or 09950)

63030 one interspace, lumbar

(63031 has been deleted. To report, use 63030 with modifier -50 or 09950

63035 each additional interspace, cervical or lumbar

(Use 63035 only for procedures 63020-63030)

63040 Laminotomy (hemilaminectomy), with decompression of nerve root(s), including partial facetectomy, foraminotomy and/or excision of herniated intervertebral disk, re-exploration; cervical

(63041 has been deleted)

63042 lumbar

(When 63001-63042 are followed by arthrodesis, see 22590-22650)

63045 Laminectomy, facetectomy and foraminotomy (unilateral or bilateral with decompression of spinal cord, cauda equina and/or nerve root(s), (eg, spinal or lateral recess stenosis), single vertebral segment; cervical

63046 thoracic

63047 lumbar

63048 each additional segment, cervical, thoracic or lumbar

(Use 63048 only for procedures 63045-63047)

(When 63001-63048 are followed by arthrodesis, see 22590-22650)

TRANSPEDICULAR OR COSTOVERTEBRAL APPROACH FOR POSTEROLATERAL EXTRADURAL EXPLORATION/ DECOMPRESSION

63055 Transpedicular approach with decompression of spinal cord, equina and/or nerve root(s) (eg, herniated intervertebral disk), single segment; thoracic

63056 lumbar

63057 each additional segment, thoracic or lumbar

(63060 has been deleted)

63064 Costovertebral approach with decompression of spinal cord or nerve root(s), (eg, herniated intervertebral disk), thoracic; single segment

(63065 has been deleted)

63066 each additional segment

(For excision of thoracic intraspinal lesions by laminectomy, see 63266, 63271, 63276, 63281, 63286)

ANTERIOR OR ANTEROLATERAL APPROACH FOR EXTRADURAL EXPLORATION/DECOMPRESSION

63075 Diskectomy, anterior, with decompression of spinal cord and/or nerve root(s), including osteophytectomy; cervical, single interspace

63076 cervical, each additional interspace

63077 thoracic, single interspace

63078 thoracic, each additional interspace

63081 Vertebral corpectomy (vertebral body resection), partial or complete, anterior approach with decompression of spinal cord and/or nerve root(s); cervical, single segment

63082 cervical, each additional segment

(For transoral approach, see 61575, 61576)

63085 Vertebral corpectomy (vertebral body resection), partial or complete, transthoracic approach with decompression of spinal cord and/or nerve root(s); thoracic, single segment

63086 thoracic, each additional segment

63087 Vertebral corpectomy (vertebral body resection), partial or complete, combined thoracolumbar approach with decompression of spinal cord, cauda equina or nerve root(s), lower thoracic or lumbar; single segment

63088 each additional segment

63090 Vertebral corpectomy (vertebral body resection), partial or complete, transperitoneal or retroperitoneal approach with decompression of spinal cord, cauda equina or nerve root(s), lower thoracic, lumbar, or sacral; single segment

63091 each additional segment

(Procedures 63081-63091 include diskectomy above and/or below vertebral segment)

(If followed by arthrodesis, see 22554-22585)

(If followed by reconstruction of spine, see 22140-22152)

INCISION

63170 Laminectomy with myelotomy (eg, Bischof or DREZ type), cervical, thoracic or thoracolumbar

63172 Laminectomy with drainage of intramedullary cyst/syrinx; to subarachnoid space

63173 to peritoneal space

63180 Laminectomy and section of dentate ligaments, with or without dural graft, cervical; one or two segments

63182 more than two segments

63185 Laminectomy with rhizotomy; one or two segments

63190 more than two segments

63191 Laminectomy with section of spinal accessory nerve

(63192 has been deleted. To report, use 63191 with modifier -50 or 09950)

(For resection of sternocleidomastoid muscle, use 21720)

63194 Laminectomy with cordotomy, with section of one spinothalamic tract, one stage; cervical

63195 thoracic

63196 Laminectomy with cordotomy, with section of both spinothalamic tracts, one stage; cervical

63197 thoracic

63198 Laminectomy with cordotomy with section of both spinothalamic tracts, two stages within 14 days; cervical

63199 thoracic

63200 Laminectomy, with release of tethered spinal cord, lumbar

EXCISION BY LAMINECTOMY OF LESION OTHER THAN HERNIATED DISK

(63210-63242 have been deleted. To report, see 63265-63290)

63250 Laminectomy for excision or occlusion of arteriovenous malformation of spinal cord; cervical

63251 thoracic

63252 thoracolumbar

63265 Laminectomy for excision or evacuation of intraspinal lesion other than neoplasm, extradural; cervical

63266 thoracic

63267 lumbar

63268 sacral

63270 Laminectomy for excision of intraspinal lesion other than neoplasm, intradural; cervical

63271 thoracic

63272 lumbar

63273 sacral

63275 Laminectomy for biopsy/excision of intraspinal neoplasm; extradural, cervical

63276 extradural, thoracic

63277 extradural, lumbar

63278 extradural, sacral

63280 intradural, extramedullary, cervical

63281 intradural, extramedullary, thoracic

63282 intradural, extramedullary, lumbar

63283 intradural, sacral

63285 intradural, intramedullary, cervical

63286 intradural, intramedullary, thoracic

63287 intradural, intramedullary, thoracolumbar

63290 combined extradural-intradural lesion, any level

(For drainage of intramedullary cyst/syrinx, use 63172, 63173)

EXCISION, ANTERIOR OR ANTEROLATERAL APPROACH, INTRASPINAL LESION

(For arthrodesis, see 22548-22650)

(For reconstruction of spine, see 22140-22152)

63300 Vertebral corpectomy (vertebral body resection), partial or complete, for excision of intraspinal lesion, single segment; extradural, cervical

63301 extradural, thoracic by transthoracic approach

63302 extradural, thoracic by thoracolumbar approach

63303 extradural, lumbar or sacral by transperitoneal or retroperitoneal approach

63304 intradural, cervical

63305 intradural, thoracic by transthoracic approach

63306 intradural, thoracic by thoracolumbar approach

63307 intradural, lumbar or sacral by transperitoneal or retroperitoneal approach

63308 each additional segment (list separately in addition to codes for single segment 63300-63307)

STEREOTAXIS

63600 Creation of lesion of spinal cord by stereotactic method, percutaneous, any modality (including stimulation and/or recording)

63610 Stereotactic stimulation of spinal cord, percutaneous, separate procedure not followed by other surgery

63615 Stereotactic biopsy, aspiration, or excision of lesion, spinal cord

NEUROSTIMULATORS, SPINAL

63650 Percutaneous implantation of neurostimulator electrodes; epidural

(63652 has been deleted)

63655 Laminectomy for implantation of neurostimulator electrodes; epidural

(63656 has been deleted)

63657 subdural

63658 subarachnoid

63660 Revision or removal of spinal neurostimulator electrodes

63685 Incision and subcutaneous placement of spinal neurostimulator pulse generator or receiver, direct or inductive coupling

63688 Revision or removal of implanted spinal neurostimulator pulse generator or receiver

63690 Electronic analysis of implanted neurostimulator pulse generator system (may include rate, pulse amplitude and duration, configuration of wave form, battery status, electrode selectability, output modulation, cycling, impedance and patient compliance measurements); without reprogramming of pulse generator

63691 with reprogramming of pulse generator

REPAIR

63700 Repair of meningocele; less than 5 cm diameter

63702 larger than 5 cm diameter

63704 Repair of myelomeningocele; less than 5 cm diameter

63706 larger than 5 cm diameter

(For complex skin closure, see Integumentary System)

63707 Repair of dural/CSF leak, not requiring laminectomy

(63708 has been deleted. To report, see 63707, 63709)

63709 Repair of dural/CSF leak or pseudomeningocele, with laminectomy

63710 Dural graft, spinal

(For laminectomy and section of dentate ligaments, with or without dural graft, cervical, see 63180, 63182)

SHUNT, SPINAL CSF

63740 Creation of shunt, lumbar, subarachnoid-peritoneal, -pleural, or other; including laminectomy

63741 percutaneous, not requiring laminectomy

63744 Replacement, irrigation or revision of lumbosubarachnoid shunt

63746 Removal of entire lumbosubarachnoid shunt system without replacement

63750 Insertion, subarachnoid catheter with reservoir and/or pump for intermittent or continuous infusion of drug, including laminectomy

63780 Insertion or replacement, subarachnoid or epidural catheter, with reservoir and/or pump for drug infusion, without laminectomy

(For pump refilling/reservoir and maintenance, see 96520, 96530)

EXTRACRANIAL NERVES, PERIPHERAL NERVES, AND AUTONOMIC NERVOUS SYSTEM

(For intracranial surgery on cranial nerves, see 61450, 61460, 61790)

INTRODUCTION/INJECTION OF ANESTHETIC AGENT (NERVE BLOCK), DIAGNOSTIC OR THERAPEUTIC

SOMATIC NERVES

64400* Injection, anesthetic agent; trigeminal nerve, any division or branch

64402* facial nerve

64405* greater occipital nerve

64408* vagus nerve

64410* phrenic nerve

64412* spinal accessory nerve

64413* cervical plexus

64415* brachial plexus

64417* axillary nerve

64418* suprascapular nerve

64420* intercostal nerve, single

64421* intercostal nerves, multiple, regional block

64425* ilioinguinal, iliohypogastric nerves

64430* pudendal nerve

64435* paracervical (uterine) nerve

64440* paravertebral nerve (thoracic, lumbar, sacral, coccygeal), single vertebral level

64441* paravertebral nerves, multiple levels (eg, regional block)

64442* paravertebral facet joint nerve, lumbar, single level

64443* paravertebral facet joint nerve, lumbar, each additional level

64445* sciatic nerve

64450* other peripheral nerve or branch

(For phenol destruction, see 64600-64640)

(For subarachnoid or subdural injection, see 62274-62277)

(For epidural or caudal injection, see 62278, 62279)

SYMPATHETIC NERVES

64505* Injection, anesthetic agent; sphenopalatine ganglion

64508* carotid sinus (separate procedure)

64510* stellate ganglion (cervical sympathetic)

64520* lumbar or thoracic (paravertebral sympathetic)

64530* celiac plexus, with or without radiologic monitoring

NEUROSTIMULATORS, PERIPHERAL NERVE

64550 Application of surface (transcutaneous) neurostimulator

64553 Percutaneous implantation of neurostimulator electrodes; cranial nerve

64555 peripheral nerve

64560 autonomic nerve

64565 neuromuscular

64573 Incision for implantation of neurostimulator electrodes; cranial nerve

64575 peripheral nerve

64577 autonomic nerve

64580 neuromuscular

64585 Revision or removal of peripheral neurostimulator electrodes

64590 Incision and subcutaneous placement of peripheral neurostimulator pulse generator or receiver, direct or inductive coupling

64595 Revision or removal of peripheral neurostimulator pulse generator or receiver

DESTRUCTION BY NEUROLYTIC AGENT (eg, CHEMICAL, THERMAL, ELECTRICAL, RADIOFREQUENCY)

SOMATIC NERVES

64600 Destruction by neurolytic agent, trigeminal nerve; supraorbital, infraorbital, mental, or inferior alveolar branch

64605 second and third division branches at foramen ovale

64610 second and third division branches at foramen ovale under radiologic monitoring

64612 Destruction by neurolytic agent (chemodenervation of muscle endplate); muscles enervated by facial nerve (eg, for blepharospasm, hemifacial spasm)

64613 cervical spinal muscles (eg, for spasmodic torticollis)

(For chemodenervation for strabismus involving the extaocular muscles, see 67345)

64620 Destruction by neurolytic agent; intercostal nerve

64622 paravertebral facet joint nerve, lumbar, single level

64623 paravertebral facet joint nerve, lumbar, each additional level

64630 pudendal nerve

64640 other peripheral nerve or branch

SYMPATHETIC NERVES

64680 Destruction by neurolytic agent, celiac plexus, with or without radiologic monitoring

NEUROPLASTY (EXPLORATION, NEUROLYSIS OR NERVE DECOMPRESSION)

Neuroplasty is the decompression or freeing of intact nerve from scar tissue, including external neurolysis and/or transposition.

(For internal neurolysis requiring use of operating microscope, use 64727)

(For facial nerve decompression, see 69720)

64702 Neuroplasty; digital, one or both, same digit

64704 nerve of hand or foot

64708 Neuroplasty, major peripheral nerve, arm or leg; other than specified

64712 sciatic nerve

64713 brachial plexus

64714 lumbar plexus

64716 Neuroplasty and/or transposition; cranial nerve (specify)

64718 ulnar nerve at elbow

64719 ulnar nerve at wrist

64721 median nerve at carpal tunnel

(For arthroscopic procedure, see 29848)

64722 Decompression; unspecified nerve(s) (specify)

64726 plantar digital nerve

64727 Internal neurolysis, requiring use of operating microscope (list separately in addition to code for neuroplasty)

(Neuroplasty includes external neurolysis)

TRANSECTION OR AVULSION OF NERVE

(For stereotactic lesion of gasserian ganglion, see 61790)

64732 Transection or avulsion of; supraorbital nerve

64734 infraorbital nerve

64736 mental nerve

64738 inferior alveolar nerve by osteotomy

64740 lingual nerve

64742 facial nerve, differential or complete

64744 greater occipital nerve

64746 phrenic nerve

(For section of recurrent laryngeal nerve, see 31595)

64752 vagus nerve (vagotomy), transthoracic

64755 vagi limited to proximal stomach (selective proximal vagotomy, proximal gastric vagotomy, parietal cell vagotomy, supra- or highly selective vagotomy)

64760 vagus nerve (vagotomy), abdominal

64761 pudendal nerve

(64762 has been deleted. To report, use 64761 with modifier -50 or 09950)

64763 Transection or avulsion of obturator nerve, extrapelvic, with or without adductor tenotomy

(64764 has been deleted. To report, use 64763 with modifier -50 or 09950)

64766 Transection or avulsion of obturator nerve, intrapelvic, with or without adductor tenotomy

(64768 has been deleted. To report, use 64766 with modifier -50 or 09950)

64771 Transection or avulsion of other cranial nerve, extradural

64772 Transection or avulsion of other spinal nerve, extradural

(For excision of tender scar, skin and subcutaneous tissue, with or without tiny neuroma, see 11400-11446, 13100-13300)

EXCISION-SOMATIC NERVES

(For Morton neurectomy, see 28080)

64774 Excision of neuroma; cutaneous nerve, surgically identifiable

64776 digital nerve, one or both, same digit

64778 digital nerve, each additional digit (list separately by this number)

64782 hand or foot, except digital nerve

64783 hand or foot, each additional nerve, except same digit (list separately by this number)

64784 major peripheral nerve, except sciatic

64786 sciatic nerve

64787 Implantation of nerve end into bone or muscle (list separately in addition to neuroma excision)

64788 Excision of neurofibroma or neurolemmoma; cutaneous nerve

64790 major peripheral nerve

64792 extensive (including malignant type)

64795 Biopsy of nerve

EXCISION-SYMPATHETIC NERVES

64802 Sympathectomy, cervical

(64803 has been deleted. To report, use 64802 with modifier -50 or 09950)

64804 Sympathectomy, cervicothoracic

(64806 has been deleted. To report, use 64804 with modifier -50 or 09950)

64809 Sympathectomy, thoracolumbar

(64811 has been deleted. To report, use 64809 with modifier -50 or 09950)

(64814 has been deleted. To report, use 64999)

64818 Sympathectomy, lumbar

(64819 has been deleted. To report, use 64818 with modifier -50 or 09950)

(64824 has been deleted. To report, use 64999)

NERVE REPAIR BY SUTURE (NEURORRHAPHY)

64830 Microdissection and/or microrepair of nerve (list separately in addition to code for nerve repair)

64831 Suture of digital nerve, hand or foot; one nerve

64832 each additional digital nerve

64834 Suture of one nerve, hand or foot; common sensory nerve

64835 median motor thenar

64836 ulnar motor

64837 Suture of each additional nerve, hand or foot

64840 Suture of posterior tibial nerve

64856 Suture of major peripheral nerve, arm or leg, except sciatic; including transposition

64857 without transposition

64858 Suture of sciatic nerve

64859 Suture of each additional major peripheral nerve

64861 Suture of; brachial plexus

64862 lumbar plexus

64864 Suture of facial nerve; extracranial

64865 intratemporal, with or without grafting

64866 Anastomosis; facial-spinal accessory

64868 facial-hypoglossal

64870 facial-phrenic

64872 Suture of nerve; requiring secondary or delayed suture (list separately in addition to code for primary neurorrhaphy)

64874 requiring extensive mobilization, or transposition of nerve (list separately in addition to code for nerve suture)

64876 requiring shortening of bone of extremity (list separately in addition to code for nerve suture)

NEURORRHAPHY WITH NERVE GRAFT

64885 Nerve graft (includes obtaining graft), head or neck; up to 4 cm in length

64886 more than 4 cm in length

64890 Nerve graft (includes obtaining graft), single strand, hand or foot; up to 4 cm length

64891 more than 4 cm length

64892 Nerve graft (includes obtaining graft), single strand, arm or leg; up to 4 cm length

64893 more than 4 cm length

64895 Nerve graft (includes obtaining graft), multiple strands (cable), hand or foot; up to 4 cm length

64896 more than 4 cm length

64897 Nerve graft (includes obtaining graft), multiple strands (cable), arm or leg; up to 4 cm length

64898 more than 4 cm length

64901 Nerve graft, each additional nerve; single strand

64902 multiple strands (cable)

64905 Nerve pedicle transfer; first stage

64907 second stage

OTHER PROCEDURES

64999 Unlisted procedure, nervous system

Eye and Ocular Adnexa

(For diagnostic and treatment ophthalmological services, see medicine, ophthalmology, and 92002 et seq)

EYEBALL

REMOVAL OF EYE

65091 Evisceration of ocular contents; without implant

65093 with implant

65101 Enucleation of eye; without implant

65103 with implant, muscles not attached to implant

65105 with implant, muscles attached to implant

(For conjunctivoplasty after enucleation, see 68320 et seq)

65110 Exenteration of orbit (does not include skin graft), removal of orbital contents; only

65112 with therapeutic removal of bone

65114 with muscle or myocutaneous flap

(For skin graft to orbit (split skin), see 15120, 15121; free, full thickness, see 15260, 15261)

(For eyelid repair involving more than skin, see 67930 et seq)

SECONDARY IMPLANT PROCEDURES

An ocular implant is an implant inside muscular cone; an orbital implant is an implant outside muscular cone.

65125 Modification of ocular implant (eg, drilling receptacle for prosthesis appendage) (separate procedure)

65130 Insertion of ocular implant secondary; after evisceration, in scleral shell

65135 after enucleation, muscles not attached to implant

65140 after enucleation, muscles attached to implant

65150 Reinsertion of ocular implant; with or without conjunctival graft

65155 with use of foreign material for reinforcement and/or attachment of muscles to implant

65175 Removal of ocular implant

(For orbital implant (implant outside muscle cone) insertion, see 67550; removal, see 67560)

REMOVAL OF OCULAR FOREIGN BODY

(For removal of implanted material: ocular implant, see 65175; anterior segment implant, see 65920; posterior segment implant, see 67120; orbital implant, see 67560)

(For diagnostic x-ray for foreign body, see 70030)

(For diagnostic echography for foreign body, see 76529)

(For removal of foreign body from orbit: frontal approach, see 67413; lateral approach, see 67430; transcranial approach, see 61334)

(For removal of foreign body from eyelid, embedded, see 67938)

(For removal of foreign body from lacrimal system, see 68530)

65205* Removal of foreign body, external eye; conjunctival superficial

65210* conjunctival embedded (includes concretions), subconjunctival, or scleral nonperforating

65220* corneal, without slit lamp

65222* corneal, with slit lamp

(For repair of corneal laceration with foreign body, see 65275)

(65230 has been deleted. To report, use 65235)

65235 Removal of foreign body, intraocular; from anterior chamber or lens

(65240, 65245 have been deleted. To report, use 65235)

(For removal of implanted material from anterior segment, see 65920)

65260 from posterior segment, magnetic extraction, anterior or posterior route

65265 from posterior segment, nonmagnetic extraction

(For removal of implanted material from posterior segment, see 67120)

REPAIR OF LACERATION OF EYEBALL

(For fracture of orbit, see 21385 et seq)

(For repair of wound of eyelid, skin, linear, simple, see 12011-12018; intermediate, layered closure, see 12051-12057; linear, complex, see 13150-13300; other, see 67930, 67935)

(For repair of wound of lacrimal system, see 68700)

(For repair of operative wound, see 66250)

65270* Repair of laceration; conjunctiva, with or without nonperforating laceration sclera, direct closure

65272 conjunctiva, by mobilization and rearrangement, without hospitalization

65273 conjunctiva, by mobilization and rearrangement, with hospitalization

65275 cornea, nonperforating, with or without removal foreign body

65280 cornea and/or sclera, perforating, not involving uveal tissue

65285 cornea and/or sclera, perforating, with reposition or resection of uveal tissue

65286 application of tissue glue, wounds of cornea and/or sclera

(Repair of laceration includes use of conjunctival flap and restoration of anterior chamber, by air or saline injection when indicated)

(For repair of iris or ciliary body, see 66680)

65290 Repair of wound, extraocular muscle, tendon and/or Tenon's capsule

ANTERIOR SEGMENT—CORNEA

EXCISION

(65300 has been deleted)

65400 Excision of lesion, cornea (keratectomy, lamellar, partial), except pterygium

65410* Biopsy of cornea

65420 Excision or transposition of pterygium; without graft

65426 with graft

REMOVAL OR DESTRUCTION

65430* Scraping of cornea, diagnostic, for smear and/or culture

65435* Removal of corneal epithelium; with or without chemocauterization (abrasion, curettage)

65436 with application of chelating agent (eg, EDTA)

(65445 has been deleted. To report, use 65450)

65450 Destruction of lesion of cornea by cryotherapy, photocoagulation or thermocauterization

(65455 has been deleted. To report, use 65450)

65600 Tattoo cornea, mechanical or chemical

KERATOPLASTY

(Keratoplasty excludes refractive keratoplasty procedures, 65760, 65765, and 65767)

(Corneal transplant includes use of fresh or preserved grafts, and preparation of donor material)

65710 Keratoplasty (corneal transplant); lamellar

(65720, 65725 have been deleted. To report, see 65710)

65730 penetrating (except in aphakia)

(65740, 65745 have been deleted. To report, see 65730)

65750 penetrating (in aphakia)

65755 penetrating (in pseudophakia)

OTHER PROCEDURES

65760 Keratomileusis

65765 Keratophakia

65767 Epikeratoplasty

65770 Keratoprosthesis

65771 Radial keratotomy

65772 Corneal relaxing incision for correction of surgically induced astigmatism

65775 Corneal wedge resection for correction of surgically induced astigmatism

(For fitting of contact lens for treatment of disease, see 92070)

(For unlisted procedures on cornea, see 66999)

ANTERIOR SEGMENT—ANTERIOR CHAMBER

INCISION

65800* Paracentesis of anterior chamber of eye (separate procedure); with diagnostic aspiration of aqueous

65805* with therapeutic release of aqueous

65810 with removal of vitreous and/or discission of anterior hyaloid membrane, with or without air injection

65815 with removal of blood, with or without irrigation and/or air injection

(For injection, see 66020-66030)

(For removal of blood clot, see 65930)

65820 Goniotomy

(65825, 65830 have been deleted)

65850 Trabeculotomy ab externo

65855 Trabeculoplasty by laser surgery, one or more sessions (defined treatment series)

(If re-treatment is necessary after several months because of disease progression, a new treatment or treatment series should be reported with a modifier, if necessary, to indicate lesser or greater complexity)

(For trabeculectomy, see 66170)

OTHER PROCEDURES

• **65860** Severing adhesions of anterior segment, laser technique (separate procedure)

65865 Severing adhesions of anterior segment of eye, incisional technique (with or without injection of air or liquid) (separate procedure); goniosynechiae

(For trabeculoplasty by laser surgery, use 65855)

65870 anterior synechiae, except goniosynechiae

65875 posterior synechiae

65880 corneovitreal adhesions

(For laser surgery, use 66821)

65900 Removal of epithelial downgrowth, anterior chamber eye

65920 Removal of implanted material, anterior segment eye

65930 Removal of blood clot, anterior segment eye

66020 Injection, anterior chamber (separate procedure); air or liquid

66030* medication

(For unlisted procedures on anterior segment, see 66999)

ANTERIOR SEGMENT—ANTERIOR SCLERA

EXCISION

(For removal of intraocular foreign body, see 65235)

(For operations on posterior sclera, see 67250, 67255)

66130 Excision of lesion, sclera

66150 Fistulization of sclera for glaucoma; trephination with iridectomy

66155 thermocauterization with iridectomy

66160 sclerectomy with punch or scissors, with iridectomy

66165 iridencleisis or iridotasis

66170 trabeculectomy ab externo

(For trabeculotomy ab externo, see 65850)

(For repair of operative wound, see 66250)

66180 Aqueous shunt to extraocular reservoir, (eg, Molteno, Schocket, Denver-Krupin)

66185 Revision of aqueous shunt to extraocular reservoir

(For removal of implanted shunt, use 67120)

REPAIR

(For scleral procedures in retinal surgery, see 67101 et seq)

66220 Repair of scleral staphyloma; without graft

66225 with graft

(For scleral reinforcement, see 67250, 67255)

REVISION OPERATIVE WOUND

66250 Revision or repair of operative wound of anterior segment, any type, early or late, major or minor procedure

OTHER PROCEDURES

(For unlisted procedures on anterior sclera, see 66999)

ANTERIOR SEGMENT—IRIS, CILIARY BODY

IRIDOTOMY, IRIDECTOMY

66500 Iridotomy by stab incision (separate procedure); except transfixion

66505 with transfixion as for iris bombe

66600 Iridectomy, with corneoscleral or corneal section; for removal of lesion

66605 with cyclectomy

66625 peripheral for glaucoma (separate procedure)

66630 sector for glaucoma (separate procedure)

66635 "optical" (separate procedure)

(For "iridotomy" by photocoagulation, see 66761)

(For "coreoplasty" by photocoagulation, see 66762)

REPAIR

66680 Repair of iris, ciliary body (as for iridodialysis)

(For reposition or resection of uveal tissue with perforating wound of cornea or sclera, see 65285)

66682 Suture of iris, ciliary body (separate procedure) with retrieval of suture through small incision (eg, McCannel suture)

DESTRUCTION

66700 Ciliary body destruction; diathermy

(66701, 66702, 66721, 66741 have been deleted. To report, see 66700, 66710, 66720, 66740)

66710 cyclophotocoagulation

66720 cryotherapy

66740 cyclodialysis

▲**66761** Iridotomy/iridectomy by laser surgery (eg, for glaucoma) (one or more sessions)

66762 Iridoplasty by photocoagulation (one or more sessions) (eg, for improvement of vision, for widening of anterior chamber angle)

66770 Destruction of cyst or lesion iris or ciliary body (nonexcisional procedure)

(For excision lesion iris, ciliary body, see 66600, 66605; for removal epithelial downgrowth, see 65900)

OTHER PROCEDURES

(For unlisted procedures on iris, ciliary body, see 66999)

ANTERIOR SEGMENT—LENS

INCISION

(66800, 66801 have been deleted. To report, use 66999)

(66802 has been deleted)

66820 Discission of secondary membraneous cataract (opacified posterior lens capsule and/or anterior hyaloid; stab incision technique (Ziegler or Wheeler knife)

66821 laser surgery (eg, YAG laser) (one or more stages)

● **66825** Repositioning of intraocular lens prosthesis, requiring an incision (separate procedure)

REMOVAL CATARACT

Lateral canthotomy, iridectomy, iridotomy, anterior capsulotomy, posterior capsulotomy, the use of viscoelastic agents, enzymatic zonulysis, use of other pharmacologic agents, and subconjunctival or sub-tenon injections are included as part of the code for the extraction of lens.

66830 Removal of secondary membranous cataract (opacified posterior lens capsule and/or anterior hyaloid) with corneo-scleral section, with or without iridectomy (iridocapsulotomy, iridocapsulectomy)

66840 Removal of lens material; aspiration technique, one or more stages

66850 phacofragmentation technique (mechanical or ultrasonic) (eg, phacoemulsification), with aspiration

66852 pars plana approach, with or without vitrectomy

(66915 has been deleted)

66920 intracapsular

66930 intracapsular, for dislocated lens

66940 extracapsular (other than 66840, 66850, 66852)

(66945 has been deleted. To report, see 66920-66940)

(For removal of intralenticular foreign body without lens extraction, see 65235)

(For repair of operative wound, see 66250)

(66980 has been deleted. To report, see 66983, 66984)

66983 Intracapsular cataract extraction with insertion of intraocular lens prosthesis (one stage procedure)

66984 Extracapsular cataract removal with insertion of intraocular lens prosthesis (one stage procedure), manual or mechanical technique (eg, irrigation and aspiration or phacoemulsification)

66985 Insertion of intraocular lens prosthesis (secondary implant), not associated with concurrent cataract removal

(To code implant at time of concurrent cataract surgery, use 66983 or 66984)

(For intraocular lens prosthesis supplied by physician, use 99070)

(For ultrasonic determination of intraocular lens power, use 76519)

(For removal of implanted material from anterior segment, use 65920)

(For secondary fixation (separate procedure), use 66682)

66986 Exchange of intraocular lens

66999 Unlisted procedure, anterior segment of eye

POSTERIOR SEGMENT—VITREOUS

67005 Removal of vitreous, anterior approach (open sky technique or limbal incision); partial removal

67010 subtotal removal with mechanical vitrectomy

(For removal of vitreous by paracentesis of anterior chamber, see 65810)

(For removal of corneovitreal adhesions, see 65880)

67015 Aspiration or release of vitreous, subretinal or choroidal fluid, pars plana approach (posterior sclerotomy)

67025 Injection of vitreous substitute, pars plana or limbal approach, (fluid-gas exchange), with or without aspiration (separate procedure)

67028 Intravitreal injection of a pharmacologic agent (separate procedure)

67030 Discission of vitreous strands (without removal), pars plana approach

67031 Severing of vitreous strands, vitreous face adhesions, sheets, membranes or opacities, laser surgery (one or more stages)

(67035 has been deleted. To report, use 67036)

67036 Vitrectomy, mechanical, pars plana approach;

67038 with epiretinal membrane stripping

67039 with focal endolaser photocoagulation

67040 with endolaser panretinal photocoagulation

(For associated lensectomy, see 66850)

(For use of vitrectomy in retinal detachment surgery, see 67108)

(For associated removal of foreign body, see 65260, 65265)

(For unlisted procedures on vitreous, see 67299)

POSTERIOR SEGMENT—RETINAL DETACHMENT

REPAIR

(If diathermy, cryotherapy and/or photocoagulation are combined, report under principal modality used)

67101 Repair of retinal detachment, one or more sessions; cryotherapy or diathermy, with or without drainage of subretinal fluid

(67102, 67103 have been deleted. To report, use 67101)

(67104, 67106 have been deleted. To report, use 67105)

67105 photocoagulation (laser or xenon arc, one or more sessions), with or without drainage of subretinal fluid

67107 scleral buckling (such as lamellar excision, imbrication or encircling procedure), with or without implant, may include procedures 67101, 67105

67108 with vitrectomy, any method, with or without air or gas tamponade, with or without focal endolaser photocoagulation, may include procedures 67101-67107 and/or removal of lens by same technique

67109 by technique other than 67101-67108 and 67110

67110 by injection of air or other gas (eg, pneumoretinopexy)

67112 previously operated upon, any technique

(For aspiration or drainage of subretinal or subchoroidal fluid, see 67015)

67115 Release of encircling material (posterior segment)

67120 Removal of implanted material, posterior segment; extraocular

67121 intraocular

(For removal from anterior segment, use 65920)

(For removal of foreign body, see 65260, 65265)

PROPHYLAXIS

Repetitive services. The services listed below are often performed in multiple sessions or groups of sessions. The methods of reporting vary. The following descriptors are intended to include all sessions in a defined treatment period.

67141 Prophylaxis of retinal detachment (eg, retinal break, lattice degeneration) without drainage, one or more sessions; cryotherapy, diathermy

(67142, 67143 have been deleted. To report, use 67141)

(67144, 67146 have been deleted. To report, use 67145)

67145 photocoagulation (laser or xenon arc)

POSTERIOR SEGMENT—OTHER PROCEDURES

DESTRUCTION—RETINA, CHOROID

67208 Destruction of localized lesion of retina (eg, maculopathy, choroidopathy, small tumors), one or more sessions; cryotherapy, diathermy

67210 photocoagulation (laser or xenon arc)

(67212, 67213 have been deleted. To report, use 67208)

(67214, 67216 have been deleted. To report, use 67210)

67218 radiation by implantation of source (includes removal of source)

(67222, 67223 have been deleted. To report, use 67227)

(67224, 67226 have been deleted. To report, use 67228)

67227 Destruction of extensive or progressive retinopathy (eg, diabetic retinopathy), one or more sessions; cryotherapy, diathermy

67228 photocoagulation (laser or xenon arc)

(For unlisted procedures on retina, see 67299)

SCLERAL REPAIR

(For excision lesion sclera, see 66130)

67250 Scleral reinforcement (separate procedure); without graft

67255 with graft

(For repair scleral staphyloma, see 66220, 66225)

67299 Unlisted procedure, posterior segment

OCULAR ADNEXA—EXTRAOCULAR MUSCLES

67311 Strabismus surgery, recession or resection procedure (patient not previously operated on); one horizontal muscle

67312 two horizontal muscles

(67313 has been deleted)

67314 one vertical muscle (excluding superior oblique)

67316 two or more vertical muscles (excluding superior oblique)

(For adjustable sutures, use 67335 in addition to primary procedure reflecting number of muscles operated on)

67318 Strabismus surgery, any procedure (patient not previously operated on), superior oblique muscle

(Use 67320, 67331, 67332, 67335, 67340, 67343 in addition to code for primary strabismus surgery (67311-67318))

67320 Transposition procedure (eg, for paretic extraocular muscle), any extraocular muscle (specify)

67331 Strabismus surgery on patient with previous eye surgery or injury that did not involve the extraocular muscles

67332 Strabismus surgery on patient with scarring of extraocular muscles (eg, prior ocular injury, strabismus or retinal detachment surgery) or restrictive myopathy (eg, dysthyroid ophthalmopathy)

67334 Strabismus surgery by posterior fixation suture technique, with or without muscle recession

67335 Placement of adjustable suture(s) during strabismus surgery, including postoperative adjustment(s) of suture(s) (Report in addition to code for specific strabismus surgery)

(Use also code for conventional muscle surgery, 67311-67334, to identify number of muscles involved)

67340 Strabismus surgery involving exploration and/or repair of detached extraocular muscle(s)

67343 Release of extensive scar tissue without detaching extraocular muscle (separate procedure)

67345 Chemodenervation of extraocular muscle

(For chemodenervation for blepharospasm and other neurological disorders, see 64612 and 64613)

OTHER PROCEDURES

67350 Biopsy of extraocular muscle

(For repair of wound, extraocular muscle, tendon or Tenon's capsule, see 65290)

67399 Unlisted procedure, ocular muscle

OCULAR ADNEXA—ORBIT

EXPLORATION, EXCISION, DECOMPRESSION

67400 Orbitotomy without bone flap (frontal or transconjunctival approach); for exploration, with or without bone biopsy

67405 with drainage only

67412 with removal of lesion

67413 with removal of foreign body

67414 with removal of bone for decompression

67415 Fine needle aspiration of orbital contents

(For exenteration, enucleation, and repair, see 65101 et seq; for optic nerve decompression, see 67570)

67420 Orbitotomy with bone flap or window, lateral approach (eg, Kroenlein); with removal of lesion

67430 with removal of foreign body

67440 with drainage

67445 with removal of bone for decompression

(For optic nerve sheath decompression, see 67570)

67450 for exploration, with or without biopsy

(For orbitotomy, transcranial approach, see 61330-61334)

(For orbital implant, see 67550, 67560)

(For removal of eyeball or for repair after removal, see 65091-65175)

OTHER PROCEDURES

67500* Retrobulbar injection; medication (separate procedure, does not include supply of medication)

67505 alcohol

(67510 has been deleted. To report, use 67599)

67515* Injection of therapeutic agent into Tenon's capsule

(For subconjunctival injection, see 68200)

67550 Orbital implant (implant outside muscle cone); insertion

67560 removal or revision

(For ocular implant (implant inside muscle cone), see 65093-65105, 65130-65175)

(For treatment of fractures of malar area, orbit, see 21355 et seq)

67570 Optic nerve decompression (eg, incision or fenestration of optic nerve sheath)

67599 Unlisted procedure, orbit

OCULAR ADNEXA—EYELIDS

INCISION

67700* Blepharotomy, drainage of abscess, eyelid

67710* Severing of tarsorrhaphy

67715* Canthotomy (separate procedure)

(For canthoplasty, see 67950)

(For division of symblepharon, see 68340)

EXCISION OR REMOVAL OF LESION INVOLVING MORE THAN SKIN (ie, INVOLVING LID MARGIN, TARSUS, AND/OR PALPEBRAL CONJUNCTIVA)

(For removal of lesion, involving mainly skin of eyelid, see 11440-11446; 11640-11646; 17000-17010)

(For repair of wounds, blepharoplasty, grafts, reconstructive surgery, see 67930-67975)

67800 Excision of chalazion; single

67801 multiple, same lid

67805 multiple, different lids

67808 under general anesthesia and/or requiring hospitalization, single or multiple

67810* Biopsy of eyelid

67820* Correction of trichiasis; epilation, by forceps only

67825* epilation, (eg, by electrosurgery or cryotherapy)

67830 incision of lid margin

67835 incision of lid margin, with free mucous membrane graft

67840* Excision of lesion of eyelid (except chalazion) without closure or with simple direct closure

(For excision and repair of eyelid by reconstructive surgery, see 67961, 67966)

67850* Destruction of lesion of lid margin (up to 1 cm)

(For chemosurgery technique of malignancies of skin, see 17304-17310)

(For initiation or follow-up care of topical chemotherapy (eg, 5-FU or similar agents), see appropriate office visits)

TARSORRHAPHY

67875 Temporary closure of eyelids by suture (eg, Frost suture)

67880 Construction of intermarginal adhesions, median tarsorrhaphy, or canthorrhaphy;

67882 with transposition of tarsal plate

(For severing of tarsorrhaphy, see 67710)

(For canthoplasty, reconstruction canthus, see 67950)

(For canthotomy, see 67715)

REPAIR OF BROW PTOSIS, BLEPHAROPTOSIS, LID RETRACTION

67900 Repair of brow ptosis (supraciliary, mid-forehead or coronal approach)

(For forehead rhytidectomy, see 15824)

67901 Repair of blepharoptosis; frontalis muscle technique with suture or other material

67902 frontalis muscle technique with fascial sling (includes obtaining fascia)

67903 (tarso)levator resection or advancement, internal approach

67904 (tarso)levator resection or advancement, external approach

67906 superior rectus technique with fascial sling (includes obtaining fascia)

(67907 has been deleted. To report, use 67999)

67908 conjunctivo-tarso-Muller's muscle-levator resection (eg, Fasanella-Servat type)

67909 Reduction of overcorrection of ptosis

67911 Correction of lid retraction

(For obtaining autogenous graft materials, see 20920, 20922 or 20926)

REPAIR ECTROPION, ENTROPION

(For correction trichiasis by mucous membrane graft, see 67835)

67914 Repair of ectropion; suture

67915 thermocauterization

67916 blepharoplasty, excision tarsal wedge

67917 blepharoplasty, extensive (eg, Kuhnt-Szymanowski or tarsal strip operations)

(For correction of everted punctum, see 68705)

67921 Repair of entropion; suture

67922 thermocauterization

67923 blepharoplasty, excision tarsal wedge

67924 blepharoplasty, extensive (eg, Wheeler operation)

(For repair of cicatricial ectropion or entropion requiring scar excision or skin graft, see also 67961 et seq)

RECONSTRUCTIVE SURGERY, BLEPHAROPLASTY INVOLVING MORE THAN SKIN (ie, INVOLVING LID MARGIN, TARSUS, AND/OR PALPEBRAL CONJUNCTIVA)

67930 Suture of recent wound, eyelid, involving lid margin, tarsus, and/or palpebral conjunctiva) direct closure; partial thickness

67935 full thickness

67938 Removal of embedded foreign body, eyelid

(For repair of skin of eyelid, see 12011-12018; 12051-12057; 13150, 13152, 13300)

(For tarsorrhaphy, canthorrhaphy, see 67880, 67882)

(For repair of blepharoptosis and lid retraction, see 67901-67911)

(For blepharoplasty for entropion, ectropion, see 67916, 67917, 67923, 67924)

(For correction of blepharochalasis (blepharorhytidectomy), see 15820-15823)

(For repair of skin of eyelid, adjacent tissue transfer, see 14060, 14061; preparation for graft, see 15000; free graft, see 15120, 15121, 15260, 15261)

(For excision of lesion of eyelid, see 67800 et seq)

(For repair of lacrimal canaliculi, see 68700)

67950 Canthoplasty (reconstruction of canthus)

67961 Excision and repair of eyelid, involving lid margin, tarsus, conjunctiva, canthus, or full thickness, may include preparation for skin graft or pedicle flap with adjacent tissue transfer or rearrangement; up to one-fourth of lid margin

67966 over one-fourth of lid margin

(For canthoplasty, see 67950)

(For free skin grafts, see 15120, 15121, 15260, 15261)

(For tubed pedicle flap preparation, see 15576; for delay, see 15630; for attachment, see 15630)

67971 Reconstruction of eyelid, full thickness by transfer of tarsoconjunctival flap from opposing eyelid; up to two-thirds of eyelid, one stage or first stage

67973 total eyelid, lower, one stage or first stage

67974 total eyelid, upper, one stage or first stage

67975 second stage

OTHER PROCEDURES

67999 Unlisted procedure, eyelids

OCULAR ADNEXA—CONJUNCTIVA

(For removal of foreign body, see 65205 et seq)

INCISION, DRAINAGE

68020 Incision of conjunctiva, drainage of cyst

68040 Expression of conjunctival follicles, eg, for trachoma

EXCISION, DESTRUCTION

68100 Biopsy of conjunctiva

68110 Excision of lesion, conjunctiva; up to 1 cm

68115 over 1 cm

68130 with adjacent sclera

68135* Destruction of lesion, conjunctiva

INJECTION

(For injection into Tenon's capsule or retrobulbar injection, see 67500-67515)

68200* Subconjunctival injection

CONJUNCTIVOPLASTY

(For wound repair, see 65270-65273)

68320 Conjunctivoplasty; with conjunctival graft or extensive rearrangement

68325 with buccal mucous membrane graft (includes obtaining graft)

68326 Conjunctivoplasty, reconstruction cul-de-sac; with conjunctival graft or extensive rearrangement

68328 with buccal mucous membrane graft (includes obtaining graft)

68330 Repair of symblepharon; conjunctivoplasty, without graft

68335 with free graft conjunctiva or buccal mucous membrane (includes obtaining graft)

68340 division of symblepharon, with or without insertion of conformer or contact lens

OTHER PROCEDURES

68360 Conjunctival flap; bridge or partial (separate procedure)

68362 total (such as Gunderson thin flap or purse string flap)

(For conjunctival flap for perforating injury, see 65280, 65285)

(For repair of operative wound, see 66250)

(For removal of conjunctival foreign body, see 65205, 65210)

68399 Unlisted procedure, conjunctiva

OCULAR ADNEXA—LACRIMAL SYSTEM

INCISION

68400 Incision, drainage of lacrimal gland

68420 Incision, drainage of lacrimal sac (dacryocystotomy or dacryocystostomy)

68440* Snip incision of lacrimal punctum

EXCISION

68500 Excision of lacrimal gland (dacryoadenectomy), except for tumor; total

68505 partial

68510 Biopsy of lacrimal gland

68520 Excision of lacrimal sac (dacryocystectomy)

68525 Biopsy of lacrimal sac

68530 Removal of foreign body or dacryolith, lacrimal passages

68540 Excision of lacrimal gland tumor; frontal approach

68550 involving osteotomy

REPAIR

68700 Plastic repair of canaliculi

68705 Correction of everted punctum, cautery

68720 Dacryocystorhinostomy (fistulization of lacrimal sac to nasal cavity)

68745 Conjunctivorhinostomy (fistulization of conjunctiva to nasal cavity); without tube

68750 with insertion of tube or stent

▲**68760** Closure of the lacrimal punctum; by thermocauterization, ligation, or laser surgery

● **68761** by plug, each

68770 Closure of lacrimal fistula (separate procedure)

PROBING AND RELATED PROCEDURES

68800* Dilation of lacrimal punctum, with or without irrigation, unilateral or bilateral

68820* Probing of nasolacrimal duct, with or without irrigation, unilateral or bilateral;

68825 requiring general anesthesia

(See also 92018)

68830 with insertion of tube or stent

68840* Probing of lacrimal canaliculi, with or without irrigation

68850* Injection of contrast medium for dacryocystography

(For radiological supervision and interpretation, see 70170)

OTHER PROCEDURES

68899 Unlisted procedure, lacrimal system

Auditory System

(For diagnostic services (eg, audiometry, vestibular tests), see 92502 et seq)

EXTERNAL EAR

INCISION

69000* Drainage external ear, abscess or hematoma; simple

69005 complicated

69020* Drainage external auditory canal, abscess

69090 Ear piercing

EXCISION

69100 Biopsy external ear

69105 Biopsy external auditory canal

69110 Excision external ear; partial, simple repair

69120 complete amputation

(For reconstruction of ear, see 15120 et seq)

69140 Excision exostosis(es), external auditory canal

69145 Excision soft tissue lesion, external auditory canal

69150 Radical excision external auditory canal lesion; without neck dissection

69155 with neck dissection

(For resection of temporal bone, see 69535)

(For skin grafting, see 15000-15261)

REMOVAL FOREIGN BODY

69200 Removal foreign body from external auditory canal; without general anesthesia

69205 with general anesthesia

69210 Removal impacted cerumen (separate procedure), one or both ears

69220 Debridement, mastoidectomy cavity, simple (eg, routine cleaning)

(69221 has been deleted. To report, use 69220 with modifier -50 or 09950)

69222 Debridement, mastoidectomy cavity, complex (eg, with anesthesia or more than routine cleaning)

(69223 has been deleted. To report, use 69222 with modifier -50 or 09950)

REPAIR

(For suture of wound or injury of external ear, see 12011-14300)

69300 Otoplasty, protruding ear, with or without size reduction

(69301 has been deleted. To report, use 69300 with modifier -50 or 09950)

69310 Reconstruction of external auditory canal (meatoplasty) (eg, for stenosis due to trauma, infection), (separate procedure)

69320 Reconstruction external auditory canal for congenital atresia, single stage

(For combination with middle ear reconstruction, see 69631, 69641)

(For other reconstructive procedures with grafts (eg, skin, cartilage, bone), see 13150-15760, 21230-21235)

OTHER PROCEDURES

(For otoscopy under general anesthesia, see 92502)

69399 Unlisted procedure, external ear

MIDDLE EAR

INTRODUCTION

69400 Eustachian tube inflation, transnasal; with catheterization

69401 without catheterization

69405 Eustachian tube catheterization, transtympanic

69410 Focal application of phase control substance, middle ear (baffle technique)

INCISION

69420* Myringotomy including aspiration and/or eustachian tube inflation

69421* Myringotomy including aspiration and/or eustachian tube inflation requiring general anesthesia

69424 Ventilating tube removal when originally inserted by another physician

(69425 has been deleted. To report, use 69424 with modifier -50 or 09950)

(Tympanostomy 69431-69435 has been revised as 69433-69437)

69433* Tympanostomy (requiring insertion of ventilating tube), local or topical anesthesia

(69434 has been deleted. To report, use 69433 with modifier -50 or 09950)

69436 Tympanostomy (requiring insertion of ventilating tube), general anesthesia

(69437 has been deleted. To report, use 69436 with modifier -50 or 09950)

69440 Middle ear exploration through postauricular or ear canal incision

(For atticotomy, see 69601 et seq)

69450 Tympanolysis, transcanal

EXCISION

69501 Transmastoid antrotomy ("simple" mastoidectomy)

69502 Mastoidectomy; complete

69505 modified radical

69511 radical

(For skin graft, see 15000 et seq)

(For mastoidectomy cavity debridement, see 69220, 69222)

69530 Petrous apicectomy including radical mastoidectomy

69535 Resection temporal bone, external approach

(For middle fossa approach, see 69950-69970)

69540 Excision aural polyp

69550 Excision aural glomus tumor; transcanal

69552 transmastoid

69554 extended (extratemporal)

REPAIR

69601 Revision mastoidectomy; resulting in complete mastoidectomy

69602 resulting in modified radical mastoidectomy

69603 resulting in radical mastoidectomy

69604 resulting in tympanoplasty

(For planned secondary tympanoplasty after mastoidectomy, see 69631, 69632)

69605 with apicectomy

(For skin graft, see 15120, 15121, 15260, 15261)

69610 Tympanic membrane repair, with or without site preparation or perforation for closure, with or without patch

(69611 has been deleted. To report, see 69610)

69620 Myringoplasty (surgery confined to drumhead and donor area)

69631 Tympanoplasty without mastoidectomy (including canalplasty, atticotomy and/or middle ear surgery), initial or revision; without ossicular chain reconstruction

69632 with ossicular chain reconstruction (eg, postfenestration)

69633 with ossicular chain reconstruction and synthetic prosthesis (eg, partial ossicular replacement prosthesis, (PORP), total ossicular replacement prosthesis (TORP))

69635 Tympanoplasty with antrotomy or mastoidotomy (including canalplasty, atticotomy, middle ear surgery, and/or tympanic membrane repair); without ossicular chain reconstruction

69636 with ossicular chain reconstruction

69637 with ossicular chain reconstruction and synthetic prosthesis (eg, partial ossicular replacement prosthesis, (PORP), total ossicular replacement prosthesis (TORP))

69641 Tympanoplasty with mastoidectomy (including canalplasty, middle ear surgery, tympanic membrane repair); without ossicular chain reconstruction

69642 with ossicular chain reconstruction

69643 with intact or reconstructed wall, without ossicular chain reconstruction

69644 with intact or reconstructed canal wall, with ossicular chain reconstruction

69645 radical or complete, without ossicular chain reconstruction

69646 radical or complete, with ossicular chain reconstruction

69650 Stapes mobilization

69660 Stapedectomy or stapedotomy with reestablishment of ossicular continuity, with or without use of foreign material;

69661 with footplate drill out

69662 Revision of stapedectomy or stapedotomy

69666 Repair oval window fistula

69667 Repair round window fistula

69670 Mastoid obliteration (separate procedure)

(69675 Tympanic neurectomy has been revised as 69676)

69676 Tympanic neurectomy

(69677 has been deleted. To report, use 69676 with modifier -50 or 09950)

OTHER PROCEDURES

69700 Closure postauricular fistula, mastoid (separate procedure)

69710 Implantation or replacement of electromagnetic bone conduction hearing device in temporal bone

(Replacement procedure includes removal of old device)

69711 Removal or repair of electromagnetic bone conduction hearing device in temporal bone

69720 Decompression facial nerve, intratemporal; lateral to geniculate ganglion

69725 including medial to geniculate ganglion

69740 Suture facial nerve, intratemporal, with or without graft or decompression; lateral to geniculate ganglion

69745 including medial to geniculate ganglion

(For extracranial suture of facial nerve, see 64864)

69799 Unlisted procedure, middle ear

INNER EAR

INCISION, DESTRUCTION

69801 Labyrinthotomy, with or without cryosurgery or other nonexcisional destructive procedures or tack procedure; transcanal

69802 with mastoidectomy

69805 Endolymphatic sac operation; without shunt

69806 with shunt

69820 Fenestration semicircular canal

69840 Revision fenestration operation

EXCISION

69905 Labyrinthectomy; transcanal

69910 with mastoidectomy

69915 Vestibular nerve section, translabyrinthine approach

(For transcranial approach, see 69950)

INSERTION

69930 Cochlear device implantation, with or without mastoidectomy

OTHER PROCEDURES

69949 Unlisted procedure, inner ear

TEMPORAL BONE, MIDDLE FOSSA APPROACH

(For external approach, see 69535)

69950 Vestibular nerve section, transcranial approach

69955 Total facial nerve decompression and/or repair (may include graft)

69960 Decompression internal auditory canal

(69965 has been deleted. To report, use 69979)

69970 Removal of tumor, temporal bone

OTHER PROCEDURES

69979 Unlisted procedure, temporal bone, middle fossa approach

Radiology

(Including Nuclear Medicine and Diagnostic Ultrasound)

Guidelines

Items used by all physicians in reporting their services are presented in the **INTRODUCTION.** Some of the commonalities are repeated here for the convenience of those physicians referring to this section on **RADIOLOGY (INCLUDING NUCLEAR MEDICINE AND DIAGNOSTIC ULTRASOUND).** Other definitions and items unique to Radiology are also listed.

1. **SUBJECT LISTINGS** apply when radiological services are performed by or under the responsible supervision of a physician.

2. **MULTIPLE PROCEDURES:** It is appropriate to designate multiple procedures that are rendered on the same date by separate entries. This can be reported by using the multiple procedure modifier (-51 or 09951). See item 8 below for modifier definitions.

3. **SEPARATE PROCEDURES:** Some of the listed procedures are commonly carried out as an integral part of a total service, and as such, do not warrant a separate identification. When, however, such a procedure is performed independently of, and is not immediately related to, other services, it may be listed as a "separate procedure." Thus, when a procedure that is ordinarily a component of a larger procedure is performed alone for a specific purpose, it may be reported as a separate procedure.

4. **SUBSECTION INFORMATION:** Several of the subheadings or subsections have special needs or instructions unique to that section. Where these are indicated (eg, "Radiation Oncology") special **"NOTES"** will be presented preceding those procedural terminology listings, referring to that subsection specifically. If there is an "Unlisted Procedure" code number (see item 5 below) for the individual subsection, it will be shown. Those subsections with **"NOTES"** are as follows:

Subsection	Code Numbers
Diagnostic Ultrasound	76506-76999
Radiation Oncology	77261-77799
Nuclear Medicine	78000-79999

5. **UNLISTED SERVICE OR PROCEDURE:** A service or procedure may be provided that is not listed in this edition of CPT. When reporting such a service, the appropriate "Unlisted Procedure" code may be used to indicate the service, identifying it by "Special Report" as discussed in item 6. The "Unlisted Procedures" and accompanying codes for **RADIOLOGY (INCLUDING NUCLEAR MEDICINE AND DIAGNOSTIC ULTRASOUND)** are as follows:

   76499 Unlisted diagnostic radiologic procedure
   76999 Unlisted diagnostic ultrasound procedure
   77299 Unlisted procedure, therapeutic radiology, clinical treatment planning
   77399 Unlisted procedure, medical radiation physics, dosimetry and treatment devices
   77499 Unlisted procedure, therapeutic radiology clinical treatment management
   77799 Unlisted procedure, clinical brachytherapy
   78099 Unlisted endocrine procedure, diagnostic nuclear medicine
   78199 Unlisted hematopoietic, reticuloendothelial and lymphatic procedure, diagnostic nuclear medicine
   78299 Unlisted gastrointestinal procedure, diagnostic nuclear medicine
   78399 Unlisted musculoskeletal procedure, diagnostic nuclear medicine
   78499 Unlisted cardiovascular procedure, diagnostic nuclear medicine
   78599 Unlisted respiratory procedure, diagnostic nuclear medicine
   78699 Unlisted nervous system procedure, diagnostic nuclear medicine
   78799 Unlisted genitourinary procedure, diagnostic nuclear medicine
   78999 Unlisted miscellaneous procedure, diagnostic nuclear medicine
   79999 Unlisted radionuclide therapeutic procedure

6. **SPECIAL REPORT:** A service that is rarely provided, unusual, variable, or new may require a special report in determining medical appropriateness of the service. Pertinent information should include an adequate definition or description of the nature, extent, and need for the procedure; and the time, effort, and equipment necessary to provide the service. Additional items which may be included are:

   Complexity of symptoms, final diagnosis, pertinent physical findings, diagnostic and therapeutic procedures, concurrent problems, and follow-up care.

7. **SUPERVISION AND INTERPRETATION:** When a procedure is performed by two physicians, the radiologic portion of the procedure is designated as "radiological supervision and interpretation." When a physician performs both the procedure and provides imaging supervision and interpretation, a combination of procedure codes outside the 70000 series and imaging supervision and interpretation codes are to be used.

   (The Radiological Supervision and Interpretation codes are not applicable to the Radiation Oncology subsection.)

8. **MODIFIERS:** Listed services and procedures may be modified under certain circumstances. When applicable, the modifying circumstances should be identified by the addition of the appropriate modifier code, which may be reported in either of two ways. The modifier may be reported by a two digit number placed after the usual procedure number from which it is separated by a hyphen. Or the modifier may be reported by a separate five digit code that is used in addition to the procedure code. If more than one modifier is used, place the "Multiple Modifiers" code immediately after the procedure code. This indicates that one or more additional modifier codes will follow. Modifiers commonly used in **RADIOLOGY (INCLUDING NUCLEAR MEDICINE AND DIAGNOSTIC ULTRASOUND)** are as follows:

-22 Unusual Procedural Services: When the service(s) provided is greater than that usually required for the listed procedure, it may be identified by adding modifier '-22' to the usual procedure number or by use of the separate five digit modifier code 09922. A report may also be appropriate. Note: Modifier '-22' or 09922 may be utilized with computerized tomography numbers when additional slices are required or a more detailed examination is necessary.

-26 Professional Component: Certain procedures are a combination of a physician component and a technical component. When the physician component is reported separately, the service may be identified by adding the modifier '-26' to the usual procedure number or the service may be reported by use of the five digit modifier code 09926.

-32 Mandated Services: Services related to *mandated* consultation and/or related services (eg, PRO, 3rd party payor) may be identified by adding the modifier '-32' to the basic procedure or the service may be reported by use of the five digit modifier 09932.

-51 Multiple Procedures: When multiple procedures are performed on the same day or at the same session, the major procedure or service may be reported as listed. The secondary additional, or lesser procedure(s) or service(s) may be identified by adding the modifier '-51' to the secondary procedure or service code(s) or by use of the separate five digit modifier code 09951. This modifier may be used to report multiple medical procedures performed at the same session, as well as a combination of medical and surgical procedures, or several surgical procedures performed at the same operative session.

-52 Reduced Services: Under certain circumstances a service or procedure is partially reduced or eliminated at the physician's election. Under these circumstances the service provided can be identified by its usual procedure number and the addition of the modifier '-52,' signifying that the service is reduced. This provides a means of reporting reduced services without disturbing the identification of the basic service. Modifier code 09952 may be used as an alternative to modifier '-52.'

Note: Modifier '-52' or 09952 may be utilized with computerized tomography numbers for a limited study or a follow-up study.

-62 Two Surgeons: Under certain circumstances the skills of two surgeons (usually with different skills) may be required in the management of a specific surgical procedure. Under such circumstances the separate services may be identified by adding the modifier '-62' to the procedure number used by each surgeon for reporting his services. Modifier code 09962 may be used as an alternative to modifier '-62.'

-66 Surgical Team: Under some circumstances, highly complex procedures (requiring the concomitant services of several physicians, often of different specialties, plus other highly skilled, specially trained personnel and various types of complex equipment) are carried out under the "surgical team" concept. Such circumstances may be identified by each participating physician with the addition of the modifier '-66' to the basic procedure number used for reporting services. Modifier code 09966 may be used as an alternative to modifier '-66'.

-76 Repeat Procedure by Same Physician: The physician may need to indicate that a procedure or service was repeated subsequent to the original service. This circumstance may be reported by adding the modifier '-76' to the repeated service or the separate five digit modifier code 09976 may be used.

-77 Repeat Procedure by Another Physician: The physician may need to indicate that a basic procedure performed by another physician had to be repeated. This situation may be reported by adding modifier '-77' to the repeated service or the separate five digit modifier code 09977 may be used.

-78 Return to the Operating Room for a Related Procedure During the Postoperative Period: The physician may need to indicate that another procedure was performed during the postoperative period of the initial procedure. When this subsequent procedure is related to the first, and requires the use of the operating room, it may be reported by adding the modifier '-78' to the related procedure, or by using the separate five digit modifier 09978. (For repeat procedures on the same day, see -76).

-79 Unrelated Procedure or Service by the Same Physician During the Postoperative Period: The physician may need to indicate that the performance of a procedure or service during the postoperative period was unrelated to the original procedure. This circumstance may be reported by using the modifier '-79' or by using the separate five digit modifier 09979. (For repeat procedures on the same day, see -76).

-80 Assistant Surgeon: Surgical assistant services may be identified by adding the modifier '-80' to the usual procedure number(s) or by use of the separate five digit modifier code 09980.

-90 Reference (Outside) Laboratory: When laboratory procedures are performed by a party other than the treating or reporting physician, the procedure may be identified by adding the modifier '-90' to the usual procedure number or by using the separate five digit modifier code 09990.

-99 Multiple Modifiers: Under certain circumstances two or more modifiers may be necessary to completely delineate a service. In such situations modifier '-99' should be added to the basic procedure, and other applicable modifiers may be listed as part of the description of the service. Modifier code 09999 may be used as an alternative to modifier '-99.'

9. **WRITTEN REPORT(S):** A written report, signed by the interpreting physician, should be considered an integral part of a radiologic procedure or interpretation.

RADIOLOGY
(INCLUDING NUCLEAR MEDICINE AND DIAGNOSTIC ULTRASOUND)

Procedures

Diagnostic Radiology (Diagnostic Imaging)

HEAD AND NECK

(70002, 70003 have been deleted. To report, use 76499)

70010 Myelography, posterior fossa, radiological supervision and interpretation

(70011 (complete procedure) has been deleted, see 61055, 62284, 70010)

70015 Cisternography, positive contrast, radiological supervision and interpretation

(70016 (complete procedure) has been deleted, see 61055, 62284, 70015)

(70020, 70021 have been deleted. To report, use 76499)

(70022 has been deleted. To report CT guidance for stereotactic localization, use 76355)

70030 Radiologic examination, eye, for detection of foreign body

(70040, 70050 have been deleted)

70100 Radiologic examination, mandible; partial, less than four views

70110 complete, minimum of four views

70120 Radiologic examination, mastoids; less than three views per side

70130 complete, minimum of three views per side

70134 Radiologic examination, internal auditory meati, complete

70140 Radiologic examination, facial bones; less than three views

70150 complete, minimum of three views

70160 Radiologic examination, nasal bones, complete, minimum of three views

70170 Dacryocystography, nasolacrimal duct, radiological supervision and interpretation

(70171 (complete procedure) has been deleted, see 68850, 70170)

70190 Radiologic examination; optic foramina

70200 orbits, complete, minimum of four views

70210 Radiologic examination, sinuses, paranasal, less than three views

70220 Radiologic examination, sinuses, paranasal, complete, minimum of three views

(70230, 70231 have been deleted. To report, use 76499)

70240 Radiologic examination, sella turcica

70250 Radiologic examination, skull; less than four views, with or without stereo

70260 complete, minimum of four views, with or without stereo

70300 Radiologic examination, teeth; single view

70310 partial examination, less than full mouth

70320 complete, full mouth

70328 Radiologic examination, temporomandibular joint, open and closed mouth; unilateral

70330 bilateral

70332 Temporomandibular joint arthrography, radiological supervision and interpretation

(70333 (complete procedure) has been deleted, see 21116, 70332)

70336 Magnetic resonance (eg, proton) imaging, temporomandibular joint

70350 Cephalogram, orthodontic

70355 Orthopantogram

70360 Radiologic examination; neck, soft tissue

70370 pharynx or larynx, including fluoroscopy and/or magnification technique

70371 Complex dynamic pharyngeal and speech evaluation by cine or video recording

70373 Laryngography, contrast, radiological supervision and interpretation

(70374 (complete procedure) has been deleted, see 31708, 70373)

70380 Radiologic examination, salivary gland for calculus

70390 Sialography, radiological supervision and interpretation

(70391 (complete procedure) has been deleted, see 42550, 70390)

(70400, 70401 have been deleted. To report, use 76499)

70450 Computerized axial tomography, head or brain; without contrast material

70460 with contrast material(s)

70470 without contrast material, followed by contrast material(s) and further sections

(For coronal, sagittal, and/or oblique sections, see 76375)

70480 Computerized axial tomography, orbit, sella, or posterior fossa or outer, middle, or inner ear; without contrast material

70481 with contrast material(s)

70482 without contrast material, followed by contrast material(s) and further sections

(For coronal, sagittal, and/or oblique sections, see 76375)

70486 Computerized axial tomography, maxillofacial area; without contrast material

70487 with contrast material(s)

70488 without contrast material, followed by contrast material(s) and further sections

(For coronal, sagittal, and/or oblique sections, see 76375)

70490 Computerized axial tomography, soft tissue neck; without contrast material

70491 with contrast material(s)

70492 without contrast material followed by contrast material(s) and further sections

(For coronal, sagittal, and/or oblique sections, see 76375)

(For cervical spine, see 72125, 72126)

70540 Magnetic resonance (eg, proton) imaging; orbit, face, and neck

(70550 has been deleted. To report, use 70551)

70551 Magnetic resonance (eg, proton) imaging, brain (including brain stem); without contrast material

70552 with contrast material(s)

70553 without contrast material, followed by contrast material(s) and further sequences

Diagnostic Radiology

CHEST

(71000 has been deleted)

71010 Radiologic examination, chest; single view, frontal

71015 stereo, frontal

71020 Radiologic examination, chest, two views, frontal and lateral;

71021 with apical lordotic procedure

71022 with oblique projections

71023 with fluoroscopy

71030 Radiologic examination, chest, complete, minimum of four views;

71034 with fluoroscopy

(For separate chest fluoroscopy, see 76000)

71035 Radiologic examination, chest, special views (eg, lateral decubitus, Bucky studies)

71036 Needle biopsy of intrathoracic lesion, including follow-up films; fluoroscopic localization only, radiological supervision and interpretation

(71037 (complete procedure) has been deleted, see 32400, 32405, 71036)

71038 Fluoroscopic localization for transbronchial biopsy or brushing

71040 Bronchography, unilateral, radiological supervision and interpretation

(71041 (complete procedure) has been deleted, see 31656, 31708, 31710, 31715, 71040)

71060 Bronchography, bilateral, radiological supervision and interpretation

(71061 (complete procedure) has been deleted, see 31656, 31708, 31710, 31715, 71060)

71090 Insertion pacemaker, fluoroscopy and radiography, radiological supervision and interpretation

71100 Radiologic examination, ribs, unilateral; two views

71101 including posteroanterior chest, minimum of three views

71110 Radiologic examination, ribs, bilateral; three views

71111 including posteroanterior chest, minimum of four views

71120 Radiologic examination; sternum, minimum of two views

71130 sternoclavicular joint or joints, minimum of three views

71250 Computerized axial tomography, thorax; without contrast material

71260 with contrast material(s)

71270 without contrast material, followed by contrast material(s) and further sections

(For coronal, sagittal, and/or oblique sections, see 76375)

71550 Magnetic resonance (eg, proton) imaging, chest (eg, for evaluation of hilar and mediastinal lymphadenopathy)

SPINE AND PELVIS

72010 Radiologic examination, spine, entire, survey study, anteroposterior and lateral

72020 Radiologic examination, spine, single view, specify level

72040 Radiologic examination, spine, cervical; anteroposterior and lateral

72050 minimum of four views

72052 complete, including oblique and flexion and/or extension studies

72069 Radiologic examination, spine, thoracolumbar, standing (scoliosis)

72070 Radiologic examination, spine; thoracic, anteroposterior and lateral

72072 thoracic, anteroposterior and lateral, including swimmer's view of the cervicothoracic junction

72074 thoracic, complete, including obliques, minimum of four views

72080 thoracolumbar, anteroposterior and lateral

72090 scoliosis study, including supine and erect studies

72100 Radiologic examination, spine, lumbosacral; anteroposterior and lateral

72110 complete, with oblique views

72114 complete, including bending views

72120 Radiologic examination, spine, lumbosacral, bending views only, minimum of four views

Contrast material in CT of spine is either by intrathecal or intravenous injection. For intrathecal injection, use also 61055 or 62284. IV injection of contrast material is part of the CT procedure.

72125 Computerized axial tomography, cervical spine; without contrast material

72126 with contrast material

72127 without contrast material, followed by contrast material(s) and further sections

(For intrathecal injection procedure, see 61055, 62284)

72128 Computerized axial tomography, thoracic spine; without contrast material

72129 with contrast material

(For intrathecal injection procedure, see 61055, 62284)

72130 without contrast material, followed by contrast material(s) and further sections

(For intrathecal injection procedure, see 61055, 62284)

72131 Computerized axial tomography, lumbar spine; without contrast material

72132 with contrast material

72133 without contrast material, followed by contrast material(s) and further sections

(For intrathecal injection procedure, see 61055, 62284)

(For coronal, sagittal, and/or oblique sections, see 76375)

(72140 has been deleted. To report, see 72141-72149)

72141 Magnetic resonance (eg, proton) imaging, spinal canal and contents, cervical; without contrast material

72142 with contrast material(s)

(For cervical spinal canal imaging without contrast material followed by contrast material, use 72156)

(72143 has been deleted. To report, see 72146, 72147)

(72144 has been deleted. To report, see 72148, 72149)

(72145 has been deleted. To report, see 72125-72133)

72146 Magnetic resonance (eg, proton) imaging, spinal canal and contents, thoracic; without contrast material

72147 with contrast material(s)

(For thoracic spinal canal imaging without contrast material followed by contrast material, use 72157)

72148 Magnetic resonance (eg, proton) imaging, spinal canal and contents, lumbar; without contrast material

72149 with contrast material(s)

(For lumbar spinal canal imaging without contrast material followed by contrast material, use 72158)

72156 Magnetic resonance (eg, proton) imaging, spinal canal and contents, without contrast material, followed by contrast material(s) and further sequences; cervical

72157 thoracic

72158 lumbar

72170 Radiologic examination, pelvis; anteroposterior only

(72180 has been deleted. To report, use 72170)

72190 complete, minimum of three views

(For pelvimetry, see 74710)

72192 Computerized axial tomography, pelvis; without contrast material

72193 with contrast material(s)

72194 without contrast material, followed by contrast material(s) and further sections

(For coronal, sagittal, and/or oblique sections, see 76375)

72196 Magnetic resonance (eg, proton) imaging, pelvis

72200 Radiologic examination, sacroiliac joints; less than three views

72202 three or more views

72220 Radiologic examination, sacrum and coccyx, minimum of two views

72240 Myelography, cervical, radiological supervision and interpretation

(72241 (complete procedure) has been deleted, see 61055, 62284, 72240)

72255 Myelography, thoracic, radiological supervision and interpretation

(72256 (complete procedure) has been deleted, see 61055, 62284, 72255)

72265 Myelography, lumbosacral, radiological supervision and interpretation

(72266 (complete procedure) has been deleted, see 61055, 62284, 72265)

72270 Myelography, entire spinal canal, radiological supervision and interpretation

(72271 (complete procedure) has been deleted, see 61055, 62284, 72270)

72285 Diskography, cervical, radiological supervision and interpretation

(72286 (complete procedure) has been deleted, see 62291, 72285)

72295 Diskography, lumbar, radiological supervision and interpretation

(72296 (complete procedure) has been deleted, see 62290, 72295)

UPPER EXTREMITIES

73000 Radiologic examination; clavicle, complete

73010 scapula, complete

73020 Radiologic examination, shoulder; one view

73030 complete, minimum of two views

73040 Radiologic examination, shoulder, arthrography, radiological supervision and interpretation

(73041 (complete procedure) has been deleted, see 23350, 73040)

73050 Radiologic examination; acromioclavicular joints, bilateral, with or without weighted distraction

73060 humerus, minimum of two views

73070 Radiologic examination, elbow; anteroposterior and lateral views

73080 complete, minimum of three views

73085 Radiologic examination, elbow, arthrography, radiological supervision and interpretation

(73086 (complete procedure) has been deleted, see 24220, 73085)

73090 Radiologic examination; forearm, anteroposterior and lateral views

73092 upper extremity, infant, minimum of two views

73100 Radiologic examination, wrist; anteroposterior and lateral views

73110 complete, minimum of three views

73115 Radiologic examination, wrist, arthrography, radiological supervision and interpretation

(73116 (complete procedure) has been deleted, see 25246, 73115)

73120 Radiologic examination, hand; two views

73130 minimum of three views

73140 Radiologic examination, finger or fingers, minimum of two views

73200 Computerized axial tomography, upper extremity; without contrast material

73201 with contrast material(s)

73202 without contrast material, followed by contrast material(s) and further sections

(For coronal, sagittal, and/or oblique sections, see 76375)

73220 Magnetic resonance (eg, proton) imaging, upper extremity, other than joint

73221 Magnetic resonance (eg, proton) imaging, any joint of upper extremity

LOWER EXTREMITIES

73500 Radiologic examination, hip; unilateral, one view

73510 complete, minimum of two views

73520 Radiologic examination, hips, bilateral, minimum of two views of each hip, including anteroposterior view of pelvis

73525 Radiologic examination, hip, arthrography, radiological supervision and interpretation

(73526 (complete procedure) has been deleted, see 27093, 27095, 73525)

73530 Radiologic examination, hip, during operative procedure

(73531 has been deleted. To report, use 73530)

73540 Radiologic examination, pelvis and hips, infant or child, minimum of two views

73550 Radiologic examination, femur, anteroposterior and lateral views

73560 Radiologic examination, knee; anteroposterior and lateral views

73562 anteroposterior and lateral, with oblique(s), minimum of three views

73564 complete, including oblique(s), and tunnel, and/or patellar and/or standing views

73565 both knees, standing, anteroposterior

(73570 has been deleted. To report, use 73562, 73564)

73580 Radiologic examination, knee, arthrography, radiological supervision and interpretation

(73581 (complete procedure) has been deleted, see 27370, 73580)

73590 Radiologic examination; tibia and fibula, anteroposterior and lateral views

73592 lower extremity, infant, minimum of two views

73600 Radiologic examination, ankle; anteroposterior and lateral views

73610 complete, minimum of three views

73615 Radiologic examination, ankle, arthrography, radiological supervision and interpretation

(73616 (complete procedure) has been deleted, see 27648, 73615)

73620 Radiologic examination, foot; anteroposterior and lateral views

73630 complete, minimum of three views

73650 Radiologic examination; calcaneus, minimum of two views

73660 toe or toes, minimum of two views

73700 Computerized axial tomography, lower extremity; without contrast material

73701 with contrast material(s)

73702 without contrast material, followed by contrast material(s) and further sections

(For coronal, sagittal, and/or oblique sections, see 76375)

73720 Magnetic resonance (eg, proton) imaging, lower extremity, other than joint

73721 Magnetic resonance (eg, proton) imaging, any joint of lower extremity

ABDOMEN

74000 Radiologic examination, abdomen; single anteroposterior view

74010 anteroposterior and additional oblique and cone views

74020 complete, including decubitus and/or erect views

74022 complete acute abdomen series, including supine, erect, and/or decubitus views, upright PA chest

74150 Computerized axial tomography, abdomen; without contrast material

74160 with contrast material(s)

74170 without contrast material, followed by contrast material(s) and further sections

(For coronal, sagittal, and/or oblique sections, see 76375)

74181 Magnetic resonance (eg, proton) imaging, abdomen

GASTROINTESTINAL TRACT

(For percutaneous placement of gastrostomy tube, see 43750)

74210 Radiologic examination; pharynx and/or cervical esophagus

74220 esophagus

74230 Swallowing function, pharynx and/or esophagus, with cineradiography and/or video

74235 Removal of foreign body(s), esophageal, with use of balloon catheter, radiological supervision and interpretation

(For procedure, see 43215, 43247)

74240 Radiologic examination, gastrointestinal tract, upper; with or without delayed films, without KUB

74241 with or without delayed films, with KUB

74245 with small bowel, includes multiple serial films

74246 Radiological examination, gastrointestinal tract, upper, air contrast, with specific high density barium, effervescent agent, with or without glucagon; with or without delayed films, without KUB

74247 with or without delayed films, with KUB

74249 with small bowel follow-through

74250 Radiologic examination, small bowel, includes multiple serial films

74260 Duodenography, hypotonic

74270 Radiologic examination, colon; barium enema

(74275 has been deleted. To report, use 76499)

74280 air contrast with specific high density barium, with or without glucagon

74283 Barium enema, therapeutic, for reduction of intussusception

(74285 has been deleted. To report, see 74270, 74280)

74290 Cholecystography, oral contrast;

74291 additional or repeat examination or multiple day examination

74300 Cholangiography and/or pancreatography; during surgery

74301 additional set during surgery

74305 postoperative

(For biliary duct stone extraction, percutaneous, see 47630, 74327)

(74310, 74315 have been deleted. To report, use 76499)

74320 Cholangiography, percutaneous, transhepatic, radiological supervision and interpretation

(74321 (complete procedure) has been deleted, see 47500, 74320)

(74325, 74326 have been deleted. To report, use 76499)

74327 Postoperative biliary duct stone removal, percutaneous via T-tube tract, basket or snare (eg, Burhenne technique), radiological supervision and interpretation

(For procedure, see 47630)

74328 Endoscopic catheterization of the biliary ductal system, radiological supervision and interpretation

(For procedure, see 43260-43272 as appropriate)

74329 Endoscopic catheterization of the pancreatic ductal system, radiological supervision and interpretation

(For procedure, see 43260-43272 as appropriate)

74330 Combined endoscopic catheterization of the biliary and pancreatic ductal systems, radiological supervision and interpretation

(For procedure, see 43260-43272 as appropriate)

(74331 has been deleted. To report, see 43262)

74340 Introduction of long gastrointestinal tube (eg, Miller-Abbott), with multiple fluoroscopies and films

74350 Percutaneous placement of gastrostomy tube, radiological supervision and interpretation

(74351 (complete procedure) has been deleted, see 43246, 43750, 74350)

74355 Percutaneous placement of enteroclysis tube, radiological supervision and interpretation

(74356 (complete procedure) has been deleted, see 44015, 74355)

74360 Intraluminal dilation of strictures and/or obstructions (eg, esophagus), radiological supervision and interpretation

(74361 (complete procedure) has been deleted, see 43220, 43455, 74360)

74363 Percutaneous transhepatic dilatation of biliary duct stricture with or without placement of stent, radiological supervision and interpretation

(For procedure, see 47510, 47511, 47555, 47556)

URINARY TRACT

▲**74400** Urography (pyelography), intravenous, with or without KUB, with or without tomography;

74405 with special hypertensive contrast concentration and/or clearance studies

74410 Urography, infusion, drip technique and/or bolus technique;

74415 with nephrotomography

74420 Urography, retrograde, with or without KUB

74425 Urography, antegrade, (pyelostogram, nephrostogram, loopogram), radiological supervision and interpretation

(74426 (complete procedure) has been deleted, see 50394, 50684, 50690, 74425)

74430 Cystography, minimum of three views, radiological supervision and interpretation

(74431 (complete procedure) has been deleted, see 51600, 51605, 74430)

74440 Vasography, vesiculography, or epididymography, radiological supervision and interpretation

(74441 (complete procedure) has been deleted, see 52010, 55300, 74440)

74445 Corpora cavernosography, radiological supervision and interpretation

(74446 (complete procedure) has been deleted, use 54230, 74445)

74450 Urethrocystography, retrograde, radiological supervision and interpretation

(74451 (complete procedure) has been deleted, see 51610, 74450)

74455 Urethrocystography, voiding, radiological supervision and interpretation

(74456 (complete procedure) has been deleted, see 51600, 74455)

(74460, 74461 have been deleted. To report, use 76499)

74470 Radiologic examination, renal cyst study, translumbar, contrast visualization, radiological supervision and interpretation

(74471 (complete procedure) has been deleted, see 50390, 74470)

74475 Introduction of intracatheter or catheter into renal pelvis for drainage and/or injection, percutaneous, radiological supervision and interpretation

(74476 (complete procedure) has been deleted, see 50392-50398, 74475)

74480 Introduction of ureteral catheter or stent into ureter through renal pelvis for drainage and/or injection, percutaneous, radiological supervision and interpretation

(74481 (complete procedure) has been deleted, see 50392-50398, 74480)

(For transurethral surgery (ureter and pelvis), see 52320-52338)

74485 Dilation of nephrostomy, ureters, or urethra, radiological supervision and interpretation

(74486 (complete procedure) has been deleted, see 50395, 53600-53621, 74485)

(For dilation of ureter without radiologic guidance, use 52335)

(For change of nephrostomy or pyelostomy tube, use 50398)

GYNECOLOGICAL AND OBSTETRICAL

(For abdomen and pelvis, see 72170-72190, 74000-74170)

74710 Pelvimetry, with or without placental localization

(74720, 74725 have been deleted. To report, see 74000)

(74730, 74731 have been deleted. To report, use 76499)

74740 Hysterosalpingography, radiological supervision and interpretation

(74741 (complete procedure) has been deleted, see 58340, 74740)

• **74742** Transcervical catheterization of fallopian tube, radiological supervision and interpretation

(For procedure, see 58345)

(74760, 74761, 74770, 74771 have been deleted. To report, use 76499)

74775 Perineogram (eg, vaginogram, for sex determination or extent of anomalies)

Diagnostic Radiology (Diagnostic Imaging)

HEART

(For separate injection procedures for vascular radiology, see Surgery section, 36000-36299)

(For cardiac fluoroscopy, see 93280)

(For cardiac catheterization procedures, see 93501-93562)

75500 Angiocardiography by cineradiography, radiological supervision and interpretation

(75501 (complete procedure) has been deleted, see 93501-93536, 93542, 93543, 75500)

75505 Angiocardiography by serialography, single plane, radiological supervision and interpretation

(75506 (complete procedure) has been deleted, see 36400-36425 for intravenous procedure, 36100-36248 for intra-arterial procedure and 93501-93536, 93542, 93543, 75505)

75507 Angiocardiography by serialography, multi-plane, radiological supervision and interpretation

(75509 (complete procedure) has been deleted, see 36400-36425 for intravenous procedure, 36100-36248 for intra-arterial procedure and 93501-93536, 93542, 93543, 75507)

(75510, 75511 have been deleted. To report, use 76499)

75519 Cardiac radiography, selective cardiac catheterization, right side, radiological supervision and interpretation

(75520 (complete procedure) has been deleted, see 36400-36425 for intravenous procedure, 36100-36248 for intra-arterial procedure, and 93501, 93542, 75519)

75523 Cardiac radiography, selective cardiac catheterization, left side, radiological supervision and interpretation

(75524 (complete procedure) has been deleted, see 36400-36425 for intravenous procedure, 36100-36248 for intra-arterial procedure, and 93510-93514, 93524, 93543, 93546, 75523)

75527 Cardiac radiography, selective cardiac catheterization, right and left side, radiological supervision and interpretation

(75528 (complete procedure) has been deleted, see 36400-36425 for intravenous procedure, 36100-36248 for intra-arterial procedure, and 93526-93529, 93542, 93543, 75527)

75552 Magnetic resonance (eg, proton) imaging, myocardium

AORTA AND ARTERIES

Selective vascular catheterizations should be coded to include introduction and all lesser order selective catheterizations used in the approach (eg, the description for a selective right middle cerebral artery catheterization includes the introduction and placement catheterization of the right common and internal carotid arteries). Additional second and/or third order arterial catheterizations within the same family of arteries supplied by a single first order artery should be expressed by 36218 or 36248. Additional first order or higher catheterizations in vascular families supplied by a first order vessel different from a previously selected and coded family should be separately coded using the conventions described above.

(For intravenous procedure, see 36000-36013, 36400-36425 and 36100-36248 for intra-arterial procedure)

(For radiological supervision and interpretation, see 75600-75978)

75600 Aortography, thoracic, without serialography, radiological supervision and interpretation

(75601 (complete procedure) has been deleted, see 36000-36013, 36400-36425 for intravenous procedure, and 36100-36200 for intra-arterial procedure and 75600)

(For injection procedure, see 93544)

75605 Aortography, thoracic, by serialography, radiological supervision and interpretation

(75606 (complete procedure) has been deleted, see 36000-36013, 36400-36425 for intravenous procedure, and 36100-36200 for intra-arterial procedure and 75605)

(For injection procedure, see 93544)

(75620, 75621, 75622, 75623 have been deleted. To report, use 76499)

75625 Aortography, abdominal, by serialography, radiological supervision and interpretation

(75626, 75627 and 75628 have been deleted, see 36000-36013, 36400-36425 for intravenous procedure, and 36100-36200 for intra-arterial procedure and 75625)

(For injection procedure, see 93544)

75630 Aortography, abdominal plus bilateral iliofemoral lower extremity, catheter, by serialography, radiological supervision and interpretation

(75631 (complete procedure) has been deleted, see 36000-36013, 36400-36425 for intravenous procedure, and 36100-36200 and 36245-36248 for intra-arterial procedure and 75630)

75650 Angiography, cervicocerebral, catheter, including vessel origin, radiological supervision and interpretation

(75651-75657 (complete procedure) have been deleted, see 36000-36013, 36400-36425 for intravenous procedure, and 36100-36218 for intra-arterial procedure and 75650, 75660-75685 as appropriate)

75658 Angiography, brachial, retrograde, radiological supervision and interpretation

(75659 (complete procedure) has been deleted, see 36000-36013, 36400-36425 for intravenous procedure, and 36100-36218 for intra-arterial procedure and 75658)

75660 Angiography, external carotid, unilateral, selective, radiological supervision and interpretation

(75661 (complete procedure) has been deleted, see 36000-36013, 36400-36425 for intravenous procedure, and 36100-36218 and 75660)

75662 Angiography, external carotid, bilateral, selective, radiological supervision and interpretation

(75663 (complete procedure) has been deleted, see 36000-36013, 36400-36425 for intravenous procedure, and 36100-36218 for intra-arterial procedure and 75662)

75665 Angiography, carotid, cerebral, unilateral, radiological supervision and interpretation

(75667, 75669 (complete procedure) have been deleted, see 36000-36013, 36400-36425 for intravenous procedure, and 36100-36218 for intra-arterial procedure and 75665)

75671 Angiography, carotid, cerebral, bilateral, radiological supervision and interpretation

(75672, 75673 (complete procedure) have been deleted, see 36000-36013, 36400-36425 for intravenous procedure, and 36100-36218 for intra-arterial procedure and 75671)

75676 Angiography, carotid, cervical, unilateral, radiological supervision and interpretation

(75677, 75678 (complete procedure) have been deleted, see 36000-36013, 36400-36425 for intravenous procedure, and 36100-36218 for intra-arterial procedure and 75676)

75680 Angiography, carotid, cervical, bilateral, radiological supervision and interpretation

(75681, 75682 (complete procedure) have been deleted, see 36000-36013, 36400-36425 for intravenous procedure, and 36100-36218 for intra-arterial procedure and 75680)

75685 Angiography, vertebral, cervical, and/or intracranial, radiological supervision and interpretation

(75686 has been deleted)

(75687 (complete procedure) has been deleted, see 36000-36013, 36400-36425 for intravenous procedure, and 36100-36218 for intra-arterial procedure and 75685)

(75691 has been deleted)

(75690, 75692 (complete procedure) have been deleted, see 36000-36013, 36400-36425 for intravenous procedure, and 36100-36218 for intra-arterial procedure and 75685)

(75695, 75697 (complete procedure) have been deleted, see 36000-36013, 36400-36425 for intravenous procedure, and 36100-36218 for intra-arterial procedure and 75685)

(75696 has been deleted)

75705 Angiography, spinal, selective, radiological supervision and interpretation

(75706 (complete procedure) has been deleted, see 36000-36013, 36400-36425 for intravenous procedure, and 36100-36248 for intra-arterial procedure and 75705)

75710 Angiography, extremity, unilateral, radiological supervision and interpretation

(75711, 75712 (complete procedure) have been deleted, see 36000-36013, 36400-36425 for intravenous procedure, and 36100-36248 for intra-arterial procedure and 75710)

75716 Angiography, extremity, bilateral, radiological supervision and interpretation

(75717, 75718 (complete procedure) have been deleted, see 36000-36013, 36400-36425 for intravenous procedure, and 36100-36248 for intra-arterial procedure and 75716)

75722 Angiography, renal, unilateral, selective (including flush aortogram), radiological supervision and interpretation

(75723 (complete procedure) has been deleted, see 36000-36013, 36400-36425 for intravenous procedure, and 36100-36200 and 36245-36248 for intra-arterial procedure and 75722)

75724 Angiography, renal, bilateral, selective (including flush aortogram), radiological supervision and interpretation

(75725 (complete procedure) has been deleted, see 36000-36013, 36400-36425 for intravenous procedure, and 36100-36200 and 36245-36248 for intra-arterial procedure and 75724)

75726 Angiography, visceral, selective or supraselective, (with or without flush aortogram) radiological supervision and interpretation

(For selective angiography, each additional visceral vessel studied after basic examination, see 75774)

(75727, 75728 (complete procedure) have been deleted, see 36000-36013, 36400-36425 for intravenous procedure, and 36100-36248 for intra-arterial procedure and 75726)

75731 Angiography, adrenal, unilateral, selective, radiological supervision and interpretation

(75732 (complete procedure) has been deleted, see 36000-36013, 36400-36425 for intravenous procedure, and 36100-36200 and 36245-36248 for intra-arterial procedure and 75731)

75733 Angiography, adrenal, bilateral, selective, radiological supervision and interpretation

(75734 (complete procedure) has been deleted, see 36000-36013, 36400-36425 for intravenous procedure, and 36100-36200 and 36245-36248 for intra-arterial procedure and 75733)

75736 Angiography, pelvic, selective or supraselective, radiological supervision and interpretation

(75737, 75738 (complete procedure) have been deleted, see 36000-36013, 36400-36425 for intravenous procedure, and 36100-36200 and 36245-36248 for intra-arterial procedure and 75736)

75741 Angiography, pulmonary, unilateral, selective, radiological supervision and interpretation

(75742 (complete procedure) has been deleted, see 36000-36015, 36400-36425 for intravenous procedure and 75741)

(For injection procedure, see 93541)

75743 Angiography, pulmonary, bilateral, selective, radiological supervision and interpretation

(75744 (complete procedure) has been deleted, see 36000-36015, 36400-36425 for intravenous procedure and 75743)

(For injection procedure, see 93541)

75746 Angiography, pulmonary, by nonselective catheter or venous injection, radiological supervision and interpretation

(75747, 75748 (complete procedure) have been deleted, see 36000-36013, 36400-36425 for intravenous procedure, and 36100-36200 for intra-arterial procedure and 75746)

(For injection procedure, see 93541)

75750 Angiography, coronary, root injection, radiological supervision and interpretation

(75751 (complete procedure) has been deleted, see 36000-36013, 36400-36425 for intravenous procedure, and 36100-36200 for intra-arterial procedure and 75750)

(For introduction of catheter, injection procedure, see 93545, 93501-93536, 93546-93553)

75752 Angiography, coronary, unilateral selective injection, including left ventricular and supravalvular angiogram and pressure recording, radiological supervision and interpretation

(75753 (complete procedure) has been deleted, see 36100-36230 for intra-arterial procedure and 75752)

(For introduction of catheter, injection procedure, see 93501-93536, 93545-93553)

75754 Angiography, coronary, bilateral selective injection, including left ventricular and supravalvular angiogram and pressure recording, radiological supervision and interpretation

(75755 (complete procedure) has been deleted, see 36100-36230 for intra-arterial procedure and 75754)

(For introduction of catheter, injection procedure, see 93545, 93501-93536, 93546-93553)

75756 Angiography, internal mammary, radiological supervision and interpretation

(75757 (complete procedure) has been deleted, see 36000-36013, 36400-36425 for intravenous procedure, and 36100-36218 for intra-arterial procedure and 75756)

75762 Angiography, coronary bypass, unilateral selective injection, radiological supervision and interpretation

(75764 (complete procedure) has been deleted, see 36000-36013, 36400-36425 for intravenous procedure, and 36100-36230 for intra-arterial procedure and 75762)

(For introduction of catheter, injection procedure, see 93501-93536, 93545-93553)

75766 Angiography, coronary bypass, multiple selective injection, radiological supervision and interpretation

(75767 (complete procedure) has been deleted, see 36000-36013, 36400-36425 for intravenous procedure, and 36100-36230 for intra-arterial procedure and 75766)

(For introduction of catheter, injection procedure, see 93501-93536, 93545-93553)

(75772, 75773 have been deleted. To report, see 75774)

75774 Angiography, selective, each additional vessel studied after basic examination, radiological supervision and interpretation

(75775 (complete procedure) has been deleted, see 36000-36015, 36400-36425 for intravenous procedure, and 36100-36248 for intra-arterial procedure and 75774)

(For introduction of catheter, injection procedure, see 93501-93536, 93545-93553)

75790 Angiography, arteriovenous shunt (eg, dialysis patient), radiological supervision and interpretation

(For introduction of catheter, see 36140, 36215-36217, 36245-36247)

VEINS AND LYMPHATICS

(For injection procedure for venous system, see 36000-36015, 36400-36510)

(For injection procedure for lymphatic system, see 38790)

75801 Lymphangiography, extremity only, unilateral, radiological supervision and interpretation

(75802 (complete procedure) has been deleted, see 38790, 75801)

75803 Lymphangiography, extremity only, bilateral, radiological supervision and interpretation

(75804 (complete procedure) has been deleted, see 38790, 75803)

75805 Lymphangiography, pelvic/abdominal, unilateral, radiological supervision and interpretation

(75806 (complete procedure) has been deleted, see 38790, 75805)

75807 Lymphangiography, pelvic/abdominal, bilateral, radiological supervision and interpretation

(75808 (complete procedure) has been deleted, see 38790, 75807)

• **75809** Shuntogram for investigation of previously placed indwelling nonvascular shunt (eg, LeVeen shunt, ventriculoperitoneal shunt), radiological supervision and interpretation

(For procedure, see 49427 or 61070)

75810 Splenoportography, radiological supervision and interpretation

(75811 (complete procedure) has been deleted, see 38200, 75810)

75820 Venography, extremity, unilateral, radiological supervision and interpretation

(75821 (complete procedure) has been deleted, see 36000, 36406, 36410, 36420, 36425, 75820)

75822 Venography, extremity, bilateral, radiological supervision and interpretation

(75823 (complete procedure) has been deleted, see 36000, 36406, 36410, 36420, 36425, 75822)

75825 Venography, caval, inferior, with serialography, radiological supervision and interpretation

(75826 (complete procedure) has been deleted, see 36010, 75825)

75827 Venography, caval, superior, with serialography, radiological supervision and interpretation

(75828 (complete procedure) has been deleted, see 36010, 75827)

75831 Venography, renal, unilateral, selective, radiological supervision and interpretation

(75832 (complete procedure) has been deleted, see 36000-36012, 75831)

75833 Venography, renal, bilateral, selective, radiological supervision and interpretation

(75834 (complete procedure) has been deleted, see 36000-36012, 75833)

75840 Venography, adrenal, unilateral, selective, radiological supervision and interpretation

(75841 (complete procedure) has been deleted, see 36000-36012, 75840)

75842 Venography, adrenal, bilateral, selective, radiological supervision and interpretation

(75843 (complete procedure) has been deleted, see 36000-36012, 75842)

(75845, 75846, 75847, 75850, 75851 have been deleted)

75860 Venography, sinus or jugular, catheter, radiological supervision and interpretation

(75861 (complete procedure) has been deleted, see 36000-36012 for intravenous procedure and 36100-36218 for intra-arterial procedure, 75860)

75870 Venography, superior sagittal sinus, radiological supervision and interpretation

(75871 (complete procedure) has been deleted, see 36000-36012 for intravenous procedure and 36100-36218 for intra-arterial procedure, 75870)

75872 Venography, epidural, radiological supervision and interpretation

(75873 (complete procedure) has been deleted, see 36000-36012 for intravenous procedure and 36100-36218 for intra-arterial procedure, 75872)

75880 Venography, orbital, radiological supervision and interpretation

(75881 (complete procedure) has been deleted, see 36000-36012 for intravenous procedure and 36100-36218 for intra-arterial procedure, 75880)

75885 Percutaneous transhepatic portography with hemodynamic evaluation, radiological supervision and interpretation

(75886 (complete procedure) has been deleted, see 36011, 36012, 36481, 75885)

75887 Percutaneous transhepatic portography without hemodynamic evaluation, radiological supervision and interpretation

(75888 (complete procedure) has been deleted, see 36011, 36012, 36481, 75887)

75889 Hepatic venography, wedged or free, with hemodynamic evaluation, radiological supervision and interpretation

(75890 (complete procedure) has been deleted, see 36000-36012, 75889)

75891 Hepatic venography, wedged or free, without hemodynamic evaluation, radiological supervision and interpretation

(75892 (complete procedure) has been deleted, see 36000-36012, 75891)

75893 Venous sampling through catheter, with or without angiography (eg, for parathyroid hormone, renin), radiological supervision and interpretation

(For procedure, see 36500)

TRANSCATHETER THERAPY AND BIOPSY

75894 Transcatheter therapy, embolization, any method, radiological supervision and interpretation

(75895 (complete procedure) has been deleted, see 37204, 61624, 61626, 75894)

75896 Transcatheter therapy, infusion, any method (eg, thrombolysis other than coronary), radiological supervision and interpretation

(75897 (complete procedure) has been deleted, see 37201, 37202, 75896)

(Infusion for coronary disease, see 92975, 92977)

75898 Angiogram through existing catheter for follow-up study for transcatheter therapy, embolization or infusion

75940 Percutaneous placement of IVC filter, radiological supervision and interpretation

(75941 (complete procedure) has been deleted, see 37620, 75940)

(75950, 75951, 75955, 75956 (complete procedure) have been deleted, see 37204, 61624, 61626, 75894)

● **75960** Transcatheter introduction of intravascular stent(s), (non-coronary vessel), percutaneous and/or open, radiological supervision and interpretation, each vessel

(For procedure, see 37205-37208)

75961 Transcatheter retrieval, percutaneous, of intravascular foreign body (eg, fractured venous or arterial catheter), radiological supervision and interpretation

(For procedure see 37203)

▲ **75962** Transluminal balloon angioplasty, peripheral artery, radiological supervision and interpretation

(75963 (complete procedure) has been deleted, see 35450-35460 or 35470-35476 and 75962)

▲75964 Transluminal balloon angioplasty, each additional peripheral artery, radiological supervision and interpretation

(75965 (complete procedure) has been deleted, see 35450-35460 or 35470-35476 and 75964)

▲75966 Transluminal balloon angioplasty, renal or other visceral artery, radiological supervision and interpretation

(75967 (complete procedure) has been deleted, see 35450-35460 or 35470-35476 and 75966)

▲75968 Transluminal balloon angioplasty, each additional visceral artery, radiological supervision and interpretation

(75969 (complete procedure) has been deleted, see 35450-35460 or 35470-35476 and 75968)

(For percutaneous transluminal coronary angioplasty, see 92982-92984)

75970 Transcatheter biopsy, radiological supervision and interpretation

(For injection procedure only for transcatheter therapy or biopsy, see 36100-36299)

(75971 (complete procedure) has been deleted, see 37200, 75970)

(For transcatheter renal and ureteral biopsy, see 52007)

(For percutaneous needle biopsy of pancreas, see 48102; of retroperitoneal lymph node or mass, see 49180)

(75972-75977 have been deleted. To report, see 75962-75968)

▲75978 Transluminal balloon angioplasty, venous (eg, subclavian stenosis), radiological supervision and interpretation

(75979 (complete procedure) has been deleted, see 35460, 35476, 75978)

75980 Percutaneous transhepatic biliary drainage with contrast monitoring, radiological supervision and interpretation

(75981 (complete procedure) has been deleted, see 47510, 47511, 75980)

75982 Percutaneous placement of drainage catheter for combined internal and external biliary drainage or of a drainage stent for internal biliary drainage in patients with an inoperable mechanical biliary obstruction, radiological supervision and interpretation

(75983 (complete procedure) has been deleted, see 47511, 75982)

75984 Change of percutaneous drainage catheter with contrast monitoring (ie, biliary tract, urinary tract), radiological supervision and interpretation

(75985 (complete procedure) has been deleted, see 47490, 47525, 47530, 50398, 50688, 75984)

(For change of nephrostomy or pyelostomy tube only, use 50398)

(For introduction procedure only for percutaneous biliary drainage, see 47510, 47511)

(For percutaneous cholecystostomy, use 47490)

(For change of percutaneous biliary drainage catheter only, use 47525)

(For percutaneous nephrostolithotomy or pyelostolithotomy, see 50080, 50081)

75989 Radiological guidance for percutaneous drainage of abscess, or specimen collection (ie, fluoroscopy, ultrasound, or computed tomography), with or without placement of indwelling catheter, radiological supervision and interpretation

(75990 (complete procedure) has been deleted, see appropriate organ or site and 75989)

TRANSLUMINAL ATHERECTOMY

• **75992** Transluminal atherectomy, peripheral artery, radiological supervision and interpretation

(For procedure, see 35481-35485, 35491-35495)

• **75993** Transluminal atherectomy, each additional peripheral artery, radiological supervision and interpretation

(For procedure, see 35481-35485, 35491-35495)

- **75994** Transluminal atherectomy, renal, radiological supervision and interpretation

(For procedure, see 35480, 35490)

- **75995** Transluminal atherectomy, visceral, radiological supervision and interpretation

(For procedure, see 35480, 35490)

- **75996** Transluminal atherectomy, each additional visceral artery, radiological supervision and interpretation

(For procedure, see 35480, 35490)

MISCELLANEOUS

(For arthrography of shoulder, see 73040; elbow, see 73085; wrist, see 73115; hip, see 73525; knee, see 73580; ankle, see 73615)

76000 Fluoroscopy (separate procedure), up to one hour physician time, other than 71023 or 71034

76001 Fluoroscopy, physician time more than one hour, assisting a non-radiologic physician (eg, nephrostolithotomy, ERCP, bronchoscopy, transbronchial biopsy)

76003 Fluoroscopic localization for needle biopsy or fine needle aspiration

(See appropriate surgical code for location, eg, 20220, 20225, 32400, 32405, 47000, 47001, 48102, 50200, 50390, 60100)

76010 Radiologic examination from nose to rectum for foreign body, single film, child

76020 Bone age studies

76040 Bone length studies (orthoroentgenogram, scanogram)

(76060 has been deleted. See 76061, 76062)

76061 Radiologic examination, osseous survey; limited (eg, for metastases)

76062 complete (axial and appendicular skeleton)

76065 Radiologic examination osseous survey; infant

76066 Joint survey, single view, one or more joints (specify)

76070 Computerized tomography, bone density study

76080 Radiologic examination, fistula or sinus tract study, radiological supervision and interpretation

(76081 (complete procedure) has been deleted, see 20501, 76080)

76086 Mammary ductogram or galactogram, single duct, radiological supervision and interpretation

(76087 (complete procedure) has been deleted, see 19030, 76086)

76088 Mammary ductogram or galactogram, multiple ducts, radiological supervision and interpretation

(76089 (complete procedure) has been deleted, see 19030, 76088)

76090 Mammography; unilateral

76091 bilateral

76092 Screening mammography, bilateral (two view film study of each breast)

▲**76096** Preoperative placement of needle localization wire, breast, radiological supervision and interpretation

(For placement, see 19290, 19291)

(76097 has been deleted. To report, see 19291, 76096)

76098 Radiological examination, breast surgical specimen

76100 Radiologic examination, single plane body section (eg, tomography), other than with urography

76101 Radiologic examination, complex motion (ie, hypercycloidal) body section (eg, mastoid polytomography), other than with urography; unilateral

76102 bilateral

(For nephrotomography, see 74415)

76120 Cineradiography, except where specifically included

76125 Cineradiography to complement routine examination

(76127 has been deleted. The use of photographic media is not reported separately but is considered to be a component of the basic procedure)

(76130-76137 have been deleted. To report, use code for specific radiologic examination)

76140 Consultation on x-ray examination made elsewhere, written report

76150 Xeroradiography

(76150 is to be used for non-mammographic studies only)

(76300 has been deleted. To report, use 76499)

76350 Subtraction in conjunction with contrast studies

76355 Computerized tomography guidance for stereotactic localization

76360 Computerized tomography guidance for needle biopsy, radiological supervision and interpretation

(76361 (complete procedure) has been deleted, see appropriate organ or site and 76360)

76365 Computerized tomography guidance for cyst aspiration, radiological supervision and interpretation

(76366 (complete procedure) has been deleted, see appropriate organ or site and 76365)

76370 Computerized tomography guidance for placement of radiation therapy fields

76375 Computerized tomography, coronal, sagittal, multiplanar, oblique and/or 3-dimensional reconstruction

76380 Computerized tomography, limited or localized follow-up study

76400 Magnetic resonance (eg, proton) imaging, bone marrow blood supply

76499 Unlisted diagnostic radiologic procedure

Diagnostic Ultrasound

A-mode: Implies a one-dimensional ultrasonic measurement procedure.

M-mode: Implies a one-dimensional ultrasonic measurement procedure with movement of the trace to record amplitude and velocity of moving echo-producing structures.

B-scan: Implies a two-dimensional ultrasonic scanning procedure with a two-dimensional display.

Real-time scan: Implies a two-dimensional ultrasonic scanning procedure with display of both two-dimensional structure and motion with time.

HEAD AND NECK

(76500, 76505 have been deleted. To report, use 76999)

76506 Echoencephalography, B-scan and/or real time with image documentation (gray scale) (for determination of ventricular size, delineation of cerebral contents and detection of fluid masses or other intracranial abnormalties), including A-mode encephalography as secondary component where indicated

76511 Ophthalmic ultrasound, echography, diagnostic; A-scan only, with amplitude quantification

76512 contact B-scan (with or without simultaneous A-scan)

76513 immersion (water bath) B-scan

(76515 has been deleted. To report, use 76999)

76516 Ophthalmic biometry by ultrasound echography, A-scan;

(76517 has been deleted. To report, use 76999)

76519 with intraocular lens power calculation

76529 Ophthalmic ultrasonic foreign body localization

(76530 has been deleted. To report, use 76999)

(76535 has been deleted. To report, use 76536)

76536 Echography, soft tissues of head and neck (eg, thyroid, parathyroid, parotid), B-scan and/or real time with image documentation

(76550 has been deleted. To report, see 93880-93888)

CHEST

(76601 has been deleted. To report, use 76999)

76604 Echography, chest, B-scan (includes mediastinum) and/or real time with image documentation

(76620, 76625 have been deleted)

(76627, 76628 have been deleted. To report, see 93307, 93308)

(76629 has been deleted)

(76632 has been deleted. To report, see 93320, 93321)

(76640 has been deleted. To report, use 76999)

76645 Echography, breast(s) (unilateral or bilateral), B-scan and/or real time with image documentation

ABDOMEN AND RETROPERITONEUM

76700 Echography, abdominal, B-scan and/or real time with image documentation; complete

76705 limited (eg, single organ, quadrant, follow-up)

76770 Echography, retroperitoneal (eg, renal, aorta, nodes), B-scan and/or real time with image documentation; complete

76775 limited

76778 Echography of transplanted kidney, B-scan and/or real time with image documentation, with or without duplex Doppler studies

SPINAL CANAL

76800 Echography, spinal canal and contents

PELVIS

76805 Echography, pregnant uterus, B-scan and/or real time with image documentation; complete (complete fetal and maternal evaluation)

76810 complete (complete fetal and maternal evaluation), multiple gestation, after the first trimester

76815 limited (gestational age, heart beat, placental location, fetal position, or emergency in the delivery room)

76816 follow-up or repeat

76818 Fetal biophysical profile

▲**76825** Echocardiography, fetal, cardiovascular system, real time with image documentation (2D) with or without M-mode recording;

● **76826** follow-up or repeat study

● **76827** Doppler echocardiography, fetal, cardiovascular system, pulsed wave and/or continuous wave with spectral display; complete

● **76828** follow-up or repeat study

(To report the use of color mapping, see 93325)

76830 Echography, transvaginal

(76855 has been deleted. To report, see 93975-93979)

76856 Echography, pelvic (nonobstetric), B-scan and/or real time with image documentation; complete

76857 limited or follow-up (eg, for follicles)

GENITALIA

76870 Echography, scrotum and contents

▲**76872** Echography, transrectal

EXTREMITIES

76880 Echography, extremity, non-vascular, B-scan and/or real time with image documentation

VASCULAR STUDIES

(76900-76920 have been deleted. To report, see 93920-93971; for cerebrovascular studies, see 93875-93888)

(76925 has been deleted. To report, see 93920-93931 or 93965-93971)

(76926 has been deleted. To report, see 93875-93888 or 93975-93979)

ULTRASONIC GUIDANCE PROCEDURES

76930 Ultrasonic guidance for pericardiocentesis, radiological supervision and interpretation

(76931 (complete procedure) has been deleted, see 33010, 33011, 76930)

76932 Ultrasonic guidance for endomyocardial biopsy, radiological supervision and interpretation

(76933 (complete procedure) has been deleted, see 93505, 76932)

76934 Ultrasonic guidance for thoracentesis or abdominal paracentesis, radiological supervision and interpretation

(76935 (complete procedure) has been deleted, see 32000, 76934)

76938 Ultrasonic guidance for cyst (any location), or renal pelvis aspiration, radiological supervision and interpretation

(76939 (complete procedure) has been deleted, see appropriate organ or site and 76938)

76942 Ultrasonic guidance for needle biopsy, radiological supervision and interpretation

(76943 (complete procedure) has been deleted, see appropriate organ or site and 76942)

(76944, 76945 have been deleted. To report, see 75989)

76946 Ultrasonic guidance for amniocentesis, radiological supervision and interpretation

(76947 (complete procedure) has been deleted, see 59000, 76946)

76948 Ultrasonic guidance for aspiration of ova, radiological supervision and interpretation

(76949 (complete procedure) has been deleted, see 58970, 76948)

76950 Echography for placement of radiation therapy fields, B-scan

76960 Ultrasonic guidance for placement of radiation therapy fields, except for B-scan echography

MISCELLANEOUS

76970 Ultrasound study follow-up (specify)

(76980 has been deleted. To report, use code for specific ultrasound examination)

(76985 has been deleted. To report, use 76986)

76986 Echography, intraoperative

(76990 has been deleted. To report, use 76999)

(76991 has been deleted. To report, see 76830, 76872)

76999 Unlisted ultrasound procedure

Radiation Oncology

Listings for Radiation Oncology provide for teletherapy and brachytherapy to include initial consultation, clinical treatment planning, simulation, medical radiation physics, dosimetry, treatment devices, special services, and clinical treatment management procedures. They include normal follow-up care during course of treatment and for three months following its completion.

When a service or procedure is provided that is not listed in this edition of CPT it should be identified by a Special Report (see page 600) and one of the unlisted procedure codes listed below:

77299 Unlisted procedure, therapeutic radiology clinical treatment planning

77399 Unlisted procedure, medical radiation physics, dosimetry and treatment devices

77499 Unlisted procedure, therapeutic radiology clinical treatment management

77799 Unlisted procedure, clinical brachytherapy

(For treatment by injectable or ingestible isotopes, see subsection NUCLEAR MEDICINE)

CONSULTATION: CLINICAL MANAGEMENT

Preliminary consultation, evaluation of patient prior to decision to treat, or full medical care (in addition to treatment management) when provided by the therapeutic radiologist may be identified by the appropriate procedure codes from Evaluation and Management, Medicine or Surgery sections.

CLINICAL TREATMENT PLANNING (EXTERNAL AND INTERNAL SOURCES)

The clinical treatment planning process is a complex service including interpretation of special testing, tumor localization, treatment volume determination, treatment time/dosage determination, choice of treatment modality, determination of number and size of treatment ports, selection of appropriate treatment devices, and other procedures.

DEFINITIONS:

Simple—planning requiring single treatment area of interest encompassed in a single port or simple parallel opposed ports with simple or no blocking.

Intermediate—planning requiring three or more converging ports, two separate treatment areas, multiple blocks, or special time dose constraints.

Complex—planning requiring highly complex blocking, custom shielding blocks, tangential ports, special wedges or compensators, three or more separate treatment areas, rotational or special beam considerations, combination of therapeutic modalities.

(77260, 77265, 77270, 77275 have been deleted. To report, use 77261-77263)

77261 Therapeutic radiology treatment planning; simple

77262 intermediate

77263 complex

Simple—simulation of a single treatment area with either a single port or parallel opposed ports. Simple or no blocking.

Intermediate—simulation of three or more converging ports, two separate treatment areas, multiple blocks.

Complex—simulation of tangential portals, three or more treatment areas, rotation or arc therapy, complex blocking, custom shielding blocks, brachytherapy source verification, hyperthermia probe verification, any use of contrast materials.

Simulation may be carried out on a dedicated simulator, a radiation therapy treatment unit, or diagnostic x-ray machine.

77280 Therapeutic radiology simulation-aided field setting; simple

77285 intermediate

77290 complex

77299 Unlisted procedure, therapeutic radiology clinical treatment planning

MEDICAL RADIATION PHYSICS, DOSIMETRY, TREATMENT DEVICES AND SPECIAL SERVICES

77300 Basic radiation dosimetry calculation, central axis depth dose, TDF, NSD, gap calculation, off axis factor, tissue inhomogeneity factors, as required during course of treatment, only when prescribed by the treating physician

77305 Teletherapy, isodose plan (whether hand or computer calculated); simple (one or two parallel opposed unmodified ports directed to a single area of interest)

77310 intermediate (three or more treatment ports directed to a single area of interest)

77315 complex (mantle or inverted Y, tangential ports, the use of wedges, compensators, complex blocking, rotational beam, or special beam considerations)

(Only one teletherapy isodose plan may be reported for a given course of therapy to a specific treatment area)

(77320, 77325, 77330, 77335, 77340 have been deleted. To report, use 77300-77399)

77321 Special teletherapy port plan, particles, hemi-body, total body

77326 Brachytherapy isodose calculation; simple (calculation made from single plane, one to four sources/ribbon application, remote afterloading brachytherapy, 1 to 8 sources)

(For definition of source/ribbon, see page 449)

77327 intermediate (multiplane dosage calculations, application involving five to ten sources/ribbons, remote afterloading brachytherapy, 9 to 12 sources)

77328 complex (multiplane isodose plan, volume implant calculations, over ten sources/ribbons used, special spatial reconstruction, remote afterloading brachytherapy, over 12 sources)

77331 Special dosimetry (eg, TLD, microdosimetry) (specify), only when prescribed by the treating physician

77332 Treatment devices, design and construction; simple (simple block, simple bolus)

77333 intermediate (multiple blocks, stents, bite blocks, special bolus)

77334 complex (irregular blocks, special shields, compensators, wedges, molds or casts)

77336 Continuing medical radiation physics consultation in support of therapeutic radiologist including continuing quality assurance reported per week of therapy

(77345-77360 have been deleted. To report, use 77300-77399)

77370 Special medical radiation physics consultation

77399 Unlisted procedure, medical radiation physics, dosimetry and treatment devices

RADIATION TREATMENT DELIVERY

Radiation treatment delivery (77401-77414) recognizes the technical component and the various energy levels.

(77400 has been deleted)

77401 Radiation treatment delivery, superficial and/or ortho voltage

77402 Radiation treatment delivery, single treatment area, single port or parallel opposed ports, simple blocks or no blocks; up to 5 MeV

77403 6-10 MeV

77404 11-19 MeV

(77405 has been deleted)

77406 20 MeV or greater

77407 Radiation treatment delivery, two separate treatment areas, three or more ports on a single treatment area, use of multiple blocks; up to 5 MeV

77408 6-10 MeV

77409 11-19 MeV

(77410 has been deleted)

77411 20 MeV or greater

77412 Radiation treatment delivery, three or more separate treatment areas, custom blocking, tangential ports, wedges, rotational beam, compensators, special particle beam (eg, electron or neutrons); up to 5 MeV

77413 6-10 MeV

77414 11-19 MeV

77416 20 MeV or greater

(77415 has been deleted. To report, see 77417)

77417 Therapeutic radiology port film(s)

CLINICAL TREATMENT MANAGEMENT

Weekly clinical management is based on five fractions delivered comprising one week regardless of the time interval separating the delivery of treatments.

DEFINITIONS:

Simple—single treatment area, single port or parallel opposed ports, simple blocks.

Intermediate—two separate treatment areas, three or more ports on a single treatment area, use of special blocks.

Complex—three or more separate treatment areas, highly complex blocking (mantle, inverted Y), tangential ports, wedges, rotational compensators or other special beam considerations.

77420 Weekly radiology therapy management; simple

77425 intermediate

77430 complex

77431 Radiation therapy management with complete course of therapy consisting of one or two fractions only

(77431 is not to be used to fill in the last week of a long course of therapy)

(77435-77460 have been deleted. To report use 77400-77499)

(77465 has been deleted)

77470 Special treatment procedure (eg, total body irradiation, hemibody irradiation, per oral, vaginal cone irradiation)

(77470 assumes that the procedure is performed one or more times during the course of therapy, in addition to daily or weekly patient management)

77499 Unlisted procedure, therapeutic radiology clinical treatment management

HYPERTHERMIA

Hyperthermia treatments as listed in this section include external (superficial and deep), interstitial, and intracavitary. Radiation therapy when given concurrently is listed separately.

Hyperthermia is used only as an adjunct to radiation therapy or chemotherapy. It may be induced by a variety of sources (eg, microwave, ultrasound, low energy radio-frequency conduction, or by probes).

The listed treatments include management during the course of therapy and follow-up care for three months after completion. Preliminary consultation is not included (see Evaluation and Management 99241-99263). Physics planning and interstitial insertion of temperature sensors, and use of external or interstitial heat generating sources are included.

The following descriptors are included in the treatment schedule:

77600 Hyperthermia, externally generated; superficial (ie, heating to a depth of 4 cm or less)

77605 deep (ie, heating to depths greater than 4 cm)

77610 Hyperthermia generated by interstitial probe(s); 5 or fewer interstitial applicators

77615 more than 5 interstitial applicators

CLINICAL INTRACAVITARY HYPERTHERMIA

77620 Hyperthermia generated by intracavitary probe(s)

CLINICAL BRACHYTHERAPY

Clinical brachytherapy requires the use of either natural or man-made radioelements applied into or around a treatment field of interest. The supervision of radioelements and dose interpretation are performed solely by the therapeutic radiologist. When a procedure requires the service of a surgeon in addition, either modifier '-66' or 09966 or modifier '-80' or 09980 may be used (see modifiers in Radiology Guidelines, page 401).

Services 77750-77799 include admission to the hospital and daily visits.

DEFINITIONS:

(Sources refer to intracavitary placement or permanent interstitial placement; ribbons refer to temporary interstitial placement)

Simple—application with one to four sources/ribbons

Intermediate—application with five to ten sources/ribbons

Complex—application with greater than ten sources/ribbons

(77700-77749 have been deleted. To report, see 77761-77799)

77750 Infusion or instillation of radioelement solution

(77755, 77760, have been deleted. To report, see 77761-77799)

77761 Intracavitary radioelement application; simple

77762 intermediate

77763 complex

(77765, 77770, 77775 have been deleted. To report, see 77761-77799)

77776 Interstitial radioelement application; simple

77777 intermediate

77778 complex

(77780 has been deleted. To report, see 77761-77799)

77781 Remote afterloading high intensity brachytherapy; 1-4 source positions or catheters

77782 5-8 source positions or catheters

77783 9-12 source positions or catheters

77784 over 12 source positions or catheters

(77785 has been deleted. To report, see 77761-77799)

77789 Surface application of radioelement

77790 Supervision, handling, loading of radioelement

77799 Unlisted procedure, clinical brachytherapy

(77800 has been deleted. To report, use 77331)

(77805-77810 have been deleted. To report, use 77305-77321 or 77326-77328)

(77850 has been deleted. To report, use 77300, 77336, 77370)

(77860 has been deleted. To report, use 77336)

(77999 has been deleted. To report, use 77399)

Nuclear Medicine

Listed procedures may be performed independently or in the course of overall medical care. If the physician providing these services is also responsible for diagnostic work-up and/or follow-up care of patient, see appropriate sections also.

Radioimmunoassay tests are found in the Clinical Pathology section (codes 82000-84999). These codes can be appropriately used by any specialist performing such tests in a laboratory licensed and/or certified for radioimmunoassays. The reporting of these tests is not confined to clinical pathology laboratories alone.

The services listed do not include the provision of radium or other radioelements. Those materials supplied by the physician should be listed separately and identified by the code 78990 for diagnostic radionuclide(s) and 79900 for therapeutic radionuclide.

DIAGNOSTIC

ENDOCRINE SYSTEM

78000 Thyroid uptake; single determination

78001 multiple determinations

78003 stimulation, suppression or discharge (not including initial uptake studies)

78006 Thyroid imaging, with uptake; single determination

78007 multiple determinations

78010 Thyroid imaging; only

78011 with vascular flow

78015 Thyroid carcinoma metastases imaging; limited area (eg, neck and chest only)

78016 with additional studies (eg, urinary recovery)

78017 multiple areas

78018 whole body

(For triiodothyronine (true TT-3), RIA, see 84480)

(For calcitonin, RIA, see 82308)

(For triiodothyronine, free (FT-3), RIA (unbound T-3 only), see 84481)

(For TT-4 thyroxine, RIA, see 84436)

(For T-4 thyroxine, neonatal, see 84437)

(For FT-4 thyroxine, free, RIA (unbound T-4 only), see 84439)

78070 Parathyroid imaging

(For parathormone (parathyroid hormone), RIA, see 83970)

78075 Adrenal imaging, cortex and/or medulla

(For adrenal cortex antibodies, RIA, see 86255, 86256)

(For cortisol, RIA, plasma or urine, see 82533)

(For aldosterone, double isotope technique, see 82088)

(For aldosterone, RIA, blood or urine, see 82088)

(For 17-ketosteroids, RIA, see 83586)

(For 17-OH ketosteroids, RIA, see 83586)

(For 17-hydroxycorticosteroids, RIA, see 83491)

(For insulin, RIA, see 83525)

(For insulin antibodies, RIA, see 86337)

(For insulin factor antibodies, RIA, see 86337)

(For proinsulin, RIA, see 84206)

(For glucagon, RIA, see 82943)

(For adrenocorticotropic hormone (ACTH), RIA, see 82024)

(For human growth hormone (HGH), (somatotropin), RIA, see 83003)

(For human growth antibody, RIA, see 86277)

(For thyroglobulin antibody, RIA, see 86800)

(For thyroid microsomal antibody, RIA, see 86376)

(For thyroid stimulating hormone (TSH), RIA, see 84443)

(For thyrotropin releasing factor, RIA, see 84444)

(For thyroid stimulating immunoglobulins (TSI), see 84445)

(For follicle stimulating hormone (FSH component of pituitary gonadotropin), RIA, see 83001)

(For luteinizing hormone (LH component of pituitary gonadotropin), (ICSH), RIA, see 83002)

(For luteinizing releasing factor (LRH), RIA, see 83727)

(For prolactin level (mammotropin), RIA, see 84146)

(For vasopressin level (antidiuretic hormone), RIA, see 84588)

(For estradiol, RIA, see 82670)

(For progesterone, RIA, see 84144)

(For testosterone, blood or urine, RIA, see 84403)

(For etiocholanolone, RIA, see 82696)

78099 Unlisted endocrine procedure, diagnostic nuclear medicine

(For chemical analysis, RIA tests, see Chemistry section)

HEMATOPOIETIC, RETICULOENDOTHELIAL AND LYMPHATIC SYSTEM

78102 Bone marrow imaging; limited area

78103 multiple areas

78104 whole body

78110 Plasma volume, radionuclide volume-dilution technique (separate procedure); single sampling

78111 multiple samplings

78120 Red cell volume determination (separate procedure); single sampling

78121 multiple samplings

78122 Whole blood volume determination, including separate measurement of plasma volume and red cell volume (radionuclide volume-dilution technique)

78130 Red cell survival study;

78135 differential organ/tissue kinetics, (eg, splenic and/or hepatic sequestration)

78140 Labeled red cell sequestration, differential organ/tissue, (eg, splenic and/or hepatic)

78160 Plasma radioiron disappearance (turnover) rate

78162 Radioiron oral absorption

78170 Radioiron red cell utilization

78172 Chelatable iron for estimation of total body iron

(78180 has been deleted. To report, use 78199)

(For hemosiderin, RIA, see 83071)

(For intrinsic factor antibodies, RIA, see 83528)

(For cyanocobalamin (vitamin B-12), RIA, see 82607)

(For folic acid (folate) serum, RIA, see 82746)

(For human hepatitis antigen, hepatitis associated agent, (Australian antigen) (HAA), RIA, see 86287)

(For hepatitis A antibody (HAAb), RIA, see 86296)

(For hepatitis A virus antibody (HAVAb), see 86296)

(For hepatitis B core antibody (HBcAb), RIA, see 86289)

(For hepatitis B surface antigen (HBsAb), RIA, see 86287)

(For hepatitis B surface antibody (HBsAb), RIA, see 86291)

(For hepatitis Be antigen (HBeAg), RIA, see 86293)

(For hepatitis Be antibody (HBeAb), RIA, see 86295)

78185 Spleen imaging only, with or without vascular flow

(If combined with liver study, use procedures 78215 and 78216)

(78186 has been deleted)

78190 Kinetics, study of platelet survival, with or without differential organ/tissue localization

78191 Platelet survival study

78192 White blood cell localization; limited area scanning

78193 whole body

78195 Lymphatics and lymph glands imaging

78199 Unlisted hematopoietic, reticuloendothelial and lymphatic procedure, diagnostic nuclear medicine

(For chemical analysis, RIA tests, see Chemistry section)

GASTROINTESTINAL SYSTEM

78201 Liver imaging; static only

78202 with vascular flow

(For spleen imaging only, use 78185)

78205 Liver imaging (SPECT)

78215 Liver and spleen imaging; static only

78216 with vascular flow

78220 Liver function study with hepatobiliary agents, with serial images

(78221 has been deleted. To report, use 78299)

78223 Hepatobiliary ductal system imaging, including gallbladder, with or without pharmacologic intervention, with or without quantitative measurement of gallbladder function

(78225 has been deleted)

78230 Salivary gland imaging;

78231 with serial images

78232 Salivary gland function study

(78240 has been deleted. To report pancreas imaging, use 78299)

78258 Esophageal motility

78261 Gastric mucosa imaging

78262 Gastroesophageal reflux study

78264 Gastric emptying study

78270 Vitamin B-12 absorption study (eg, Schilling test); without intrinsic factor

78271 with intrinsic factor

78272 Vitamin B-12 absorption studies combined, with and without intrinsic factor

78276 Gastrointestinal aspirate blood loss localization

78278 Acute gastrointestinal blood loss imaging

78280 Gastrointestinal blood loss study (eg, stool counting)

78282 Gastrointestinal protein loss

(78285, 78286 have been deleted. To report, use 78299)

(For gastrin, RIA, see 82941)

(For intrinsic factor level, see 83528)

(For carcinoembryonic antigen level (CEA), RIA, see 82378)

78290 Bowel imaging (eg, ectopic gastric mucosa, Meckel's localization, volvulus)

78291 Peritoneal-venous shunt patency test (eg, for LeVeen, Denver shunt)

78299 Unlisted gastrointestinal procedure, diagnostic nuclear medicine

(For chemical analysis, RIA tests, see Chemistry section)

MUSCULOSKELETAL SYSTEM

Bone and joint imaging can be used in the diagnosis of a variety of infectious inflammatory diseases (eg, osteomyelitis), as well as for localization of primary and/or metastatic neoplasms.

78300 Bone and/or joint imaging; limited area

78305 multiple areas

78306 whole body

78310 vascular flow only

78315 three phase study

78320 tomographic (SPECT)

78350 Bone density (bone mineral content) study; single photon absorptiometry

78351 dual photon absorptiometry

(78380, 78381 have been deleted. To report, see 78300, 78305)

78399 Unlisted musculoskeletal procedure, diagnostic nuclear medicine

CARDIOVASCULAR SYSTEM

(78401-78412 have been deleted. To report, see 78472-78483)

78414 Determination of central c-v hemodynamics (non-imaging) (eg, ejection fraction with probe technique) with or without pharmacologic intervention or exercise, single or multiple determinations

(78415 has been deleted. To report, see 78472)

(78418-78424 have been deleted. To report, see 78460-78469)

(78425 has been deleted. To report, see 78472)

78428 Cardiac shunt detection

(78435 has been deleted. To report, see 78481)

78445 Vascular flow imaging (ie, angiography, venography)

78455 Venous thrombosis study (eg, radioactive fibrinogen)

78457 Venous thrombosis imaging (eg, venogram); unilateral

78458 bilateral

78460 Myocardial perfusion imaging; single study, resting or stress (exercise and/or pharmacologic), quantitative or qualitative

78461 multiple studies, resting and/or stress (exercise and/or pharmacologic), and redistribution and/or rest injection, qualitative or quantitative

(78462, 78463 have been deleted. To report, see 78460, 78461)

78464 tomographic (SPECT), single study at rest or stress (exercise and/or pharmacologic), with or without quantitation

78465 tomographic (SPECT), multiple studies, resting and/or stress (exercise and/or pharmacologic) and redistribution and/or rest injection, qualitative or quantitative

78466 Myocardial imaging, infarct avid, planar; qualitative or quantitative

(78467 has been deleted. To report, see 78466)

78468 with ejection fraction by first pass technique

78469 tomographic SPECT with or without quantitation

(78470 has been deleted. To report, see 78472, 78473 or 78481)

(78471 has been deleted. To report, see 78472)

78472 Cardiac blood pool imaging, gated equilibrium; single study at rest, wall motion study plus ejection fraction, with or without additional quantitative processing

78473 multiple studies, wall motion study plus ejection fraction, resting and stress (with exercise and/or pharmacologic), with or without additional quantification

(78474 has been deleted. To report, see 78472)

(78475-78477 have been deleted. To report, see 78473)

78478 Myocardial perfusion study with wall motion, qualitative or quantitative study (list separately in addition to code for primary procedure) (Use only for codes 78460, 78461, 78464, 78465)

(78479 has been deleted)

78480 Myocardial perfusion study with ejection fraction (list separately in addition to code for primary procedure) (Use only for codes 78460, 78461, 78464, 78465)

78481 Cardiac blood pool imaging, first pass technique; single study, at rest, wall motion study, with ejection fraction

78483 multiple studies, resting and with stress (exercise and/or pharmacologic), with or without additional quantification

(78484 has been deleted. To report, see 78481)

(78485, 78486 have been deleted. To report, see 78483)

(78487 and 78489 have been deleted. To report, see 78483)

(78490 has been deleted. To report, use 78499)

(For digoxin, RIA, see 80162)

(For cerebral blood flow study, see 78615)

78499 Unlisted cardiovascular procedure, diagnostic nuclear medicine

(For chemical analysis, RIA tests, see Chemistry section)

RESPIRATORY SYSTEM

78580 Pulmonary perfusion imaging; particulate

78581 gaseous

78582 gaseous, with ventilation, rebreathing and washout

78584 Pulmonary perfusion imaging, particulate, with ventilation; single breath

78585 rebreathing and washout, with or without single breath

78586 Pulmonary ventilation imaging, aerosol; single projection

78587 multiple projections (eg, anterior, posterior, lateral views)

78591 Pulmonary ventilation imaging, gaseous, single breath, single projection

78593 Pulmonary ventilation imaging, gaseous, with rebreathing and washout with or without single breath; single projection

78594 multiple projections (eg, anterior, posterior, lateral views)

78596 Pulmonary quantitative differential function (ventilation/perfusion) study

78599 Unlisted respiratory procedure, diagnostic nuclear medicine

NERVOUS SYSTEM

78600 Brain imaging, limited procedure; static

78601 with vascular flow

78605 Brain imaging, complete study; static

78606 with vascular flow

78607 tomographic (SPECT)

78610 Brain imaging, vascular flow only

78615 Cerebral blood flow

78630 Cerebrospinal fluid flow, imaging (not including introduction of material); cisternography

(For injection procedure, see 61000-61070, 62270-62294)

78635 ventriculography

(For injection procedure, see 61000-61070, 62270-62294)

(78640 has been deleted. To report, use 78699)

78645 shunt evaluation

(For injection procedure, see 61000-61070, 62270-62294)

78650 CSF leakage detection and localization

(For injection procedure, see 61000-61070, 62270-62294)

78652 tomographic (ECT)

(For myelin basic protein, CSF, RIA, see 83873)

78655 Radionuclide identification of eye tumor

78660 Radionuclide dacryocystography

78699 Unlisted nervous system procedure, diagnostic nuclear medicine

GENITOURINARY SYSTEM

78700 Kidney imaging; static only

78701 with vascular flow

78704 with function study (ie, imaging renogram)

78707 with vascular flow and function study

(For introduction of radioactive substance in association with renal endoscopy, see 50559, 50578)

78710 Kidney imaging (SPECT)

78715 Kidney vascular flow only

(78720 has been deleted. To report, use 78704)

78725 Kidney function study without pharmacologic intervention

78726 Kidney function study including pharmacologic intervention

(For renin (angiotensin I), RIA, see 84244)

(For angiotensin II, RIA, see 82163)

(For beta-2 microglobulin, RIA, see 82232)

78727 Kidney transplant evaluation

78730 Urinary bladder residual study

(For introduction of radioactive substance in association with cystotomy or cystostomy, see 51020; in association with cystourethroscopy, see 52250)

78740 Ureteral reflux study (radionuclide voiding cystogram)

(For estradiol, RIA, see 82670)

(For estriol, RIA, see 82677)

(For progesterone, RIA, see 84144)

(For prostatic acid phosphatase, RIA, see 84066)

78760 Testicular imaging;

78761 with vascular flow

(For testosterone, blood or urine, RIA, see 84403)

(For introduction of radioactive substance in association with ureteral endoscopy, see 50959, 50978)

(78770, 78775 have been deleted. To report, use 78799)

(For lactogen, human placental (HPL) chorionic somatomammotropin, RIA, see 83632)

(For chorionic gonadotropin, RIA or beta subunit, see 84702, 84703)

(For pregnanediol, RIA, see 84135)

(For pregnanetriol, RIA, see 84138)

78799 Unlisted genitourinary procedure, diagnostic nuclear medicine

(For chemical analysis, RIA tests, see Chemistry section)

MISCELLANEOUS STUDIES

(For specific organ, see appropriate heading)

(For radiophosphorus tumor identification, ocular, see 78655)

78800 Radionuclide localization of tumor; limited area

(For specific organ, see appropriate heading)

(For eye tumor identification, see 78655)

78801 multiple areas

78802 whole body

78803 Tumor localization (SPECT)

78805 Radionuclide localization of abscess; limited area

78806 whole body

(For imaging bone infectious inflammatory disease, see 78300-78381)

(For Rast, see 86421, 86422)

(For gamma-E immunoglobulin, RIA, see 82785)

(For gamma-G immunoglobulin, see 82784)

(For alpha-1 antitrypsin, RIA, see 82103)

(For alpha-1 fetoprotein, RIA, see 82105, 82106)

(For antinuclear antibodies, RIA, see 86038)

(For lactic dehydrogenase, RIA, see 83615)

(For amikacin, see 80150)

(For aminophylline, see 84420)

(For amitriptyline, see 80152)

(For amphetamine, chemical quantitative, see 82145)

(For chlordiazepoxide, see code for specific method)

(For chlorpromazine, see phenothiazine, urine 84022)

(For clonazepam, see 80154)

(For cocaine, quantitative, see 82520)

(For diazepam, see 80154)

(For dihydromorphinone, quantitative, see 82649)

(For phenytoin (diphenylhydantoin), see 80185)

(For flucytosine, see 82741)

(For gentamicin, see 80170)

(For lysergic acid diethylamide (LSD), RIA see 80100-80103, 80299)

(For morphine (heroin), RIA, see 80100-80103, 83925)

(For phencyclidine (PCP), see 80100-80103, 83992)

(For phenobarbital, see barbiturates 82205, 82210)

(For tobramycin, see 80200)

78890 Generation of automated data: interactive process involving nuclear physician and/or allied health professional personnel; simple manipulations and interpretation, not to exceed 30 minutes

78891 complex manipulations and interpretation, exceeding 30 minutes

(Use 78890 or 78891 in addition to primary procedure)

(78895 has been deleted)

78990 Provision of diagnostic radionuclide(s)

78999 Unlisted miscellaneous procedure, diagnostic nuclear medicine

THERAPEUTIC

79000 Radionuclide therapy, hyperthyroidism; initial, including evaluation of patient

79001 subsequent, each therapy

(For follow-up visit, see 99211-99215)

79020 Radionuclide therapy, thyroid suppression (euthyroid cardiac disease), including evaluation of patient

79030 Radionuclide ablation of gland for thyroid carcinoma

79035 Radionuclide therapy for metastases of thyroid carcinoma

79100 Radionuclide therapy, polycythemia vera, chronic leukemia, each treatment

79200 Intracavitary radioactive colloid therapy

79300 Interstitial radioactive colloid therapy

79400 Radionuclide therapy, nonthyroid, nonhematologic

79420 Intravascular radionuclide therapy, particulate

79440 Intra-articular radionuclide therapy

79900 Provision of therapeutic radionuclide(s)

79999 Unlisted radionuclide therapeutic procedure

Pathology and Laboratory

Guidelines

Items used by all physicians in reporting their services are presented in the **INTRODUCTION.** Some of the commonalities are repeated here for the convenience of those physicians referring to this section on **PATHOLOGY AND LABORATORY.** Other definitions and items unique to Pathology and Laboratory are also listed.

1. **SERVICES IN PATHOLOGY AND LABORATORY** are provided by the pathologist or by technologists under responsible supervision of a physician.

2. **SEPARATE OR MULTIPLE PROCEDURES:** It is appropriate to designate multiple procedures that are rendered on the same date by separate entries.

3. **SUBSECTION INFORMATION:** Several of the subheadings or subsections have special needs or instructions unique to that section. Where these are indicated, (eg, "Panel Tests"), special **"NOTES"** will be presented preceding those procedural terminology listings referring to that subsection specifically. If there is an "Unlisted Procedure" code number (see item 4 below) for the individual subsection, it will also be shown. Those subsections with **"NOTES"** are as follows:

Subsection	**Code Numbers**
Automated, multichannel tests	80002-80019
Chemistry	82000-84999
Surgical pathology	88300-88399

4. **UNLISTED SERVICE OR PROCEDURE:** A service or procedure may be provided that is not listed in this edition of CPT. When reporting such a service, the appropriate "Unlisted Procedure" Code may be used to indicate the service, identifying it by "Special Report" as discussed in item 5 below. The "Unlisted Procedures" and accompanying codes for **PATHOLOGY AND LABORATORY** are as follows:

80299	Unlisted quantitation of drug
81099	Unlisted urinalysis procedure
84999	Unlisted chemistry procedure
85999	Unlisted hematology procedure
86849	Unlisted immunology procedure
86999	Unlisted transfusion medicine procedure
87999	Unlisted microbiology procedure
88099	Unlisted necropsy (autopsy) procedure
88199	Unlisted cytopathology procedure
88299	Unlisted cytogenetic study
88399	Unlisted surgical pathology procedure
89399	Unlisted miscellaneous pathology test

5. **SPECIAL REPORT:** A service that is rarely provided, unusual, variable, or new may require a special report in determining medical appropriateness of the service. Pertinent information should include an adequate definition or description of the nature, extent, and need for the procedure; and the time, effort, and equipment necessary to provide the service. Additional items which may be included are:

   Complexity of symptoms, final diagnosis, pertinent physical findings, diagnostic and therapeutic procedures, concurrent problems, and follow-up care.

6. **MODIFIERS:** Listed services and procedures may be modified under certain circumstances. When applicable, the modifying circumstances should be identified by the addition of the appropriate modifier code, which may be reported in either of two ways. The modifier may be reported by a two digit number placed after the usual procedure number from which it is separated by a hyphen. Or the modifier may be reported by a separate five digit code that is used in addition to the procedure code. If more than one modifier is used, place the "Multiple Modifiers" code immediately after the procedure code. This indicates that one or more additional modifier codes will follow. Modifiers commonly used in **PATHOLOGY AND LABORATORY** are as follows:

   -22 Unusual Procedural Services: When the service(s) provided is greater than that usually required for the listed procedure, it may be identified by adding modifier '-22' to the usual procedure number or by use of the separate five digit modifier code 09922. A report may also be appropriate.

-26 Professional Component: Certain procedures are a combination of a physician component and a technical component. When the physician component is reported separately, the service may be identified by adding the modifier '-26' to the usual procedure number or the service may be reported by use of the five digit modifier code 09926.

-32 Mandated Services: Services related to *mandated* consultation and/or related services (eg, PRO, 3rd party payor) may be identified by adding the modifier '-32' to the basic procedure or the service may be reported by use of the five digit modifier 09932.

-52 Reduced Services: Under certain circumstances a service or procedure is partially reduced or eliminated at the physician's election. Under these circumstances the service provided can be identified by its usual procedure number and the addition of the modifier '-52,' signifying that the service is reduced. This provides a means of reporting reduced services without disturbing the identification of the basic service. Modifier code 09952 may be used as an alternative to modifier '-52.'

-90 Reference (Outside) Laboratory: When laboratory procedures are performed by a party other than the treating or reporting physician, the procedure may be identified by adding the modifier '-90' to the usual procedure number or by using the separate five digit modifier code 09990.

PATHOLOGY AND LABORATORY

Procedures

Automated, Multichannel Tests

The following list contains those tests that can be and are frequently done as groups and combinations ("profiles") on automated multichannel equipment. For any combination of tests among those listed immediately below, use the appropriate number 80002-80019. Groups of the tests listed here are distinguished from multiple tests performed individually for immediate or "stat" reporting. (For handling of specimen, see 99000 and 99001)

Alanine aminotransferase (ALT, SGPT)

Albumin

Aspartate aminotransferase (AST, SGOT)

Bilirubin, direct

Bilirubin, total

Calcium

Carbon dioxide content

Chloride

Cholesterol

Creatinine

Glucose

Lactate dehydrogenase (LD)

Phosphatase, alkaline

Phosphorus (inorganic phosphate)

Potassium

Protein, total

Sodium

Urea Nitrogen (BUN)

Uric acid

80002 Automated multichannel test; 1 or 2 clinical chemistry test(s)

80003 3 clinical chemistry tests

80004 4 clinical chemistry tests

80005 5 clinical chemistry tests

80006 6 clinical chemistry tests

80007 7 clinical chemistry tests

80008 8 clinical chemistry tests

80009 9 clinical chemistry tests

80010 10 clinical chemistry tests

80011 11 clinical chemistry tests

80012 12 clinical chemistry tests

80016 13-16 clinical chemistry tests

80018 17-18 clinical chemistry tests

▲**80019** 19 or more clinical chemistry tests

(80031-80034 have been deleted. To report, see Therapeutic Drug Assays)

(80040 has been deleted. To report, use 83520)

(80042 has been deleted. For serum cidal level, see 87197)

Organ or Disease Oriented Panels

These panels were developed for coding purposes only and should not be interpreted as clinical parameters. The tests listed with each panel, identify the defined components of that panel. These panel components are not intended to limit the performance of other tests. If one performs tests in addition to those specifically indicated for a particular panel, those tests should be reported separately in addition to the panel code.

▲**80050** General health panel

This panel must include the following:

Automated chemistries, 12 or more (80012-80019)

Hematocrit, hemogram, automated, and manual differential WBC count (CBC) (85022) **OR**

Hematocrit, hemogram and platelet count, automated, and automated complete differential WBC count (CBC) (85025)

Thyroid stimulating hormone (TSH) (84443)

(80052 has been deleted. To report, see codes for specific tests)

(80053 has been deleted. To report, see 80050 and codes for individual tests)

▲**80055** Obstetric panel

This panel must include the following:

Hematocrit, hemogram, automated, and manual differential WBC count (CBC) (85022) **OR**

Hematocrit, hemogram and platelet count, automated, and automated complete differential WBC count (CBC) (85025)

Hepatitis B surface antigen (HBsAg) (86287)

Antibody, rubella (86762)

Syphilis test, qualitative (eg, VDRL, RPR, ART) (86592)

Antibody screen, RBC, each serum technique (86850)

Blood typing, ABO (86900) AND

Blood typing, Rh (D) (86901)

(80056 has been deleted. To report, see codes for specific tests)

(80057 has been deleted. To report, see codes for specific tests)

▲80058 Hepatic function panel

This panel must include the following:

Albumin, serum (82040)

Bilirubin, total or direct (82250)

Phosphatase, alkaline (84075)

Transferase, aspartate amino (AST) (SGOT) (84450)

Transferase, alanine amino (ALT) (SGPT) (84460)

▲80059 Hepatitis panel

This panel must include the following:

Hepatitis B surface antigen (HBsAg) (86287)

Hepatitis B surface antibody (HBsAb) (86291)

Hepatitis B core antibody (HBcAb), IgG and IgM (86289)

Hepatitis A antibody (HAAb), IgG and IgM (86296)

Hepatitis C antibody (86302)

(80060 has been deleted. To report, see codes for specific tests)

▲80061 Lipid panel

This panel must include the following:

Cholesterol, serum, total (82465)

Lipoprotein, direct measurement, high density cholesterol (HDL cholesterol) (83718)

Triglycerides (84478)

(80062 has been deleted. To report, see 80061 and/or codes for specific tests)

(80063 has been deleted. To report, see codes for specific tests)

(80064 has been deleted. To report, see codes for specific tests)

(80065 has been deleted. To report, see codes for specific tests)

(80066 has been deleted. To report, see codes for specific tests)

(80067 has been deleted. To report, see codes for specific tests)

(80068 has been deleted. To report, see codes for specific tests)

(80070 has been deleted. To report, see 80091)

(80071 has been deleted. To report, see codes for specific tests)

▲80072 Arthritis panel

This panel must include the following:

Uric acid, blood, chemical (84550)

Sedimentation rate, erthrocyte, non-automated (85651)

Fluorescent antibody, screen, each antibody (86255)

Rheumatoid factor, qualitative (86430)

(80073 has been deleted. To report, see automated multichannel test codes (80002-80019))

(80075 has been deleted. To report, see codes for specific tests)

(80080 has been deleted. To report PSA, see 84153)

(80082 has been deleted. To report, see codes for specific tests)

(80084 has been deleted. To report, see codes for specific tests)

(80085 has been deleted. To report, see codes for specific tests)

(80086 has been deleted. To report, see codes for specific tests)

(80088 has been deleted. To report, see codes for specific tests)

(80089 has been deleted. To report, see codes for specific tests)

▲80090 TORCH antibody panel

This panel must include the following tests:

Antibody, cytomegalovirus (CMV) (86644)

Herpes simplex, non-specific type test (86694)

Antibody, rubella (86762)

Antibody, toxoplasma (86777)

● 80091 Thyroid panel;

This panel must include the following tests:

Thyroxine, total (84436)

Triodothyroine (T-3), resin uptake (84479)

● 80092 with thyroid stimulating hormone (TSH) (84443)

(80099 has been deleted. To report, use codes for specific tests)

Drug Testing

The following list contains examples of drugs or classes of drugs that are commonly assayed by qualitative screen, followed by confirmation with a second method. if a drug is present

Alcohols

Amphetamines

Barbiturates

Benzodiazepines

Cocaine and Metabolites

Methadones

Methaqualones

Opiates

Phencyclidines

Phenothiazines

Propoxyphenes

Tetrahydrocannabinoids

Tricyclic Antidepressants

Confirmed drugs may also be quantitated. Qualitative screening tests are coded by procedure, not method or analyte. For example, if chromatography is being used, code each combination of stationary and mobile phases separately using 80100 if the analysis is designed to detect multiple drug classes or 80101 if the procedure is capable of detecting a single class of drugs.

Use 80102 for each procedure necessary for confirmation, eg, if confirmation of three drugs by chromatography requires three stationary or mobile phases, use 80102 three (3) times. However, if multiple drugs can be confirmed using a single analysis, use 80102 only once.

For quantitation of drugs screened, use appropriate code in Chemistry section (82000-84999) or Therapeutic Drug Assay section (80150-80299).

The following codes (80100-80103) should be used for testing of other drugs which may not be listed above:

• **80100** Drug, screen; multiple drug classes, each procedure

• **80101** single drug class, each drug class

• **80102** Drug, confirmation, each procedure

Therapeutic Drug Assays

The material for examination may be from any source. Examination is quantitative. For nonquantitative testing, see Drug Testing (80100-80103).

• **80150** Amikacin

• **80152** Amitriptyline

- • **80154** Benzodiazepines
- • **80156** Carbamazepine
- • **80158** Cyclosporine
- • **80160** Desipramine
- • **80162** Digoxin
- • **80164** Dipropylacetic acid (valproic acid)
- • **80166** Doxepin
- • **80168** Ethosuximide
- • **80170** Gentamicin
- • **80172** Gold
- • **80174** Imipramine
- • **80176** Lidocaine
- • **80178** Lithium
- • **80182** Nortriptyline
- • **80184** Phenobarbital
- • **80185** Phenytoin; total
- • **80186** free
- • **80188** Primidone
- • **80190** Procainamide;
- • **80192** with metabolites (eg, n-acetyl procainamide)
- • **80194** Quinidine
- • **80196** Salicylate
- • **80198** Theophylline
- • **80200** Tobramycin
- • **80202** Vancomycin
- • **80299** Quantitation of drug, not elsewhere specified

Consultations (Clinical Pathology)

A clinical pathology consultation is a service, including a written report, rendered by the pathologist in response to a request from an attending physician in relation to a test result(s) requiring additional medical interpretive judgment. Reporting of a test result(s) without medical interpretive judgment is not considered a clinical pathology consultation.

80500 Clinical pathology consultation; limited, without review of patient's history and medical records

80502 comprehensive, for a complex diagnostic problem, with review of patient's history and medical records

(These codes may also be used for pharmacokinetic consultations)

(For consultations involving the examination and evaluation of the patient, see 99241-99275)

Urinalysis

(For specific analyses, see appropriate section)

▲**81000** Urinalysis, by dip stick or tablet reagent for bilirubin, glucose, hemoglobin, ketones, leukocytes, nitrite, pH, protein, specific gravity, urobilinogen, any number of these constituents; with microscopy

▲**81002** without microscopy, non-automated

● **81003** without microscopy, automated

(81004 has been deleted. To report, see 81000)

▲**81005** Urinalysis; qualitative or semiquantitative, except immunoassays

(For non-immunoassay reagent strip urinalysis, see 81000, 81002)

(For immunoassay, qualitative or semiquantitative, see 83518)

(81006 has been deleted. To report, use 81099)

(For microalbumin, see 82043, 82044)

81007 bacteriuria screen, by non-culture technique, commercial kit (specify type)

(81010, 81011, and 81012 have been deleted)

81015 microscopic only

(81020 has been deleted)

● **81025** Urine pregnancy test, by visual color comparison methods

(81030 has been deleted)

● **81050** Volume measurement for timed collection, each

81099 Unlisted urinalysis procedure

Chemistry

The material for examination may be from any source. Examination is quantitative unless specified. (For list of automated, multichannel tests, see 80002-80019).

Clinical information derived from the results of laboratory data that is mathematically calculated (eg, free thyroxine index (T7)) is considered part of the test procedure and therefore is not a separately reportable service.

82000 Acetaldehyde, blood

▲**82003** Acetaminophen

(82005 has been deleted)

▲**82009** Acetone or other ketone bodies, serum; qualitative

82010 quantitative

(82011 has been deleted. To report, use 80196)

(82012 has been deleted)

82013 Acetylcholinesterase

(Acid, gastric, see gastric acid, 82926, 82928)

(Acid phosphatase, see 84060-84066)

(82015 has been deleted)

▲**82024** Adrenocorticotropic hormone (ACTH)

▲**82030** Adenosine; 5'-monophosphate, cyclic (cyclic AMP)

(82035 has been deleted)

82040 Albumin; serum

▲**82042** urine, quantitative

● **82043** urine, microalbumin, quantitative

● **82044** urine, microalbumin, semiquantitative (eg, reagent strip assay)

(For prealbumin, see 84134)

▲**82055** Alcohol (ethanol); any specimen except breath

(For other volatiles, alcohol, see 84600)

(82060, 82065, 82070 have been deleted. To report, use 82055)

(82072 has been deleted)

▲**82075** breath

(82076, 82078 have been deleted. For ethanol, see 82055; for volatiles, see 84600)

▲**82085** Aldolase

(82086 has been deleted. To report, use 82085)

(82087 has been deleted. To report, use 82088)

▲**82088** Aldosterone;

(82089 has been deleted. To report, use 82088)

82091 saline infusion test

(Alkaline phosphatase, see 84075, 84080)

(82095 has been deleted. To report, use 80100, 80101 and 80103)

(82096 has been deleted. To report, use code for specific drug and 80103)

(82100 has been deleted. To report, use 80100 and 80101)

(Alphaketoglutarate, see 82009, 82010)

(Alpha tocopherol (Vitamin E), see 84446)

▲**82101** Alkaloids, urine, quantitative

(See also 82486-82489, 82660, 82755, 84231, 86319)

(Alphaketoglutarate, see 82009, 82010)

(Alpha tocopherol (Vitamin E), see 84446)

● **82103** Alpha-1-antitrypsin; total

● **82104** phenotype

● **82105** Alpha-fetoprotein; serum

● **82106** amniotic fluid

▲ **82108** Aluminum

(82112 has been deleted. To report, see 80150)

(82126 has been deleted)

82128 Amino acids, qualitative

82130 Amino acids, urine or plasma, chromatographic fractionation and quantitation, one or more

● **82131** Amino acids, fractionation and quantitation, each

(82134 has been deleted)

82135 Aminolevulinic acid, delta (ALA)

(82137 has been deleted. To report, use 84420)

(82138 has been deleted. To report, use 80152)

▲ **82140** Ammonia

(82141 has been deleted. To report, use 82140)

(82142 has been deleted)

82143 Amniotic fluid scan (spectrophotometric)

(For L/S ratio, see 83661)

(Amobarbital, see 80101-80103 for qualitative analysis, 82205 for quantitative analysis)

▲ **82145** Amphetamine or methamphetamine

(For qualitative analysis, see 80101-80103)

▲ **82150** Amylase

(82155 has been deleted)

(82156 has been deleted. To report, use 82150)

▲**82157** Androstenedione

(82159 has been deleted. To report, use 82160)

▲**82160** Androsterone

▲**82163** Angiotensin II

▲**82164** Angiotensin I - converting enzyme (ACE)

(82165 has been deleted)

(Antidiuretic hormone (ADH), see 84588)

(82168 has been deleted. For antihistamines, see code for specific method)

(82170 has been deleted. To report, use 83015, 83018)

(Antimony, see 83015)

(Antitrypsin, alpha-1-, see 82103, 82104)

▲**82172** Apolipoprotein, each

82173 Arginine tolerance test

▲**82175** Arsenic

(For heavy metal screening, see 83015)

82180 Ascorbic acid (Vitamin C), blood

(Aspirin, see acetylsalicylic acid, 82011)

(Atherogenic index, blood, ultracentrifugation, quantitative, see 83717)

● **82190** Atomic absorption spectroscopy, each analyte

▲**82205** Barbiturates, not elsewhere specified

(For qualitative analysis, see 80100-80103)

(82210 has been deleted. To report, see 80100-80103, 82205)

(82225, 82230 have been deleted. To report, see 83015, 83018)

(82231 has been deleted. To report, use 82232)

▲**82232** Beta-2 microglobulin

(82235, 82236 have been deleted)

(Bicarbonate, see 82374)

● **82239** Bile acids; total

▲**82240** cholylglycine

(For bile pigments, urine, see 81000-81005)

(82245 has been deleted. To report, see 81000, 81002, 81005)

▲**82250** Bilirubin; total OR direct

▲**82251** total AND direct

82252 feces, qualitative

(82260 has been deleted. To report, use 82250)

(82265 has been deleted. To report spectrophotometric scan, see 82143)

(82268 has been deleted. To report, see 83015, 83018)

82270 Blood, occult; feces screening

▲**82273** other sources, qualitative

(Blood urea nitrogen (BUN), see 84520, 84525)

(82280, 82285 have been deleted. To report, see code for specific method)

82286 Bradykinin

(82290, 82291 have been deleted. To report, use 84311)

▲**82300** Cadmium

(82305 has been deleted. To report, see 82486, 82491)

▲**82306** Calcifediol (25-OH Vitamin D-3)

▲**82307** Calciferol (Vitamin D)

(For 1,25-Dihydroxyvitamin D, use 82652)

▲**82308** Calcitonin

▲**82310** Calcium; total

(82315, 82320, 82325 have been deleted. To report, use 82310)

▲**82330** ionized

82331 after calcium infusion test

(82335 has been deleted)

▲**82340** urine quantitative, timed specimen

(82345 has been deleted)

▲**82355** Calculus (stone); qualitative analysis, chemical

▲**82360** quantitative analysis, chemical

(Carbamates, see individual listings)

82365 infrared spectroscopy

82370 x-ray diffraction

(82372 has been deleted. To report, use 80156)

▲**82374** Carbon dioxide (bicarbonate)

(See also 82802, 82803)

82375 Carbon monoxide, (carboxyhemoglobin); quantitative

82376 qualitative

● **82378** Carcinoembryonic antigen (CEA)

▲**82380** Carotene

▲**82382** Catecholamines; total urine

82383 blood

82384 fractionated

(For urine metabolites, see 83835, 84585)

● **82387** Cathepsin-D

▲**82390** Ceruloplasmin

● **82397** Chemiluminescent assay

(82400 has been deleted. To report, use code for specific method)

(82405 has been deleted)

▲**82415** Chloramphenicol

(82418, 82420, 82425 have been deleted. To report, use code for specific method)

▲**82435** Chloride; blood

▲**82436** urine

(82437 has been deleted)

(For sweat chloride with iontophoresis, see 89360)

82438 spinal fluid

82441 Chlorinated hydrocarbons, screen

(82443 has been deleted. To report, use code for specific method)

(Chlorpromazine, see 84022)

(Cholecalciferol (Vitamin D), see 82307)

82465 Cholesterol, serum, total

(For high density lipoprotein (HDL), see 83718)

(82470 has been deleted)

82480 Cholinesterase; serum

82482 RBC

(82484 has been deleted. To report, use 82480 and 82482)

82485 Chondroitin B sulfate, quantitative

(Chorionic gonadotropin, see gonadotropin, 84702, 84703)

▲**82486** Chromatography, qualitative; column (eg, gas liquid or high performance liquid chromatography), analyte not elsewhere specified

▲**82487** paper, 1-dimensional, analyte not elsewhere specified

▲**82488** paper, 2-dimensional, analyte not elsewhere specified

▲82489 thin layer, analyte not elsewhere specified

(82490 has been deleted)

● 82491 Chromotography, quantitative; column (eg, gas liquid or high performance liquid chromatography), analyte not elsewhere specified

▲82495 Chromium

(82505 has been deleted)

82507 Citrate

(82512 has been deleted. To report, use 80154)

▲82520 Cocaine or metabolite

(Cocaine, qualitative analysis, see 80100-80103)

(Codeine, qualitative analysis, see 80100-80103)

(Codeine, quantitative analysis, see 82101)

(Complement, see 86160-86162)

▲82525 Copper

(82526 has been deleted. To report, use 82525)

(Coproporphyrin, see 84119, 84120)

(Corticosteroids, see 83491)

▲82528 Corticosterone

(82529 has been deleted. To report, use 82533)

● 82530 Cortisol; free

(82531, 82532 have been deleted)

▲82533 total

(82534 has been deleted. To report, use 82533)

82536 after adrenocorticotropic hormone (ACTH) administration

82537 48 hours after continuous ACTH infusion

82538 after metyrapone tartrate administration

82539 dexamethasone suppression test, plasma and/or urine

(C-peptide, use 84681)

▲**82540** Creatine

(82545 has been deleted. To report, use 82540)

(82546 has been deleted. To report, use 82540 and 82565)

▲**82550** Creatine kinase (CK), (CPK); total

82552 isoenzymes

• **82553** MB fraction only

• **82554** isoforms

(82555 has been deleted)

▲**82565** Creatinine;

82570 urine

82575 clearance

▲**82585** Cryofibrinogen

▲**82595** Cryoglobulin

(Crystals, pyrophosphate vs. urate, see 89060)

▲**82600** Cyanide

(82601 has been deleted. To report, use 80103, 82600)

(82606 has been deleted)

▲**82607** Cyanocobalamin (Vitamin B-12);

82608 unsaturated binding capacity

(Cyclic AMP, see 82030)

(Cyclic GMP, see 83008)

(Cyclosporine, use 80158)

(82614 has been deleted)

82615 Cystine and homocystine, urine, qualitative

(82620 has been deleted. For cystine and homocystine, quantitative, see 82130)

(82624 has been deleted)

(Delta-aminolevulinic acid (ALA), see 82135)

▲**82626** Dehydroepiandrosterone (DHEA)

● **82627** Dehydroepiandrosterone-sulfate (DHEA-S)

(82628 has been deleted. To report, see 80100-80103 for qualitative analysis; see 80299 for quantitative analysis)

▲**82633** Desoxycorticosterone, 11-

▲**82634** Deoxycortisol, 11-

(Dexamethasone suppression test, see 82539)

(82635 has been deleted)

(Diastase, urine, see 82150)

(82636 has been deleted. To report, see 80100-80103, 80154)

82638 Dibucaine number

(82639 has been deleted. To report, use code for specific method)

(Dichloroethane, see 84600)

(Dichloromethane, see 84600)

(Diethylether, see 84600)

(82640, 82641 have been deleted)

(82643 has been deleted. To report, use 80162)

82646 Dihydrocodeinone

(For qualitative analysis, see 80100-80103)

▲**82649** Dihydromorphinone

(For qualitative analysis, see 80100-80103)

82651 Dihydrotestosterone (DHT)

82652 Dihydroxyvitamin D, 1,25-

(Diphenylhydantoin, see 80185)

(Dipropylacetic acid, see 80164)

82654 Dimethadione

(For qualitative analysis, see 80100-80103)

(Diphenylhydantoin, see 84045)

(Dopamine, see 82382-82384)

(82656 has been deleted. To report, use 80166)

(Duodenal contents, see individual enzymes; for intubation and collection, see 89100)

(82660 has been deleted. To report, see 80100, 80101)

(82662 has been deleted. To report, see 80100-80103)

82664 Electrophoretic technique, not elsewhere specified

(Endocrine receptor assays, see 84233-84235)

82666 Epiandrosterone

(Epinephrine, see 82382-82384)

▲**82668** Erythropoietin

▲**82670** Estradiol

82671 Estrogens; fractionated

82672 total

(82673, 82674, 82676 have been deleted. To report, use 82677)

▲**82677** Estriol

(Estrogen receptor assay, see 84233)

(82678 has been deleted. To report, use 82679)

▲**82679** Estrone

(Ethanol, see 82055 and 82075)

▲**82690** Ethchlorvynol

(82691 has been deleted. To report, see 82690)

(82692 has been deleted. To report, use 80168)

(Ethyl alcohol, see 82055 and 82075)

● **82693** Ethylene glycol

(82694 has been deleted. To report, use 82696)

▲ **82696** Etiocholanolone

(For fractionation of ketosteroids, see 83593)

▲ **82705** Fat or lipids, feces; qualitative

▲ **82710** quantitative

82715 Fat differential, feces, quantitative

(82720 has been deleted)

▲ **82725** Fatty acids, nonesterified

(82727 has been deleted. To report ferric chloride test, urine, use 81005)

▲ **82728** Ferritin

(Fetal hemoglobin, see hemoglobin 83030, 83033, and 85460)

(Fetoprotein, alpha-1, see 82105, 82106)

(82730 has been deleted. To report fibrinogen, see 85384, 85385)

▲ **82735** Fluoride

(82740 has been deleted. To report, use 82735)

(82741 has been deleted. To report, see code for specific method)

82742 Flurazepam

(For qualitative analysis, see 80100-80103)

(Foam stability test, see 83662)

(82745 has been deleted)

▲ **82746** Folic acid; serum

● **82747** RBC

(Follicle stimulating hormone (FSH), see 83001)

(82750 has been deleted. To report, use code for specific method)

(82755, 82756 have been deleted)

82757 Fructose, semen

(Fructosamine, see 82985)

(Fructose, TLC screen, see 84375)

82759 Galactokinase, RBC

▲**82760** Galactose

(82763 has been deleted. To report, use 82760 and codes for administration)

(82765 has been deleted. To report, use 82760)

82775 Galactose-1-phosphate uridyl transferase; quantitative

82776 screen

(82780 has been deleted. To report gallium, use code for specific method)

▲**82784** Gammaglobulin; IgA, IgD, IgG, IgM, each

▲**82785** IgE

(82786 has been deleted)

● **82787** immunoglobulin subclasses, (IgG1, 2, 3, and 4)

(Gamma-glutamyltransferase (GGT), see 82977)

(82790, 82791 have been deleted)

▲**82792** Gases, blood, oxygen saturation quantification

(82793, 82795 have been deleted)

82800 Gases, blood; pH only

82801 pCO_2

82802 pH, pCO_2 by electrode

82803 pH, pCO_2, pO_2 simultaneous

82804 pO_2 by electrode

82812 pO_2 by manometry

82817 pH, pCO_2 by tonometry

(For arterial puncture, see 36600)

(For blood gas studies as a part of pulmonary function studies, see 94680-94690)

● **82820** Hemoglobin-oxygen affinity (PO_2 for 50% hemoglobin saturation with oxygen)

▲ **82926** Gastric acid, free and total; each specimen

(82927 has been deleted. To report, use 82926)

▲ **82928** Gastric acid, free or total; each specimen

(82929, 82931 and 82932 have been deleted. To report, use 82928)

▲ **82938** Gastrin after secretin stimulation

▲ **82941** Gastrin

(Gentamicin, see 80170)

(GGT, see 82977)

(GLC, gas liquid chromatography, see 82486)

(82942 has been deleted)

▲ **82943** Glucagon

(82944 has been deleted)

82946 Glucagon tolerance test

▲ **82947** Glucose; quantitative

▲ **82948** blood, reagent strip

(82949 has been deleted)

82950 post glucose dose (includes glucose)

82951 tolerance test (GTT), three specimens (includes glucose)

82952 tolerance test, each additional beyond three specimens

(For intravenous glucose tolerance test, see 82961)

82953 tolbutamide tolerance test

(For insulin tolerance test, see 83526)

(For leucine tolerance test, see 83681)

(82954 has been deleted. To report, use 82947)

(For semiquantitative urine glucose, see 81000, 81002, 81005, 81099)

82955 Glucose-6-phosphate dehydrogenase (G6PD); quantitative

82960 screen

82961 Glucose tolerance test, intravenous

(For glucose tolerance test with medication, use 90784 in addition)

● **82962** Glucose, blood, by glucose monitoring device(s) cleared by the FDA specifically for home use

82963 Glucosidase, beta

▲ **82965** Glutamate dehydrogenase

▲ **82975** Glutamine (glutamic acid amide)

▲ **82977** Glutamyltransferase, gamma (GGT)

82978 Glutathione

82979 Glutathione reductase, RBC

82980 Glutethimide

(Glycohemoglobin, see 83036)

▲ **82985** Glycated protein

(82995 has been deleted. To report, use 80172)

(82996-82998 have been deleted. To report, see 84702, 84703)

(Gonadotropin, chorionic, see 84702, 84703)

(83000 has been deleted)

▲ **83001** Gonadotropin; follicle stimulating hormone (FSH)

▲83002 luteinizing hormone (LH)

(For luteinizing releasing factor (LRH), see 83727)

▲83003 Growth hormone, human (HGH) (somatotropin);

83004 after glucose tolerance test

(For growth hormone secretion after arginine tolerance test, see 82173)

(For antibody to human growth hormone, see 86277)

(83005 has been deleted)

▲83008 Guanosine monophosphate (GMP), cyclic

▲83010 Haptoglobin; quantitative

(83011 has been deleted. To report, use 83010)

▲83012 phenotypes

▲83015 Heavy metal (arsenic, barium, beryllium, bismuth, antimony, mercury); screen

▲83018 quantitative, each

▲83020 Hemoglobin, electrophoresis (eg, A2, S, C)

• 83026 Hemoglobin; by copper sulfate method, non-automated

83030 F(fetal), chemical

83033 F(fetal), qualitative (APT) test, fecal

▲83036 glycated

(83040 has been deleted. To report, see 83050)

83045 methemoglobin, qualitative

83050 methemoglobin, quantitative

83051 plasma

(83052, 83053 have been deleted. To report, use 85660)

83055 sulfhemoglobin, qualitative

83060 sulfhemoglobin, quantitative

83065 thermolabile

83068 unstable, screen

83069 urine

▲**83070** Hemosiderin; qualitative

▲**83071** quantitative

(Heroin, see 80100-80103)

(HIAA, see 83497)

(High performance liquid chromatography (HPLC), see 82486)

(83086, 83087 have been deleted. To report, use 82128)

83088 Histamine

(Hollander test, see 91052)

(Homocystine, see 82128, 82130)

(83093-83095 have been deleted. For homogentisic acid, qualitative urine screen, see 81005. For quantitative assay, see code for specific method)

▲**83150** Homovanillic acid (HVA)

(Hormones, see individual alphabetic listings in Chemistry section)

(Hydrogen breath test, see 91065)

(83485, 83486 have been deleted)

▲**83491** Hydroxycorticosteroids, 17- (17-OHCS)

(83492 has been deleted. To report, use 83491)

(83493 has been deleted)

(83494-83496 have been deleted. To report, use 83491)

(For cortisol, see 82530, 82533. For deoxycortisol, see 82634)

▲**83497** Hydroxyindolacetic acid, 5-(HIAA)

(For urine qualitative test, see 81005)

(5-Hydroxytryptamine, see 84260)

▲**83498** Hydroxyprogesterone, 17-d

83499 Hydroxyprogesterone, 20-

▲**83500** Hydroxyproline; free

▲**83505** total

(83510 has been deleted. To report, use 83500 and 83505)

• **83518** Immunoassay, for analyte other than antibody, qualitative or semiqualitative

• **83519** Immunoassay, analyte; by radionuclide technique (eg, RIA)

• **83520** not otherwise specified

(83523 has been deleted. To report, use 80174)

(Immunoglobulins, see 82784, 82785)

(83524 has been deleted)

▲**83525** Insulin

(For proinsulin, see 84206)

83526 Insulin tolerance test

▲**83528** Intrinsic factor

(For intrinsic factor antibodies, see 86340)

(83530 has been deleted)

(83533, 83534 have been deleted. To report, use 84999)

▲**83540** Iron

(83545, 83546 have been deleted. To report, use 83540)

▲**83550** Iron binding capacity

(83555, 83565 have been deleted. To report, use 83550)

▲**83570** Isocitric dehydrogenase (IDH)

(83571 has been deleted. To report, use 83570)

(Isopropyl alcohol, see 84600)

(83576 has been deleted. To report, see code for specific method)

(Isonicotinic acid hydrazide, INH, see code for specific method)

(83578 has been deleted)

▲**83582** Ketogenic steroids, fractionation

(83583, 83584 have been deleted)

(Ketone bodies for serum, see 82009, 82010; for urine, see 81000-81003)

▲**83586** Ketosteroids, 17- (17-KS); total

(83587 has been deleted. To report, use 83593)

(83588, 83589 have been deleted. To report, use 83586)

(83590 has been deleted)

▲**83593** fractionation

(83596 has been deleted)

(83597 has been deleted)

(83599 has been deleted. To report, use 83586)

(83600 has been deleted. To report, use code for specific method)

83605 Lactate (lactic acid)

(83610 has been deleted. To report, use 83615)

▲**83615** Lactate dehydrogenase (LD), (LDH);

(83620 has been deleted. To report, use 83615)

(83624 has been deleted)

▲**83625** isoenzymes, separation and quantitation

(83626 has been deleted)

(83628 has been deleted. To report, use 83625)

(83629, 83631 have been deleted. To report, use 83615)

▲**83632** Lactogen, human placental (HPL) human chorionic somatomammotropin

83633 Lactose, urine; qualitative

83634 quantitative

(For tolerance, see 82951, 82952)

(For breath hydrogen test for lactase deficiency, see 91065)

(83645 has been deleted. To report, see quantitative code or screening for toxicity)

(83650 has been deleted. To report, use 83645)

▲**83655** Lead

(For tests for lead screen, see 82135, 84202, 84203)

(83660 has been deleted. To report, use 83655)

▲**83661** Lecithin-sphingomyelin ratio (L/S ratio); quantitative

● **83662** foam stability test

▲**83670** Leucine aminopeptidase (LAP)

(83675, 83680 have been deleted. To report, see 83670)

83681 Leucine tolerance test

(83685 has been deleted. To report, use 80176)

▲**83690** Lipase

(83700, 83705 have been deleted. For cholesterol, see 82465, 83718-83721. For triglycerides, see 84478)

▲**83715** Lipoprotein, blood; electrophoretic separation and quantitation

▲**83717** ultracentrifugation and quantitation

▲**83718** Lipoprotein, direct measurement; high density cholesterol (HDL cholesterol)

▲**83719** VLDL cholesterol

(83720 has been deleted)

● **83721** LDL cholesterol

(Luteinizing hormone (LH), see 83002)

(83725 has been deleted. To report, use 80178)

▲**83727** Luteinizing releasing factor (LRH)

(For qualitative analysis, see 80100-80103)

(83728 has been deleted. To report, see 80100-80103, 80299)

(83730 has been deleted)

(Macroglobulins, alpha-2, see 86329)

▲83735 Magnesium

(83740, 83750, 83755, 83760, 83765 have been deleted. To report, use 83735)

▲83775 Malate dehydrogenase

(Maltose tolerance, see 82951, 82952)

(Mammotropin, see 84146)

▲83785 Manganese

(Marijuana, see 80100-80103)

83790 Mannitol clearance

(Marijuana, see 80100-80103, 80299)

(83795 has been deleted)

(83799 has been deleted. To report, use 83925)

▲83805 Meprobamate

(For qualitative analysis, see 80100-80103)

▲83825 Mercury, quantitative

(83830 has been deleted. To report, use 83825)

(Mercury screen, see 83015)

▲83835 Metanephrines

(For catecholamines, see 82382-82384)

83840 Methadone

(For methadone qualitative analysis, see 80100-80103)

(Methamphetamine, see 80100-80103, 82145)

(Methanol, see 84600)

(83842 has been deleted. To report, see code for specific method)

(83845 has been deleted. To report, see 80100-80103)

83857 Methemalbumin

(Methemoglobin, see hemoglobin 83045, 83050)

▲**83858** Methsuximide

(Methyl alcohol, see 84600)

(Microalbumin, see 82043 for quantitative, see 82044 for semiquantitative)

(Microglobulin, beta-2, see 82231)

(83859 has been deleted)

(83860-83862 have been deleted. To report, see 80100-80103 for qualitative analysis, 83925 for quantitative analysis)

▲**83864** Mucopolysaccharides, acid; quantitative

(83865 has been deleted. To report, use 83864)

83866 screen

(83870 has been deleted. To report, use 84999)

83872 Mucin, synovial fluid (Ropes test)

▲**83873** Myelin basic protein, CSF

(For oligoclonal bands, see 83916)

▲**83874** Myoglobin

(83875 has been deleted)

(83880 has been deleted. To report, see 83925)

• **83883** Nephelometry, each analyte not elsewhere specified

▲**83885** Nickel

83887 Nicotine

MOLECULAR DIAGNOSTICS

This series of codes 83890-83898 is intended for use with molecular diagnostic techniques for analysis of nucleic acids. These services are coded by procedure rather than analyte. Code separately for each procedure used in an analysis. For example, a procedure requiring isolation of DNA, restriction endonuclease digestion, electrophoresis, and nucleic acid probe amplification would be coded 83890, 83892, 83894, and 83898.

(For microbial identification, see 87178, 87179)

● **83890** Nuclear molecular diagnostics; molecular isolation or extraction

● **83892** enzymatic digestion

● **83894** separation (eg, dot blot, electrophoresis)

(83895 has been deleted)

● **83896** nucleic acid probe, each

● **83898** nucleic acid probe with amplification, eg, polymerase chain reaction (PCR), each

(83900 has been deleted)

(83910 has been deleted)

▲ **83912** interpretation and report

(83913 has been deleted. To report, see 83898)

83915 Nucleotidase 5'-

▲ **83916** Oligoclonal immunoglobulin (oligoclonal bands)

(83917 has been deleted)

83918 quantitative

(83920 has been deleted. To report, use code for specific method)

● **83925** Opiates, (eg, morphine, meperidine)

83930 Osmolality; blood

83935 urine

(83938 has been deleted)

▲**83945** Oxalate

(83946 has been deleted. To report, use 80154)

(83947 has been deleted. To report, see 82009, 82010)

(83948 has been deleted. To report, see 80100-80103, 83925)

(83949 has been deleted)

(83965 has been deleted. To report, use code for specific method)

▲**83970** Parathormone (parathyroid hormone)

(83971, 83972 have been deleted. To report, use code for specific method)

(83973 has been deleted. To report, use 84375)

(83974 has been deleted)

(83975, 83985 have been deleted. To report, use code for specific method)

(Pesticide, quantitative, see code for specific method. For screen for chlorinated hydrocarbons, see 82441)

83986 pH, body fluid, except blood

(For blood, see 82800-82804)

83992 Phencyclidine (PCP)

(For qualitative analysis, see 80100-80103)

(Phenobarbital, see 80184)

(83995 has been deleted. To report, use code for specific method)

(84005 has been deleted)

(84021 has been deleted. To report, see 80100, 80101, 84022)

▲**84022** Phenothiazine

(For qualitative analysis, see 80100, 80101)

▲**84030** Phenylalanine (PKU), blood

(Phenylalanine-tyrosine ratio, see 84030, 84510)

(84031 has been deleted)

(84033 has been deleted. To report, use code for specific method)

▲**84035** Phenylketones, qualitative

(84037 has been deleted. To report, use 84035)

(84038 has been deleted. To report, use code for specific method)

(84039, 84040 have been deleted)

(84045 has been deleted. To report, see 80185)

▲**84060** Phosphatase, acid; total

● **84061** forensic examination

(84065 has been deleted. To report, use 84066)

▲**84066** prostatic

▲**84075** Phosphatase, alkaline;

84078 heat stable (total not included)

▲**84080** isoenzymes

▲**84081** Phosphatidylgycerol

(84082 has been deleted)

(Phosphates inorganic, see 84100)

(Phosphates, organic, see code for specific method. For cholinesterase, see 82480, 82482)

(84083 has been deleted)

84085 Phosphogluconate, 6-, dehydrogenase, RBC

84087 Phosphohexose isomerase

(84090 has been deleted)

▲**84100** Phosphorus inorganic (phosphate);

84105 urine

(Pituitary gonadotropins, see 83000, 83002)

(PKU, see 84030, 84035)

84106 Porphobilinogen, urine; qualitative

84110 quantitative

(84118 has been deleted. To report, use 84120)

▲**84119** Porphyrins, urine; qualitative

▲**84120** quantitation and fractionation

(84121 has been deleted. To report, use 84120)

▲**84126** Porphyrins, feces; quantitative

● **84127** qualitative

(84128 has been deleted)

(Porphyrin precursors, see 82135, 84106, 84110)

(For protoporphyrin, RBC, see 84202, 84203)

▲**84132** Potassium; serum

84133 urine

● **84134** Prealbumin

(For microalbumin, see 82043, 82044)

▲**84135** Pregnanediol

(84136 has been deleted. To report, use 84135)

▲**84138** Pregnanetriol

(84139 has been deleted. To report, use 84138)

(84141 has been deleted. To report, use 80188)

(84142 has been deleted. To report, see 80190, 80192)

▲**84144** Progesterone

(Progesterone receptor assay, see 84234)

(For proinsulin, see 84206)

▲**84146** Prolactin

(84147 has been deleted. To report, see 80100-80103)

(84149 has been deleted)

▲**84150** Prostaglandin, each

● **84153** Prostate specific antigen (PSA)

▲**84155** Protein; total, except refractometry

84160 refractometric

84165 electrophoretic fractionation and quantitation

(84170 has been deleted)

▲**84175** electrophoresis, other sources requiring concentration (eg, CSF urine)

(84176 has been deleted)

(84180 has been deleted)

● **84181** Western Blot, with interpretation and report, blood or other body fluid

● **84182** Western Blot, with interpretation and report, blood or other body fluid, immunological probe for band identification, each

(For Western Blot tissue analysis, see 88371)

(84185 has been deleted)

(84190 has been deleted. To report, use 84175)

(84195 has been deleted)

(84200 has been deleted. To report, use 84175)

84201 Protirelin, thyrotropin releasing hormone (TRH) test

84202 Protoporphyrin, RBC; quantitative

84203 screen

(84205 has been deleted. To report, use code for specific method)

▲**84206** Proinsulin

(Pseudocholinesterase, see 82480)

▲**84207** Pyridoxal phosphate (Vitamin B-6)

(84208 has been deleted. To report, use 89060)

▲**84210** Pyruvate

▲**84220** Pyruvate kinase

84228 Quinine

(84230 has been deleted. To report, use 80194)

(84231 has been deleted. To report radioimmunoassay not elsewhere specified, see 83520)

(84232 has been deleted)

▲**84233** Receptor assay; estrogen

84234 progesterone

84235 endocrine, other than estrogen or progesterone (specify hormone)

(84236 has been deleted. To report, use 84233 and 84234)

84238 non-endocrine (eg, acetylcholine) (specify receptor)

▲**84244** Renin;

84246 furosemide test

(84250, 84251 have been deleted. To report, use 84479)

84252 Riboflavin (Vitamin B-2)

(Salicylates, see 82011)

(Secretin test, see 99070, 89100 and appropriate analyses)

▲**84255** Selenium

▲**84260** Serotonin

(For urine metabolites (HIAA), see 83497)

● **84270** Sex hormone binding globulin (SHBG)

▲**84275** Sialic acid

(Sickle hemoglobin, see 85660)

▲**84285** Silica

▲**84295** Sodium; serum

84300 urine

(Somatomammotropin, see 83632)

(Somatotropin, see 83003)

● **84305** Somatomedin

● **84307** Somatostatin

(84310 has been deleted)

● **84311** Spectrophotometry, analyte not elsewhere specified

84315 Specific gravity (except urine)

(For specific gravity, urine, see 81003)

(84317 has been deleted)

(84318 has been deleted)

(Stone analysis, see 82355-82370)

(84324 has been deleted. To report, use code for specific method)

84375 Sugars, chromatographic, TLC or paper chromatography

(Sulfhemoglobin, see hemoglobin, 83055, 83060)

(84382 has been deleted)

84392 Sulfate, urine

(84395 has been deleted)

(84397 has been deleted)

(T-3, see 84479-84481)

(T-4, see 84436-84439)

(84401 has been deleted)

● **84402** Testosterone; free

▲**84403** total

(84404 has been deleted)

(84405 has been deleted. To report, use 84403)

(84406 has been deleted. For testosterone binding protein, see sex hormone binding globulin, 84270)

(84407 has been deleted. To report, use code for specific method)

(84408 has been deleted. To report, see 80100-80103, 80299)

(84409, 84410 have been deleted. To report, use code for specific method)

(84420 has been deleted. To report, use 80198)

84425 Thiamine (Vitamin B-1)

▲**84430** Thiocyanate

● **84432** Thyroglobulin

(Thyroglobulin antibody, see 86800)

(84434 has been deleted. To report, use 84022)

(Thyrotropin releasing hormone (TRH) test, see 84201)

(84435 has been deleted)

▲**84436** Thyroxine; total

▲**84437** requiring elution (eg, neonatal)

▲**84439** free

(84441 has been deleted. To report, use 84436-84439)

84442 Thyroxine binding globulin (TBG)

▲**84443** Thyroid stimulating hormone (TSH)

▲**84444** Thyrotropin releasing factor (TRF)

▲**84445** Thyroid stimulating immunoglobulins (TSI)

(Tobramycin, use 80200)

84446 Tocopherol alpha (Vitamin E)

(Tolbutamide tolerance, use 82953)

(84447, 84448 have been deleted. To report, see 80100-80103)

▲**84450** Transferase; aspartate amino (AST) (SGOT)

(84455 has been deleted. To report, use 84450)

▲**84460** alanine amino (ALT) (SGPT)

(84465 has been deleted. To report, use 84460)

● **84466** Transferrin

(Iron binding capacity, see 83550)

(84472 has been deleted. To report, use code for specific method)

(84474 has been deleted. To report, use code for specific method)

(84476 has been deleted. To report, see 84022)

▲**84478** Triglycerides

▲**84479** Tridothyronine (T-3); resin uptake

▲**84480** total (TT-3)

▲**84481** free

● **84482** reverse

(84483 has been deleted. To report, see 80100-80103, 80299)

84485 Trypsin; duodenal fluid

▲**84488** feces, qualitative

▲**84490** feces, quantitative, 24-hour collection

▲**84510** Tyrosine

(Urate crystal identification, see 89060)

▲**84520** Urea nitrogen; quantitative

▲**84525** semiquantitative (eg, reagent strip test)

84540 Urea nitrogen, urine

84545 Urea nitrogen, clearance

84550 Uric acid; blood, chemical

84555 uricase, ultraviolet method

84560 Uric acid, urine

(84565, 84570, 84575 have been deleted)

84577 Urobilinogen, feces, quantitative

84578 Urobilinogen, urine; qualitative

84580 quantitative, timed specimen

84583 semiquantitative

(84584 has been deleted)

(Uroporphyrins, see 84120)

(Valproic acid (dipropylacetic acid), see 80164)

84585 Vanillylmandelic acid (VMA), urine

▲**84588** Vasopressin (antidiuretic hormone, ADH)

▲**84589** Viscosity

▲**84590** Vitamin A

(84595 has been deleted. To report, use 82380 and 84590)

(Vitamin B-1, see 84425)

(Vitamin B-2, see 84252)

(Vitamin B-6, see 84207)

(Vitamin B-12, see 82607)

(Vitamin B-12, absorption (Schilling), see 78270, 78271)

(Vitamin C, see 82180)

(Vitamin D, see 82306, 82307, 82652)

(Vitamin E, see 84446)

84597 Vitamin K

(VMA, see 84585)

▲**84600** Volatiles (eg, acetic anhydride, carbon tetrachloride, dichloroethane, dichloromethane, diethylether, isopropyl alcohol, methanol)

(For acetaldehyde, see 82000)

(84605 has been deleted)

(84610 has been deleted)

(Volume, blood, RISA or Cr-51, see 78110, 78111)

(84613 has been deleted)

(84615 has been deleted. To report, use code for specific method)

84620 Xylose absorption test, blood and/or urine

(For administration, see 99070)

▲**84630** Zinc

(84635 has been deleted. To report, use 84630)

(84645 has been deleted)

(84680 has been deleted. To report, use 82677)

▲**84681** C-peptide

(84695 has been deleted. To report, use 80170)

(84701 has been deleted. To report, see 84702-84703)

▲**84702** Gonadotropin, chorionic (hCG); quantitative

84703 qualitative

(For urine pregnancy test by visual color comparison, see 81025)

(84800 has been deleted. To report, see 84437)

(84810 has been deleted. To report, use 80200)

● **84830** Ovulation tests, by visual color comparison methods for human luteinizing hormone

▲**84999** Unlisted chemistry procedure

Hematology and Coagulation

(For blood banking procedures, see Transfusion Medicine)

(Agglutinins, see Immunology)

(Antifactor (specific coagulation factors), see 85331-85337)

(Antiplasmin, see 85410)

(Antithrombin III, see 85300, 85301)

(85000 has been deleted. To report, use 85002)

▲85002 Bleeding time

(85003 has been deleted. To report, use 85999)

(85005 has been deleted)

▲85007 Blood count; manual differential WBC count (includes RBC morphology and platelet estimation)

● 85008 manual blood smear examination without differential parameters

(See also 85585)

(For other fluids (eg, CSF), see 89050, 89051)

85009 differential WBC count, buffy coat

(85012 has been deleted)

(Eosinophils, nasal smear, see 89190)

● 85013 spun microhematocrit

▲85014 other than spun hematocrit

▲85018 hemoglobin

(For other hemoglobin determination, see 83020-83069)

85021 hemogram, automated (RBC, WBC, Hgb, Hct and indices only)

85022 hemogram, automated, and manual differential WBC count (CBC)

85023 hemogram and platelet count, automated, and manual differential WBC count (CBC)

85024 hemogram and platelet count, automated, and automated partial differential WBC count (CBC)

85025 hemogram and platelet count, automated, and automated complete differential WBC count (CBC)

85027 hemogram and platelet count, automated

(85028 has been deleted. To report, use 85023-85025)

85029 Additional automated hemogram indices (eg, red cell distribution width (RDW), mean platelet volume (MPV), red blood cell histogram, platelet histogram, white blood cell histogram); one to three indices

85030 four or more indices

85031 Blood count; hemogram, manual, complete CBC (RBC, WBC, Hgb, Hct, differential and indices)

85041 red blood cell (RBC) only

(See also 85021-85031, 89050)

85044 reticulocyte count, manual

85045 reticulocyte count, flow cytometry

85048 white blood cell (WBC)

(See also 85021-85031)

85060 Blood smear, peripheral, interpretation by physician with written report

▲**85095** Bone marrow; aspiration only

(85096 has been deleted. For interpretation of smear, use 85097; for cell block interpretation, see 88305)

85097 smear interpretation only, with or without differential cell count

(85100 has been deleted. To report, use 85095 and 85097)

(85101 has been deleted. For aspiration, see 85095)

(For special stains, see 85540, 88312, 88313)

85102 Bone marrow biopsy, needle or trocar

(For bone biopsy, use 20220)

(85103, 85105 have been deleted. For bone marrow biopsy interpretation, see 88305)

(85109 has been deleted)

(85120 has been deleted. To report, see 38230-38240)

• **85130** Chromogenic substrate assay

(85150, 85160, 85165 have been deleted)

(Circulating anti-coagulant screen (mixing studies), see 85611, 85732)

▲ **85170** Clot retraction

(85171, 85172 have been deleted)

85175 Clot lysis time, whole blood dilution

(Clotting factor I (fibrinogen), see 85384, 85385)

85210 Clotting; factor II, prothrombin, specific

(See also 85610-85613)

85220 factor V (AcG or proaccelerin), labile factor

85230 factor VII (proconvertin, stable factor)

85240 factor VIII (AHG), one stage

(85242 has been deleted)

▲ **85244** factor VIII related antigen

• **85245** factor VIII, VW factor, ristocetin cofactor

• **85246** factor VIII, VW factor antigen

• **85247** factor VIII, Von Willebrand's factor, multimetric analysis

85250 factor IX (PTC or Christmas)

85260 factor X (Stuart-Prower)

85270 factor XI (PTA)

85280 factor XII (Hageman)

85290 factor XIII (fibrin stabilizing)

85291 factor XIII (fibrin stabilizing), screen solubility

85292 prekallikrein assay (Fletcher factor assay)

85293 high molecular weight kininogen assay (Fitzgerald factor assay)

▲**85300** Clotting inhibitors or anticoagulants; antithrombin III, activity

85301 antithrombin III, antigen assay

▲**85302** protein C, antigen

• **85303** protein C, activity

▲**85305** protein S, total

• **85306** protein S, free

(85310, 85311 have been deleted)

(85320 has been deleted)

(85330 has been deleted. To report, see 85335)

• **85335** Factor inhibitor test

• **85337** Thrombomodulin

(85340, 83541 have been deleted)

85345 Coagulation time; Lee and White

85347 activated

85348 other methods

(Differential count, see 85007 et seq)

(Duke bleeding time, see 85002)

(Eosinophils, nasal smear, see 89190)

85360 Euglobulin lysis

(Fetal hemoglobin, see 83030, 83033, 85460)

▲**85362** Fibrin(ogen) degradation (split) products (FDP)(FSP); agglutination slide, semiquantitative

(85363, 85364 have been deleted)

(85365 has been deleted. To report, use 86320)

(Immunoelectrophoresis, see 86320)

● **85366** paracoagulation

(85367 has been deleted)

(85368 has been deleted. To report, use 85366)

(85369 has been deleted)

● **85370** quantitative

(83571 has been deleted. To report, see 85384, 85385)

(85372 has been deleted)

(85376, 85377 have been deleted. To report, use 85384, 85385)

● **85378** Fibrin degradation products, D-dimer; semiquantitative

● **85379** quantitative

● **85384** Fibrinogen; activity

● **85385** antigen

▲**85390** Fibrinolysins or coagulopathy screen, interpretation and report

(85392 has been deleted)

(85395 has been deleted)

(85398 has been deleted)

▲**85400** Fibrinolytic factors and inhibitors; plasmin

85410 alpha-2 antiplasmin

● **85415** plasminogen activator

85420 plasminogen, except antigenic assay

85421 plasminogen, antigenic assay

(85426 has been deleted. For von Willebrand factor assay, see 85245-85247)

(Fragility, red blood cell, see 85547, 85555-85557)

85441 Heinz bodies; direct

85445 induced, acetyl phenylhydrazine

(Hematocrit (PCV), see 85014, 85021-85031)

(Hemoglobin, see 83020-83068, 85018-85031)

85460 Hemoglobin, fetal, differential lysis (Kleihauer)

(See also 83030, 83033)

(Hemogram, see 85021-85031)

(Hemolysins, see 86006, 86281, 86282)

● **85475** Hemolysin, acid

(See also 86940, 86941)

85520 Heparin assay

● **85525** Heparin neutralization

85530 Heparin-protamine tolerance test

85535 Iron stain (RBC or bone marrow smears)

(Ivy bleeding time, see 85002)

(85538 has been deleted. For leder stain, esterase, blood or bone marrow, see 88319)

85540 Leukocyte alkaline phosphatase with count

(85544 has been deleted)

85547 Mechanical fragility, RBC

(85548 has been deleted. To report, see 85008)

▲ **85549** Muramidase

(Nitroblue tetrazolium dye test, see 86384)

▲ **85555** Osmotic fragility, RBC; unincubated

(85556 has been deleted)

▲ **85557** incubated

(Packed cell volume, see 85013)

(Partial thromboplastin time, see 85730, 85732)

(Parasites, blood (eg, malaria smears), see 87207)

(Plasmin, see 85400)

(Plasminogen, see 85420)

(Plasminogen activator, see 85415)

(85560 has been deleted. For peroxidase stain, WBC, see 88319)

▲85575 Platelet; in vitro aggregation, each agent

(85576 has been deleted. To report, see 85575)

(85577 has been deleted)

(85580 has been deleted. To report, use 85590)

85585 estimation on smear, only

(See also 85008)

▲85590 manual count

▲85595 automated count

● 85597 Platelet neutralization

85610 Prothrombin time;

● 85611 substitution, plasma fractions, each

▲85612 Russell viper venom time (includes venom); undiluted

● 85613 diluted

(85614 has been deleted)

(85615 has been deleted)

(85618 has been deleted)

(Red blood cell count, see 85021, 85031, 85041)

(85630 has been deleted. To report, use 85029, 85030)

(85632 has been deleted)

85635 Reptilase test

(Reticulocyte count, see 85044, 85045)

(85650 has been deleted)

▲85651 Sedimentation rate, erythrocyte; non-automated

85660 Sickling of RBC, reduction, slide method

(Hemoglobin electrophoresis, see 83020)

(Smears (eg, for parasites, malaria), see 87207)

(85665 has been deleted)

(85667 has been deleted)

(85700 has been deleted)

● **85705** Thromboplastin inhibition; tissue

(85710, 85711 have been deleted)

85720 all factors

(For individual clotting factors, see 85210 et seq)

85730 Thromboplastin time, partial (PTT); plasma or whole blood

85732 substitution, plasma

85810 Viscosity; blood

85820 serum or plasma

(Von Willebrand factor assay, see 85245-85247)

(WBC count, see 85021-85031, 85048, 89050)

85999 Unlisted hematology and coagulation procedure

Immunology

(Acetylcholine receptor antibody, see 86255, 86256)

(Actinomyces, antibodies to, see code for specific method)

(Adrenal cortex antibodies, see 86255, 86256)

▲ **86000** Agglutinins, febrile (eg, Brucella, Francisella, Murine typhus, Q fever, Rocky Mountain spotted fever, scrub typhus), each antigen

(86002 has been deleted)

(86004 has been deleted. To report, see 86940, 86941)

(Agglutinins and autohemolysins, see 86940, 86941)

(Alpha-1 antitrypsin, see 82103, 82104)

(Alpha-1 feto-protein, see 82105, 82106)

(Anti-AChR (acetylcholine receptor) antibody titer, see 86255, 86256)

(86006 has been deleted. To report, see 83519 and 86336 and code for specific method)

(86007, 86008, 86009 have been deleted)

(86011 has been deleted. To report, see 86021)

(86012 has been deleted. To report, see 86978)

(86013 has been deleted)

(86014 has been deleted. To report, see 86022)

(86016 has been deleted. To report, see 86850)

(86017 has been deleted. To report, see 86850 and 86901)

(86018 has been deleted)

(86019 has been deleted. To report, see 86860)

(Anticardiolipin antibody, see 86147)

(Anti-DNA, see 86225)

(Anti-deoxyribonuclease titer, see 86215)

86021 Antibody identification; leukocyte antibodies

86022 platelet antibodies

86023 platelet associated immunoglobulin assay

(86024 has been deleted. For RBC antibodies, see 86885, 86886)

(86026, 86028 have been deleted)

(86031 has been deleted. To report, see 86880)

(86032 has been deleted. To report, see 86885)

(86033 has been deleted. To report, see 86886)

(86034 has been deleted. To report, see 86880-86886 and 86971)

(86035 has been deleted. To report, use 86970)

▲**86038** Antinuclear antibodies (ANA);

• **86039** titer

(Antinuclear antibodies by fluorescent technique, see 86255, 86256)

(86045 has been deleted)

(Antistreptococcal antibody, ie, anti-DNAse, see 86215)

(Antistreptokinase titer, see 86590)

86060 Antistreptolysin 0; titer

86063 screen

(86064 has been deleted. For antitrypsin, alpha-1 see 82103, for phenotyping see 82104)

(86066, 86067 have been deleted. To report, see 82104)

(86068 has been deleted. For blood compatibility test, see 86920-86922)

(Blastomyces, antibodies to, see code for specific method)

(86069 has been deleted)

(86070 has been deleted. To report, see 86920)

(86072 has been deleted)

(86073 has been deleted. To report, see 86156, 86157, 86904)

(86074 has been deleted)

(86075, 86076 have been deleted)

86077 Blood bank physician services; difficult cross match and/or evaluation of irregular antibody(s), interpretation and written report

86078 investigation of transfusion reaction including suspicion of transmissible disease, interpretation and written report

86079 authorization for deviation from standard blood banking procedures (eg, use of outdated blood, transfusion of RH incompatible units), with written report

(86080 has been deleted. For blood typing, see 86900-86910)

(86082 has been deleted. To report, see 86900, 86901)

(86083 has been deleted. To report, see 86850 and 86901)

(86084 has been deleted. To report, see 86156, 86157)

(86085 has been deleted. To report, see 86904)

(86090 has been deleted)

(86095 has been deleted. To report, see 86905)

(86096 has been deleted)

(86100 has been deleted)

(86105 has been deleted)

(86115 has been deleted)

(86120 has been deleted. To report, use 86095)

(86128 has been deleted)

(86129 has been deleted)

(86130 has been deleted. To report, see 86891)

(86131, 86134, 86138 and 86139 have been deleted)

(Brucella, antibodies to, see code for specific method)

(Candida, antibodies to, see code for specific method. For skin testing, see 86485)

86140 C-reactive protein

(Candidiasis, see 86628)

• **86147** Cardiolipin (phospholipid) antibody

(86149 has been deleted)

(86151 has been deleted. To report, see 82378)

86155 Chemotaxis assay, specify method

(Clostridinum difficile toxin, see 87230)

(Coccidioides, antibodies to, see 86635. For skin testing, see 86490)

• **86156** Cold agglutinin; screen

• **86157** titer

(86158 has been deleted)

(86159 has been deleted. To report, see 86160 and 86161)

● **86160** Complement; antigen, each component

● **86161** functional activity, each component

▲**86162** total hemolytic (CH50)

(86163, 86164 have been deleted. To report, see 86160 and 86161)

86171 Complement fixation tests, each antigen

(Coombs test, see 86880-86886)

▲**86185** Counterimmunoelectrophoresis, each antigen

(86201, 86202 have been deleted)

(Cryptococcus, antibodies to, see code for specific method)

(86209 has been deleted. To report, use 86999)

86215 Deoxyribonuclease, antibody

▲**86225** Deoxyribonucleic acid (DNA) antibody; native or double stranded

(Echinococcus, antibodies to, see code for specific method)

(For HIV antibody tests, see 86701-86703)

● **86226** single stranded

(Anti D.S., DNA, IFA, eg, using C.Lucilae, see 86255 and 86256)

(86227, 86228 have been deleted. To report, use 86317)

(86229 has been deleted)

▲**86235** Extractable nuclear antigen, antibody to, any method (eg, nRNP, SS-A, SS-B, Sm, RNP, Sc170, J01), each antibody

(86240, 86241 have been deleted)

▲**86243** Fc receptor

(86244 has been deleted. To report, see 82105, 82106)

(86245 has been deleted)

(Filaria, antibodies to, see code for specific method)

▲**86255** Fluorescent antibody; screen, each antibody

▲**86256** titer, each antibody

(Fluorescent technique for antigen identification in tissue, see 88346; for indirect fluorescence, see 88347)

(86265 has been deleted. To report, see 86930)

(86266 has been deleted. To report, see 86931)

(FTA, see 86650)

(86267 has been deleted. To report, see 86932)

(Gel (agar) diffusion tests, see 86331)

(86272, 86273 have been deleted)

(86274 has been deleted. To report, see 90742)

▲**86277** Growth hormone, human (HGH), antibody

▲**86280** Hemagglutination inhibition test (HAI)

(For rubella, see 86762)

(86281 has been deleted. To report, see 85475)

(86282 has been deleted. To report, see 86940)

(86283 has been deleted. To report, see 86941)

(86285, 86286 have been deleted)

▲**86287** Hepatitis B surface antigen (HBsAg)

(86288 has been deleted)

▲**86289** Hepatitis B core antibody (HBcAb); IgG and IgM

▲**86290** IgM antibody

▲**86291** Hepatitis B surface antibody (HBsAb)

▲**86293** Hepatitis Be antigen (HBeAg)

▲**86295** Hepatitis Be antibody (HBeAb)

▲**86296** Hepatitis A antibody (HAAb); IgG and IgM

(86297 has been deleted. To report, use 86296)

(86298 has been deleted)

86299 IgM antibody

(86300 has been deleted. To report, see 86308)

• **86302** Hepatitis C antibody

(86305 has been deleted. To report, use 86309)

• **86306** Hepatitis, delta agent

(For hepatitis delta agent, antibody, see 86692)

• **86308** Heterophile antibodies; screening

• **86309** titer

▲**86310** titers after absorption with beef cells and guinea pig kidney

(Histoplasma, antibodies to, see 86698. For skin testing, see 86510)

▲**86311** HIV, antigen

(86312 has been deleted. To report, see 86687-86689)

(86314 has been deleted. To report, use 86689)

(Human growth hormone antibody, see 86277)

(86315 has been deleted)

▲**86316** Immunoassay for tumor antigen (eg, cancer antigen 125), each

▲**86317** Immunoassay for infectious agent antibody, quantitative, not elsewhere specified

(For immunoassays of infectious agent, see 83520)

(For particle agglutination procedures, see 86403)

▲**86318** Immunoassay to infectious agent antibody, qualitative or semiquantitative (eg, reagent strip)

(86319 has been deleted. To report immunoassays for drug, see 80100-80103)

▲**86320** Immunoelectrophoresis; serum

▲**86325** other fluids (eg, urine, CSF) with concentration

86327 crossed (2-dimensional assay)

▲**86329** Immunodiffusion; not elsewhere specified

86331 gel diffusion, qualitative (Ouchterlony), each antigen or antibody

▲**86332** Immune complex assay

(86333 has been deleted. To report, see 86332)

86334 Immunofixation electrophoresis

(86335 has been deleted)

▲**86337** Insulin antibodies

(86338 has been deleted. To report, see 86337)

▲**86340** Intrinsic factor antibodies

(Leptospira, antibodies to, see 86720)

(Leukoagglutinins, see 86021)

(86342 has been deleted. To report, see 86945)

86343 Leukocyte histamine release test (LHR)

86344 Leukocyte phagocytosis

(86345, 86346, 86347 have been deleted)

(86349 has been deleted. To report, see 86950)

(86351 has been deleted)

▲**86353** Lymphocyte transformation, mitogen (phytomitogen) or antigen induced blastogenesis

(86357 has been deleted)

(Lymphocytes immunophenotyping, see 88180 for cytometry; see 88342, 88346 for microscopic techniques)

(86358 has been deleted. To report, see 86180, 88342, 88346)

(Malaria antibodies, see 86317 for EIA; 86255 and 86256 for IFA)

(86365 has been deleted)

▲**86376** Microsomal antibodies (eg, thyroid or liver-kidney), each

(86377 has been deleted. To report, see 86376)

86378 Migration inhibitory factor test (MIF)

(Mitochondrial antibody, liver, see 86255, 86256)

(Mononucleosis, see 86308-86310)

86382 Neutralization test, viral

86384 Nitroblue tetrazolium dye test (NTD)

(Ouchterlony diffusion, see 86331)

(86385, 86386 have been deleted. To report, see 86910)

(86388, 86389, 86391 have been deleted)

(Platelet antibodies, see 86022, 86023)

(86392, 86393, 86398 have been deleted)

(86402 has been deleted)

▲**86403** Particle agglutination, antibody or antigen, each

(86404 has been deleted. To report, see 86965)

(86405 has been deleted)

(Pregnancy test, see 84702, 84703)

(86410 has been deleted. To report, see 86970)

(86411 has been deleted. To report, see 86971)

(86412 has been deleted. To report, see 86972)

(86417 has been deleted. To report, see 86975)

(86418 has been deleted. To report, see 86976)

(86419 has been deleted. To report, see 86977)

(86420 has been deleted. To report, see 86978)

▲**86421** Radioallergosorbent test, in vitro testing for allergen-specific IgE; up to 5 tests

86422 6 or more tests

(86423 has been deleted. To report, see 86421)

(Rapid plasma reagin test (RPR), see 86592, 86593)

(86424, 86425, 86426, 86427 have been deleted)

▲86430 Rheumatoid factor; qualitative

• 86431 quantitative

(86435 has been deleted. To report, use 86762)

(Serologic test for syphilis, see 86592, 86593)

(86450 has been deleted)

(86455 has been deleted. To report, use 86586)

(86450, 86460, 86470, 86480 have been deleted)

• 86485 Skin test; candida

(For antibody, candida, see 86628)

(86495, 86500, 86520, 86530 have been deleted)

86490 coccidioidomycosis

86510 histoplasmosis

(For histoplasma, antibody, see 86698)

(86540 has been deleted. For mumps, antibody, see 86735)

(86550, 86565, 86570 have been deleted)

86580 tuberculosis, intradermal

86585 tuberculosis, tine test

(For skin tests for allergy, see 95010-95199)

(Smooth muscle antibody, see 86255, 86256)

(Sporothrix, antibodies to, see code for specific method)

• 86586 unlisted antigen, each

(86587 has been deleted. To report, see 86985)

• 86588 Streptococcus, screen, direct

86590 Streptokinase, antibody

(Streptolysin O antibody, see antistreptolysin O, 86060, 86063)

86592 Syphilis test; qualitative (eg, VDRL, RPR, ART)

86593 quantitative

(Tetanus antibody, see 86774)

(Thyroglobulin antibody, see 86800)

(Thyroglobulin, see 84432)

(86594 has been deleted. To report, see 86376 and 86800)

(Thyroid microsomal antibody, see 86376)

(86595 has been deleted)

(86597 has been deleted. To report use 86812-86822)

(86600 has been deleted)

Procedures for the identification of antibodies should be coded as precisely as possible. For example, an antibody to a virus could be coded with increasing specificity for virus, family, genus, species, or type. In some cases, further precision may be added to codes by specifying the class of immunoglobulin being detected. When multiple tests are done to detect antibodies to organisms classified more precisely than the specificity allowed by available codes, it is appropriate to code each as a separate service. For example, a test for antibody to an enterovirus is coded as 86658. Coxsackie viruses are enteroviruses, but there are no codes for the individual species of enterovirus. If assays are performed for antibodies to Coxsackie A and B species, each assay should be separately coded. Similarly, if multiple assays are performed for antibodies of different immunoglobulin classes, each assay should be coded separately.

• **86602** Antibody; actinomyces

• **86603** adenovirus

• **86606** Aspirgillus

• **86609** bacterium, not elsewhere specified

• **86612** Blastomyces

• **86615** Bordetella

• **86618** Borellia Bufgdorferi (Lyme disease)

• **86619** Borrelia (relapsing fever)

• **86622** Brucella

• **86625** Campylobacter

• **86628** Candida

(For skin test, candida, see 86485)

(86630 has been deleted)

• **86631** Chlamydia

• **86632** Chlamydia, IgM

(For chlamydia antigen, see 86317)

• **86635** Coccidioides

• **86638** Coxiella Brunetii (Q fever)

• **86641** Cryptococcus

• **86644** cytomegalovirus (CMV)

(For TORCH panel, see 80090)

• **86645** cytomegalovirus (CMV), IgM

• **86648** Diptheria

(86650 has been deleted. To report, use 86781)

• **86651** encephalitis, California (La Crosse)

• **86652** encephalitis, Eastern equine

• **86653** encephalitis, St. Louis

• **86654** encephalitis, Western equine

• **86658** enterovirus (eg, coxsackie, echo, polio)

(86662 has been deleted. To report, use 86650)

(Trichinella, antibodies to, see code for specific method)

(Trypanosoma, antibodies to, see code for specific method)

(Tuberculosis, see 86580 for skin testing)

(Viral antibodies, see code for specific method)

• **86663** Epstein-Barr (EB) virus, early antigen (EA)

● **86664** Epstein-Barr (EB) virus, nuclear antigen (EBNA)

● **86665** Epstein-Barr (EB) virus, viral capsid (VCA)

● **86668** Francisella Tularensis

● **86671** fungus, not elsewhere specified

● **86674** Giardia Lamblia

● **86677** Helicobacter Pylori

(86681 has been deleted. To report, see 86255, 86256)

● **86682** helminth, not elsewhere specified

● **86684** Hemophilus influenza

(86685 has been deleted. To report, see 86255, 86256)

▲ **86687** HTLV I

● **86688** HTLV-II

▲ **86689** HTLV or HIV antibody, confirmatory test (eg, Western Blot)

● **86692** hepatitis, delta agent

(For hepatitis delta agent, antigen, see 86306)

● **86694** herpes simplex, non-specific type test

(For TORCH panel, see 80090)

● **86695** herpes simplex, type I

● **86698** histoplasma

● **86701** HIV-1

● **86702** HIV-2

● **86703** HIV-1 and HIV-2, single assay

(For HIV antigen, see 86311)

(For confirmatory test for HIV antibody (eg, Western Blot), see 86689)

● **86710** influenza virus

● **86713** Legionella

• **86717**	Leishmania
• **86720**	Leptospira
• **86723**	Listeria Monocytogenes
• **86727**	lymphocytic choriomeningitis
• **86729**	Lymphogranuloma Venereum
• **86732**	mucormycosis
• **86735**	mumps
• **86738**	Mycoplasma
• **86741**	Neisseria Meningitidis
• **86744**	Nocardia
• **86747**	parvovirus
• **86750**	Plasmodium (malaria)
• **86753**	protozoa, not elsewhere specified
• **86756**	respiratory syncytial virus
• **86759**	rotavirus
• **86762**	rubella
• **86765**	rubeola
• **86768**	Salmonella
• **86771**	Shigella
• **86774**	tetanus
• **86777**	Toxoplasma
• **86778**	Toxoplasma, IgM
• **86781**	Treponema Pallidum, confirmatory test (eg, FTA-abs)
• **86784**	trichinella
• **86787**	varicella-zoster
• **86790**	virus, not elsewhere specified
• **86793**	Yersinia

▲86800 Thyroglobulin antibody

(For thyroglobulin, see 84432)

TISSUE TYPING

(For pretransplant cross-match, use appropriate code or codes)

86805 Lymphocytotoxicity assay, visual crossmatch; with titration

86806 without titration

86807 Serum screening for cytotoxic percent reactive antibody (PRA); standard method

86808 quick method

(86810 has been deleted)

▲86812 HLA typing; A, B, or C (eg, A10, B7, B27), single antigen

▲86813 A, B, or C, multiple antigens

▲86816 DR/DQ, single antigen

▲86817 DR/DQ, multiple antigens

86821 lymphocyte culture, mixed (MLC)

86822 lymphocyte culture, primed (PLC)

• 86849 Unlisted immunology procedure

Transfusion Medicine

(For apheresis, see 36520)

(For therapeutic phlebotomy, see 99195)

• 86850 Antibody screen, RBC, each serum technique

• 86860 Antibody elution (RBC), each elution

• 86870 Antibody identification, RBC antibodies, each panel for each serum technique

• 86880 Antihuman globulin test (Coombs test); direct, each antiserum

• 86886 indirect, titer, each antiserum

• 86890 Autologous blood or component, collection processing and storage; predeposited

● **86891** intra or postoperative salvage

(For physician services to autologous donors, see 99201-99204)

● **86900** Blood typing; ABO

● **86901** Rh (D)

● **86903** antigen screening for compatible blood unit using reagent serum, per unit screened

● **86904** antigen screening for compatible unit using patient serum, per unit screened

● **86905** RBC antigens, other than ABO or Rh (D), each

● **86906** Rh phenotyping, complete

● **86910** typing for paternity testing, ABO, Rh and MN, per individual typing for paternity testing, each additional antigen system

● **86915** Bone marrow, modification or treatment to eliminate cell (eg, T-cells, metastatic carcinoma)

● **86920** Compatibility test each unit; immediate spin technique

● **86921** incubation technique

● **86922** antiglobulin technique

● **86927** Fresh frozen plasma, thawing, each unit

● **86930** Frozen blood, preparation for freezing, each unit;

● **86931** with thawing

● **86932** with freezing and thawing

● **86940** Hemolysins and agglutinins, auto, screen, each;

● **86941** incubated

● **86945** Irradiation of blood product, each unit

● **86950** Leukocyte transfusion

(For leukopheresis, see 36520)

● **86965** Pooling of platelets or other blood products

● **86970** Pretreatment of RBC's for use in RBC antibody detection, identification, and/or compatibility testing; incubation with chemical agents or drugs, each

● **86971** incubation with enzymes, each

● **86972** by density gradient separation

● **86975** Pretreatment of serum for use in RBC antibody identification; incubation with drugs, each

● **86976** by dilution

● **86977** incubation with inhibitors, each

● **86978** by differential red cell absorption using patient RBC's or RBC's of known phenotype, each absorption

● **86985** Splitting of blood or blood products, each unit

▲ **86999** Unlisted transfusion medicine procedure

Microbiology

(Includes bacteriology, mycology, parasitology, and virology)

87001 Animal inoculation, small animal; with observation

87003 with observation and dissection

87015 Concentration (any type), for parasites, ova, or tubercle bacillus (TB, AFB)

87040 Culture, bacterial, definitive; blood (includes anaerobic screen)

87045 stool

87060 throat or nose

87070 any other source

(For urine, see 87086-87088)

87072 Culture or direct bacterial identification method, each organism, by commercial kit, any source except urine

(For urine, see 87087)

87075 Culture, bacterial, any source; anaerobic (isolation)

87076 definitive identification, each anaerobic organism, including gas chromatography

(For anaerobe without GC, see 87072)

87081 Culture, bacterial, screening only, for single organisms

87082 Culture, presumptive, pathogenic organisms, screening only, by commercial kit (specify type); for single organisms

87083 multiple organisms

87084 with colony estimation from density chart

87085 with colony count

(For urine colony count, see 87086)

87086 Culture, bacterial, urine; quantitative, colony count

87087 commercial kit

87088 identification, in addition to quantitative or commercial kit

87101 Culture, fungi, isolation (with or without presumptive identification); skin

87102 other source (except blood)

87103 blood

87106 Culture, fungi, definitive identification of each fungus (use in addition to codes 87101, 87102, or 87103 when appropriate)

87109 Culture, mycoplasma, any source

87110 Culture, chlamydia

87116 Culture, tubercle or other acid-fast bacilli (eg, TB, AFB, mycobacteria); any source, isolation only

87117 concentration plus isolation

87118 Culture, mycobacteria, definitive identification of each organism

87140 Culture, typing; fluorescent method, each antiserum

87143 gas liquid chromatography (GLC) method

87145 phage method

87147 serologic method, agglutination grouping, per antiserum

87151 serologic method, speciation

87155 precipitin method, grouping, per antiserum

87158 other methods

87163 Culture, any source, additional identification methods required (use in addition to primary culture code)

87164 Dark field examination, any source (eg, penile, vaginal, oral, skin); includes specimen collection

87166 without collection

(87173 has been deleted)

87174 Endotoxin, bacterial (pyrogens); chemical

87175 biological assay (eg, Limulus lysate)

87176 homogenization, tissue, for culture

87177 Ova and parasites, direct smears, concentration and identification

(Individual smears and procedures, see 87015, 87208-87211)

(Trichrome, iron hemotoxylin and other special stains, see 88312)

87178 Microbial identification, nucleic acid probes, each probe used;

(For nucleic acid probes in cytologic material, use 88365)

87179 with amplification, eg, polymerase chain reaction (PCR)

(For molecular diagnostics, see 83890-83898)

87181 Sensitivity studies, antibiotic; agar diffusion method, per antibiotic

87184 disk method, per plate (12 or less disks)

87186 microtiter, minimum inhibitory concentration (MIC), any number of antibiotics

87187 minimum bactericidal concentration (MBC) (use in addition to 87186 or 87188)

87188 macrotube dilution method, each antibiotic

87190 tubercle bacillus (TB, AFB), each drug

87192 fungi, each drug

87197 Serum bactericidal titer (Schlicter test)

87205 Smear, primary source, with interpretation; routine stain for bacteria, fungi, or cell types

87206 fluorescent and/or acid fast stain for bacteria, fungi, or cell types

87207 special stain for inclusion bodies or intracellular parasites (eg, malaria, kala azar, herpes)

87208 direct or concentrated, dry, for ova and parasites

(For concentration, see 87015; complete examination, see 87177)

(For complex special stains, see 88312, 88313)

(For fat, meat, fibers, nasal eosinophils, and starch, see miscellaneous section)

87210 wet mount with simple stain, for bacteria, fungi, ova, and/or parasites

87211 wet and dry mount, for ova and parasites

87220 Tissue examination for fungi (eg, KOH slide)

87230 Toxin or antitoxin assay, tissue culture (eg, Clostridium difficile toxin)

87250 Virus identification; inoculation of embryonated eggs, or small animal, includes observation and dissection

87252 tissue culture inoculation and observation

87253 tissue culture, additional studies (eg, hemabsorption, neutralization) each isolate

(Electron microscopy, see 88348)

(Inclusion bodies in tissue sections, see 88304-88309; in smears, see 87207-87210; in fluids, see 88106)

(87300 has been deleted. To report, use 87999)

87999 Unlisted microbiology procedure

Anatomic Pathology

POSTMORTEM EXAMINATION

(Procedures 88000 through 88099 represent physician services only. Use modifier -90 or 09990 for outside laboratory services)

88000 Necropsy (autopsy), gross examination only; without CNS

88005 with brain

88007 with brain and spinal cord

88012 infant with brain

88014 stillborn or newborn with brain

88016 macerated stillborn

88020 Necropsy (autopsy), gross and microscopic; without CNS

88025 with brain

88027 with brain and spinal cord

88028 infant with brain

88029 stillborn or newborn with brain

88036 Necropsy (autopsy), limited, gross and/or microscopic; regional

88037 single organ

88040 Necropsy (autopsy); forensic examination

88045 coroner's call

88099 Unlisted necropsy (autopsy) procedure

CYTOPATHOLOGY

88104 Cytopathology, fluids, washings or brushings, except cervical or vaginal; smears with interpretation

88106 filter method only with interpretation

88107 smears and filter preparation with interpretation

88108 concentration technique, smears and interpretation (eg, Saccomanno technique)

(88109 has been deleted. For interpretation of smear, use 88104; for cell block interpretation, see 88305)

(For cervical or vaginal smears, see 88150-88156)

(For gastric intubation with lavage, see 89130-89141, 91055)

(For x-ray localization, see 74340)

88125 Cytopathology, forensic (eg, sperm)

88130 Sex chromatin identification; Barr bodies

88140 peripheral blood smear, polymorphonuclear "drumsticks"

(For Guard stain, see 88313)

▲**88150** Cytopathology, smears, cervical or vaginal, up to three smears; screening by technician under physician supervision

88151 requiring interpretation by physician

88155 with definitive hormonal evaluation (eg, maturation index, karyopyknotic index, estrogenic index)

● **88156** Cytopathology, smears, cervical or vaginal, the Bethesda System (TBS), up to three smears; screening by technician under physician supervision

● **88157** requiring interpretation by physician

88160 Cytopathology, any other source; screening and interpretation

88161 preparation, screening and interpretation

88162 extended study involving over 5 slides and/or multiple stains

(For obtaining specimen, see percutaneous needle biopsy under individual organ in Surgery)

(For aerosol collection of sputum, see 89350)

(For special stains, see 88312-88314)

88170 Fine needle aspiration with or without preparation of smears; superficial tissue (eg, thyroid, breast, prostate)

(For percutaneous needle biopsy, see 60100 for thyroid, 19100 for breast, 55700 for prostate)

88171 deep tissue under radiologic guidance

(For radiological supervision and interpretation, see 76003, 76360, 76942)

(For percutaneous needle biopsy, see 32405 for lung, 47000, 47001 for liver, 48102 for pancreas, 49180 for abdominal or retroperitoneal mass)

88172 Evaluation of fine needle aspirate with or without preparation of smears; immediate cytohistologic study to determine adequacy of specimen(s)

88173 interpretation and report

88180 Flow cytometry; each cell surface marker

88182 cell cycle or DNA analysis

(For tumor morphometry and DNA and ploidy analysis by imaging techniques, use 88358)

88199 Unlisted cytopathology procedure

(For electron microscopy, see 88348, 88349)

CYTOGENETIC STUDIES

(For acetylcholinesterase, see 82013)

(For alpha-fetoprotein, serum or amniotic fluid, see 82105, 82106)

88230 Tissue culture for chromosome analysis; lymphocyte

88233 skin or other solid tissue biopsy

88235 amniotic fluid or chorionic villus cells

88237 bone marrow (myeloid) cells

88239 other tissue

88245 Chromosome analysis for breakage syndromes; score 25 cells (SCE study), count 5 cells, 1 karyotype, with banding (eg, Bloom syndrome)

88248 score 100 cells, count 20 cells, 2 karyotypes, with banding (eg, ataxia telangiectasia, Fanconi anemia)

88250 Chromosome analysis for fragile X associated with fragile X-linked mental retardation, score 100 cells, count 20 cells, 2 karyotypes, with banding

88260 Chromosome analysis; count 5 cells, screening, with banding

88261 count 5 cells, 1 karyotype, with banding

88262 count 15-20 cells, 2 karyotypes, with banding

88263 count 45 cells for mosaicism, 2 karyotypes, with banding

(88265 has been deleted. To report, use 88262)

88267 Chromosome analysis, amniotic fluid or chorionic villus, count 15 cells, 1 karyotype, with banding

(88268 has been deleted. To report, see 88261)

88269 Chromosome analysis, in situ for amniotic fluid cells, count cells from 6-12 colonies, 1 karyotype, with banding

(88270 has been deleted. To report, see 88261)

88280 Chromosome analysis; additional karyotypes, each study

88283 additional specialized banding technique (eg, NOR, C-banding)

88285 additional cells counted, each study

88289 additional high resolution study

88299 Unlisted cytogenetic study

Surgical Pathology

Services 88300 through 88309 include accession, examination, and reporting. They do not include the services designated in codes 88311 through 88365 and 88399, which are coded in addition when provided.

The unit of service for codes 88300 through 88309 is the specimen. A specimen is defined as tissue or tissues that is (are) submitted for individual and separate attention, requiring individual examination and pathologic diagnosis. Two or more such specimens from the same patient (eg, separately identified endoscopic biopsies, skin lesions, etc.) are each appropriately assigned an individual code reflective of its proper level of service.

Service code 88300 is used for any specimen that in the opinion of the examining pathologist can be accurately diagnosed without microscopic examination. Service code 88302 is used when gross and microscopic examination is performed on a specimen to confirm identification and the absence of disease. Service codes 88304 through 88309 describe all other specimens requiring gross and microscopic examination, and represent additional ascending levels of physician work. Levels 88302 through 88309 are specifically defined by the assigned specimens.

Any unlisted specimen should be assigned to the code which most closely reflects the physician work involved when compared to other specimens assigned to that code.

88300 LEVEL I - Surgical pathology, gross examination only

88302 LEVEL II - Surgical pathology, gross and microscopic examination

Appendix, Incidental
Fallopian Tube, Sterilization
Fingers/Toes, Amputation, Traumatic
Foreskin, Newborn
Hernia Sac, Any Location
Hydrocele Sac
Nerve
Skin, Plastic Repair
Sympathetic Ganglion
Testis, Castration
Vaginal Mucosa, Incidental
Vas Deferens, Sterilization

88304 LEVEL III - Surgical pathology, gross and microscopic examination

Abortion, Induced
Abscess
Aneurysm - Arterial/Ventricular
Anus, Tag
Appendix, Other than Incidental
Artery, Atheromatous Plaque
Bartholin's Gland Cyst
Bone Fragment(s), Other than Pathologic Fracture
Bursa/Synovial Cyst
Carpal Tunnel Tissue
Cartilage, Shavings
Cholesteatoma
Colon, Colostomy Stoma
Conjunctiva - Biopsy/Pterygium
Cornea
Diverticulum - Esophagus/Small Bowel
Dupuytren's Contracture Tissue
Femoral Head, Other than Fracture
Fissure/Fistula
Foreskin, Other than Newborn
Gallbladder
Ganglion Cyst
Hematoma
Hemorrhoids
Hydatid of Morgagni
Intervertebral Disc
Joint, Loose Body
Meniscus
Mucocele, Salivary
Neuroma - Morton's/Traumatic
Pilonidal Cyst/Sinus
Polyps, Inflammatory - Nasal/Sinusoidal
Skin - Cyst/Tag/Debridement
Soft Tissue, Debridement
Soft Tissue, Lipoma
Spermatocele
Tendon/Tendon Sheath
Testicular Appendage
Thrombus or Embolus
Tonsil and/or Adenoids
Varicocele
Vas Deferens, Other than Sterilization
Vein, Varicosity

The level of a given specimen depends on the degree of difficulty involved in the physicians evaluation of a particular specimen -- as well as the type of tissue being examined and how the test was performed (under gross and/or microscopic examination.

88305 LEVEL IV - Surgical pathology, gross and microscopic examination

Abortion - Spontaneous/Missed
Artery, Biopsy
Bone Marrow, Biopsy
Bone Exostosis
Brain/Meninges, Other than for Tumor Resection
Breast, Biopsy
Breast, Reduction Mammoplasty
Bronchus, Biopsy
Cell Block, Any Source
Cervix, Biopsy
Colon, Biopsy
Duodenum, Biopsy
Endocervix, Curettings/Biopsy
Endometrium, Curettings/Biopsy
Esophagus, Biopsy
Extremity, Amputation, Traumatic
Fallopian Tube, Biopsy
Fallopian Tube, Ectopic Pregnancy
Femoral Head, Fracture
Fingers/Toes, Amputation, Non-traumatic
Gingiva/Oral Mucosa, Biopsy
Heart Valve
Joint, Resection
Kidney, Biopsy
Larynx, Biopsy
Leiomyoma(s), Uterine Myomectomy - without Uterus
Lip, Biopsy/Wedge Resection
Lung, Transbronchial Biopsy
Lymph Node, Biopsy
Muscle, Biopsy
Nasal Mucosa, Biopsy
Nasopharynx/Oropharynx, Biopsy
Nerve, Biopsy
Odontogenic/Dental Cyst
Omentum, Biopsy
Ovary with or without Tube, Non-neoplastic
Ovary, Biopsy/Wedge Resection
Parathyroid Gland
Peritoneum, Biopsy
Pituitary Tumor
Placenta, Other than Third Trimester
Pleura/Pericardium - Biopsy/Tissue
Polyp, Cervical/Endometrial
Polyp, Colorectal
Polyp, Stomach/Small Bowel
Prostate, Needle Biopsy
Prostate, TUR
Salivary Gland, Biopsy
Sinus, Paranasal Biopsy
Skin, Other than Cyst/Tag/Debridement/Plastic Repair
Small Intestine, Biopsy
Soft Tissue, Other than Tumor/Mass/Lipoma/Debridement
Spleen
Stomach, Biopsy
Synovium
Testis, Other than Tumor/Biopsy/Castration
Thyroglossal Duct/Brachial Cleft Cyst
Tongue, Biopsy
Tonsil, Biopsy
Trachea, Biopsy
Ureter, Biopsy
Urethra, Biopsy
Urinary Bladder, Biopsy
Uterus, with or without Tubes & Ovaries, for Prolapse
Vagina, Biopsy
Vulva/Labia, Biopsy

88307 LEVEL V - Surgical pathology, gross and microscopic examination

Adrenal, Resection
Bone - Biopsy/Curettings
Bone Fragment(s), Pathologic Fracture
Brain, Biopsy
Brain/Meninges, Tumor Resection
Breast, Mastectomy - Partial/Simple
Cervix, Conization
Colon, Segmental Resection, Other than for Tumor
Extremity, Amputation, Non-traumatic
Eye, Enucleation
Kidney, Partial/Total Nephrectomy
Larynx, Partial/Total Resection
Liver, Biopsy - Needle/Wedge
Liver, Partial Resection
Lung, Wedge Biopsy
Lymph Nodes, Regional Resection
Mediastinum, Mass
Myocardium, Biopsy
Odontogenic Tumor
Ovary with or without Tube, Neoplastic
Pancreas, Biopsy
Placenta, Third Trimester
Prostate, Except Radical Resection
Salivary Gland
Small Intestine, Resection, Other than for Tumor
Soft Tissue Mass (except Lipoma) - Biopsy/Simple Excision
Stomach - Subtotal/Total Resection, Other than for Tumor
Testis, Biopsy
Thymus, Tumor
Thyroid, Total/Lobe
Ureter, Resection
Urinary Bladder, TUR
Uterus, with or without Tubes & Ovaries, Other than Neoplastic/Prolapse

88309 LEVEL VI - Surgical pathology, gross and microscopic examination

Bone Resection
Breast, Mastectomy - with Regional Lymph Nodes
Colon, Segmental Resection for Tumor
Colon, Total Resection
Esophagus, Partial/Total Resection
Extremity, Disarticulation
Fetus, with Dissection
Larynx, Partial/Total Resection - with Regional Lymph Nodes
Lung - Total/Lobe/Segment Resection
Pancreas, Total/Subtotal Resection
Prostate, Radical Resection
Small Intestine, Resection for Tumor
Soft Tissue Tumor, Extensive Resection
Stomach - Subtotal/Total Resection for Tumor
Testis, Tumor

Tongue/Tonsil - Resection for Tumor
Urinary Bladder, Partial/Total Resection
Uterus, with or without Tubes & Ovaries, Neoplastic
Vulva, Total/Subtotal Resection

(For fine needle aspiration, preparation, and interpretation of smears, see 88170-88173)

88311 Decalcification procedure (List separately in addition to code for surgical pathology examination)

88312 Special stains (List separately in addition to code for surgical pathology examination); Group I for microorganisms (eg, Gridley, acid fast, methenamine silver), each

88313 Group II, all other, (eg, iron, trichrome), except immunocytochemistry and immunoperoxidase stains, each

(For immunocytochemistry and immunoperoxidase tissue studies, use 88342)

88314 histochemical staining with frozen section(s)

(88316 has been deleted. To report, use 99070)

(88317 has been deleted)

88318 Determinative histochemistry to identify chemical components (eg, copper, zinc)

88319 Determinative histochemistry or cytochemistry to identify enzyme constituents, each

88321 Consultation and report on referred slides prepared elsewhere

88323 Consultation and report on referred material requiring preparation of slides

88325 Consultation, comprehensive, with review of records and specimens, with report on referred material

88329 Pathology consultation during surgery;

88331 with frozen section(s), single specimen

88332 each additional tissue block with frozen section(s)

88342 Immunocytochemistry (including tissue immunoperoxidase), each antibody

(88345 has been deleted. To report, use 88346)

88346 Immunofluorescent study, each antibody; direct method

88347 indirect method

88348 Electron microscopy; diagnostic

88349 scanning

88355 Morphometric analysis; skeletal muscle

88356 nerve

88358 tumor

When semi-thin plastic-embedded sections are performed in conjunction with morphometric analysis, only the morphometric analysis should be coded; if performed as an independent procedure, see codes 88300-88309 for surgical pathology.

(88360 has been deleted. To report, use 88399)

88362 Nerve teasing preparations

(For physician interpretation of peripheral blood smear, use 85060)

88365 Tissue in situ hybridization, interpretation and report

(88370 has been deleted. To report, use 88342)

● **88371** Protein analysis of tissue by Western Blot, with interpretation and report;

● **88372** immunological probe for band identification, each

88399 Unlisted surgical pathology procedure

Miscellaneous

(Basal metabolic rate has been deleted. If necessary to report, use 89399)

(89005-89007 have been deleted)

89050 Cell count, miscellaneous body fluids (eg, CSF, joint fluid), except blood;

89051 with differential count

89060 Crystal identification by light microscopy with or without polarizing lens analysis, any body fluid (except urine)

(89070, 89080 have been deleted)

89100 Duodenal intubation and aspiration; single specimen (eg, simple bile study or afferent loop culture) plus appropriate test procedure

89105 collection of multiple fractional specimens with pancreatic or gallbladder stimulation, single or double lumen tube

(For radiological localization, see 74340)

(For chemical analyses, see Chemistry)

(Electrocardiogram, see 93000-93269)

(Esophagus acid perfusion test (Bernstein), see 91030)

89125 Fat stain, feces, urine, or sputum

89130 Gastric intubation and aspiration, diagnostic, each specimen, for chemical analyses or cytopathology;

89132 after stimulation

89135 Gastric intubation, aspiration, and fractional collections (eg, gastric secretory study); one hour

89136 two hours

89140 two hours including gastric stimulation (eg, histalog, pentagastrin)

89141 three hours, including gastric stimulation

(For gastric lavage, therapeutic, see 91105)

(For radiologic localization of gastric tube, see 74340)

(For chemical analyses, see 82926, 82928)

(Joint fluid chemistry, see Chemistry, this section)

89160 Meat fibers, feces

(89180 has been deleted. To report, use 89190)

89190 Nasal smear for eosinophils

89205 Occult blood, any source except feces

(Occult blood, feces, see 82270)

(Paternity tests, see 86910)

(89210 has been deleted)

89300 Semen analysis; presence and/or motility of sperm including Huhner test

89310 motility and count

89320 complete (volume, count, motility and differential)

(Skin tests, see 86485-86585 and 95010-95199)

(89323 has been deleted. To report, use 89325)

89325 Sperm antibodies

(For medicolegal identification of sperm, see 88125)

89329 Sperm evaluation; hamster penetration test

89330 cervical mucus penetration test, with or without spinnbarkeit test

(89345 has been deleted)

89350 Sputum, obtaining specimen, aerosol induced technique (separate procedure)

89355 Starch granules, feces

89360 Sweat collection by iontophoresis

(For chloride and sodium analysis, see 82437, 84295)

89365 Water load test

89399 Unlisted miscellaneous pathology test

Medicine

Guidelines

In addition to the definitions and commonly used terms presented in the **INTRODUCTION,** several other items unique to this section on **MEDICINE** are defined or identified here:

1. **MULTIPLE PROCEDURES:** It is appropriate to designate multiple procedures that are rendered on the same date by separate entries. For example: If individual medical psychotherapy (90841) is rendered in addition to subsequent hospital care (eg, 99231), the psychotherapy would be reported separately from the hospital visit. In this instance, both 99231 and 90841 would be reported.

2. **SEPARATE PROCEDURES:** Some of the listed procedures are commonly carried out as an integral part of a total service, and as such, do not warrant a separate identification. When, however, such a procedure is performed independently of, and is not immediately related to, other services, it may be listed as a "separate procedure." Thus, when a procedure that is ordinarily a component of a larger procedure is performed alone for a specific purpose, it may be reported as a separate procedure.

3. **SUBSECTION INFORMATION:** Several of the subheadings or subsections have special instructions unique tothat section. These special instructions will be presented preceding those procedural terminology listings, referring to that subsection specifically. If there is an "Unlisted Procedure" code number (see item 4) for the individual subsection, it will also be shown. Those subsections within the **MEDICINE** section that have special instructions are as follows:

Subsection	Code Numbers
Psychiatry	90801-90899
Ophthalmology	92002-92499
Otorhinolaryngology	92502-92599
Non-Invasive Vascular Diagnostic Studies	93875-93979

Subsection	Code Numbers
Pulmonary	94010-94799
Allergy and clinical immunology	95000-95199
Neurology and neuromuscular	95819-95999

4. **UNLISTED SERVICE OR PROCEDURE:** A service or procedure may be provided that is not listed in this edition of CPT. When reporting such a service, the appropriate "Unlisted Procedure" code may be used to indicate the service, identifying it by "Special Report" as discussed on page 600. The "Unlisted Procedures" and accompanying codes for **MEDICINE** are as follows:

90749	Unlisted immunization procedure
90799	Unlisted therapeutic or diagnostic injection
90899	Unlisted psychiatric service or procedure
90915	Unlisted biofeedback procedure
90999	Unlisted dialysis procedure, inpatient or outpatient
91299	Unlisted diagnostic gastroenterology procedure
92499	Unlisted ophthalmological service or procedure
92599	Unlisted otorhinolaryngological service or procedure
93799	Unlisted cardiovascular service or procedure
94799	Unlisted pulmonary service or procedure
95199	Unlisted allergy/clinical immunologic service or procedure
95999	Unlisted neurological or neuromuscular diagnostic procedure
96549	Unlisted chemotherapy procedure
96999	Unlisted special dermatological service or procedure
97799	Unlisted physical medicine service or procedure
99199	Unlisted special service or report

5. **SPECIAL REPORT:** A service that is rarely provided, unusual, variable, or new may require a special report in determining medical appropriateness of the service. Pertinent information should include an adequate definition or description of the nature, extent, and need for the procedure; and the time, effort, and equipment necessary to provide the service. Additional items which may be included are:

   Complexity of symptoms, final diagnosis, pertinent physical findings, diagnostic and therapeutic procedures, concurrent problems, and follow-up care.

6. **MODIFIERS:** Listed services and procedures may be modified under certain circumstances. When applicable, the modifying circumstance should be identified by the addition of the appropriate modifier code, which may be reported in either of two ways. The modifier may be reported by a two digit number placed *after* the usual procedure number from which it is separated by a hyphen. Or, the modifier may be reported by a separate five digit code that is used *in addition* to the procedure code. If more than one modifier is used, place the "Multiple Modifiers" code immediately after the procedure code. This indicates that one or more additional modifier codes will follow. Modifiers commonly used in **MEDICINE** are as follows:

-22 Unusual Procedural Services: When the service(s) provided is greater than that usually required for the listed procedure, it may be identified by adding modifier '-22' to the usual procedure number or by use of the separate five digit modifier code 09922. A report may also be appropriate.

-26 Professional Component: Certain procedures are a combination of a physician component and a technical component. When the physician component is reported separately, the service may be identified by adding the modifier '-26' to the usual procedure number or the service may be reported by use of the five digit modifier code 09926.

-32 Mandated Services: Services related to *mandated* consultation and/or related services (eg, PRO, 3rd party payor) may be identified by adding the modifier '-32' to the basic procedure or the service may be reported by use of the five digit modifier 09932.

-51 Multiple Procedures: When multiple procedures are performed on the same day or at the same session, the major procedure or service may be reported as listed. The secondary additional, or lesser procedure(s) or service(s) may be identified by adding the modifier '-51' to the secondary procedure or service code(s) or by use of the separate five digit modifier code 09951. This modifier may be used to report multiple medical procedures performed at the same session, as well as a combination of medical and surgical procedures, or several surgical procedures performed at the same operative session.

-52 Reduced Services: Under certain circumstances a service or procedure is partially reduced or eliminated at the physician's election. Under these circumstances the service provided can be identified by its usual procedure number and the addition of the modifier '-52,' signifying that the service is reduced. This provides a means of reporting reduced services without disturbing the identification of the basic service. Modifier code 09952 may be used as an alternative to modifier'-52.'

-55 Postoperative Management Only: When one physician performs the postoperative management and another physician has performed the surgical procedure, the postoperative component may be identified by adding the modifier '-55' to the usual procedure number or by use of the separate five digit modifier code 09955.

-56 Preoperative Management Only: When one physician performs the preoperative care and evaluation and another physician performs the surgical procedure, the preoperative component may be identified by adding the modifier '-56' to the usual procedure number or by use of the separate five digit modifier code 09956.

-76 Repeat Procedure by Same Physician: The physician may need to indicate that a procedure or service was repeated subsequent to the original service. This circumstance may be reported by adding the modifier '-76' to the repeated service or the separate five digit modifier code 09976 may be used.

-77 Repeat Procedure by Another Physician: The physician may need to indicate that a basic procedure performed by another physician had to be repeated. This situation may be reported by adding modifier '-77' to the repeated service or the separate five digit modifier code 09977 may be used.

-78 Return to the Operating Room for a Related Procedure During the Postoperative Period: The physician may need to indicate that another procedure was performed during the postoperative period of the initial procedure. When this subsequent procedure is related to the first, and requires the use of the operating room, it may be reported by adding the modifier '-78' to the related procedure, or by using the separate five digit modifier 09978. (For repeat procedures on the same day, see -76).

-79 Unrelated Procedure or Service by the Same Physician During the Postoperative Period: The physician may need to indicate that the performance of a procedure or service during the postoperative period was unrelated to the original procedure. This circumstance may be reported by using the modifier '-79' or by using the separate five digit modifier 09979. (For repeat procedures on the same day, see -76).

-90 Reference (Outside) Laboratory: When laboratory procedures are performed by a party other than the treating or reporting physician, the procedure may be identified by adding the modifier '-90' to the usual procedure number or by using the separate five digit modifier code 09990.

-99 Multiple Modifiers: Under certain circumstances two or more modifiers may be necessary to completely delineate a service. In such situations modifier '-99' should be added to the basic procedure, and other applicable modifiers may be listed as part of the description of the service. Modifier code 09999 may be used as an alternative to modifier '-99.'

7. **MATERIALS SUPPLIED BY PHYSICIAN:** Supplies and materials provided by the physician (eg, sterile trays/drugs), over and above those usually included with the office visit or other services rendered may be listed separately. List drugs, trays, supplies and materials provided. Identify as 99070.

MEDICINE

Procedures

(90000-90080 have been deleted. To report, see 99201-99215)

(90100-90170 have been deleted. To report, see 99341-99353)

(90200-90220 have been deleted. To report, see 99221-99223)

(90225 has been deleted. To report, use 99431)

(90240-90280 have been deleted. To report, see 99231-99233)

(90282 has been deleted. To report, see 99433)

(90292 has been deleted. To report, see 99238)

(90300-90370 have been deleted. To report, see 99301-99313)

(90400-90470 have been deleted. To report, see 99321-99333)

(90500-90580 have been deleted. To report, see 99281-99288)

(90590 has been deleted. To report, see 99288)

(90600-90630 have been deleted. To report, see 99241-99255)

(90640-90643 have been deleted. To report, see 99241-99245 or 99261-99263)

(90650-90654 have been deleted. To report, see 99271-99275)

(90699 has been deleted. To report, use 99499)

Immunization Injections

(For allergy testing, see 95004 et seq)

(For skin testing of bacterial, viral, fungal extracts, see 86485-86586)

(For therapeutic or diagnostic injections, see 90782-90799)

Immunizations are usually given in conjunction with a medical service. When an immunization is the only service performed, a minimal service may be listed in addition to the injection. Immunization procedures include the supply of materials.

(Immunizations 90720-90723 have been revised as 90701-90742)

90701 Immunization, active; diphtheria and tetanus toxoids and pertussis vaccine (DTP)

90702 diphtheria and tetanus toxoids (DT)

90703 tetanus toxoid

90704 mumps virus vaccine, live

90705 measles virus vaccine, live, attenuated

90706 rubella virus vaccine, live

90707 measles, mumps and rubella virus vaccine, live

90708 measles and rubella virus vaccine, live

90709 rubella and mumps virus vaccine, live

90712 poliovirus vaccine, live, oral (any type(s))

90713 poliomyelitis vaccine

90714 typhoid vaccine

90717 yellow fever vaccine

90718 tetanus and diphtheria toxoids absorbed, for adult use (Td)

90719 diphtheria toxoid

90724 influenza virus vaccine

90725 cholera vaccine

90726 rabies vaccine

90727 plague vaccine

90728 BCG vaccine

90731 hepatitis B vaccine

90732 pneumococcal vaccine, polyvalent

90733 meningococcal polysaccharide vaccine (any group(s))

90737 Hemophilus influenza B

90741 Immunization, passive; immune serum globulin, human (ISG)

90742 specific hyperimmune serum globulin (eg, hepatitis B, measles, pertussis, rabies, Rho(D), tetanus, vaccinia, varicella-zoster)

90749 Unlisted immunization procedure

(90750-90754 have been deleted. To report, see 99381-99387)

(90755 has been deleted. To report, use 99438)

(90757 has been deleted. To report, use 99432)

(90760-90764 have been deleted. To report, see 99391-99397)

(90774 has been deleted. To report, use 99178)

(90778 has been deleted. To report, use 94772)

Infusion Therapy (Excludes Chemotherapy)

These procedures encompass prolonged intravenous injections. These codes require the presence of the physician during the infusion. These codes are not to be used for intradermal, subcutaneous or intramuscular or routine IV drug injections. (For these services, see 90782-90788)

90780 IV infusion therapy, administered by physician or under direct supervision of physician; up to one hour

90781 each additional hour, up to eight (8) hours

Therapeutic or Diagnostic Injections

90782 Therapeutic or diagnostic injection (specify material injected); subcutaneous or intramuscular

90783 intra-arterial

90784 intravenous

(90782-90784 do not include injections for allergen immunotherapy. For allergen immunotherapy injections, see 95115-95117)

90788 Intramuscular injection of antibiotic (specify)

(90790-90796 have been deleted. To report, use 96408-96414, 96420-96425, 96440, 96450, 96530, 96545, 96549)

90798 Intravenous therapy for severe or intractable allergic disease in physician's office or institution (eg, theophyllines, corticosteroids, antihistamines)

90799 Unlisted therapeutic or diagnostic injection

(For allergy immunizations, see 95004 et seq)

Psychiatry

Hospital care by the attending physician in treating a psychiatric inpatient or partial hospitalization may be initial or subsequent in nature (see 99221-99233) and may include exchanges with nursing and ancillary personnel. Hospital care services involve a variety of responsibilities unique to the medical management of inpatients, such as physician hospital orders, interpretation of laboratory or other medical diagnostic studies and observations, review of activity therapy reports, supervision of nursing and ancillary personnel, and the programming of all hospital resources for diagnosis and treatment.

When services include not only a visit to the patient, but also activity in leadership or direction of a treatment team as related to that patient, a code may be selected based upon the services provided that day.

Some patients receive hospital evaluation and management services only and others receive evaluation and management services and other procedures. If other procedures such as electroconvulsive therapy or medical psychotherapy are rendered in addition to hospital evaluation and management services, these should be listed separately (ie, hospital care service plus electroconvulsive therapy or plus medical psychotherapy if rendered).

Psychiatric care may be reported without time dimensions according to the procedure or service as are other medical or surgical procedures. In reporting medical psychotherapy procedures, time is only one aspect and may be expressed as is customary in the local area. For example, the usual appointment length of an individual medical psychotherapy procedure may be signified by the procedure code alone. The modifier -52 or 09952 may be used to signify a service that is reduced or less extensive than the usual procedure. The modifier -22 or 09922 may be used to indicate a more extensive service. Thus, medical psychotherapy procedures may be reported by the procedure code alone or by the procedure code with a modifier. If appropriate and customary in the local area, codes 90841, 90843 or 90844 may be used.

Other evaluation and management services, such as office medical service or other patient encounters, may be described as listed in the section on Evaluation and Management, if appropriate.

General Clinical Psychiatric Diagnostic or Evaluative Interview Procedures

90801 Psychiatric diagnostic interview examination including history, mental status, or disposition (may include communication with family or other sources, ordering and medical interpretation of laboratory or other medical diagnostic studies. In certain circumstances other informants will be seen in lieu of the patient)

Consultation for psychiatric evaluation of a patient includes examination of a patient and exchange of information with primary physician and other informants such as nurses or family members, and preparation of report. These consultation services (99241-99263) are limited to initial or follow-up evaluation and do not involve psychiatric treatment. For treatment, see 99221 et seq or 90841 et seq.

Special Clinical Psychiatric Diagnostic or Evaluative Procedures

Interactive procedures are distinct forms of diagnostic procedures which predominately use physical aids and non-verbal commmunication to overcome barriers to therapeutic interaction between the physician and a patient who has lost, or has not yet developed either the expressive language communication skills to explain his/her symptoms and response to treatment or the receptive communication skills to understand the physician if he/she were to use ordinary adult language for communication.

90820 Interactive medical psychiatric diagnostic interview examination

90825 Psychiatric evaluation of hospital records, other psychiatric reports, psychometric and/or projective tests, and other accumulated data for medical diagnostic purposes

90830 Psychological testing by physician, with written report, per hour

(90831 has been deleted. To report, see 99371-99373)

PSYCHIATRIC THERAPEUTIC PROCEDURES

Interactive procedures are distinct medical psychotherapeutic procedures which predominately use physical aids and non-verbal communication to overcome barriers to therapeutic interaction between the physician and a patient who has lost, or has not yet developed either the expressive language communication skills to explain his/her symptoms and response to treatment, or the receptive communication skills to understand the physician if he/she were to use ordinary adult language for communication.

90835 Narcosynthesis for psychiatric diagnostic and therapeutic purposes (eg, sodium amobarbital (Amytal) interview)

90841 Individual medical psychotherapy by a physician, with continuing medical diagnostic evaluation, and drug management when indicated, including insight oriented, behavior modifying or supportive psychotherapy; time unspecified

90843 approximately 20 to 30 minutes

90844 approximately 45 to 50 minutes

90845 Medical psychoanalysis

90846 Family medical psychotherapy (without the patient present)

90847 Family medical psychotherapy (conjoint psychotherapy) by a physician, with continuing medical diagnostic evaluation, and drug management when indicated

(90848 has been deleted. To report, use 90847)

90849 Multiple-family group medical psychotherapy by a physician, with continuing medical diagnostic evaluation, and drug management when indicated

90853 Group medical psychotherapy (other than of a multiple-family group) by a physician, with continuing medical diagnostic evaluation and drug management when indicated

90855 Interactive individual medical psychotherapy

90857 Interactive group medical psychotherapy

PSYCHIATRIC SOMATOTHERAPY

90862 Pharmacologic management, including prescription, use, and review of medication with no more than minimal medical psychotherapy

90870 Electroconvulsive therapy (includes necessary monitoring); single seizure

90871 multiple seizures, per day

(90872 has been deleted. To report, use 90899)

OTHER PSYCHIATRIC THERAPY

90880 Medical hypnotherapy

90882 Environmental intervention for medical management purposes on a psychiatric patient's behalf with agencies, employers, or institutions

90887 Interpretation or explanation of results of psychiatric, other medical examinations and procedures, or other accumulated data to family or other responsible persons, or advising them how to assist patient

90889 Preparation of report of patient's psychiatric status, history, treatment, or progress (other than for legal or consultative purposes) for other physicians, agencies, or insurance carriers

OTHER PROCEDURES

90899 Unlisted psychiatric service or procedure

Biofeedback

90900 Biofeedback training; by electromyogram application (eg, in tension headache, muscle spasm)

90902 in conduction disorder (eg, arrhythmia)

90904 regulation of blood pressure (eg, in essential hypertension)

90906 regulation of skin temperature or peripheral blood flow

90908 by electroencephalogram application (eg, in anxiety, insomnia)

90910 by electro-oculogram application (eg, in blepharospasm)

90915 other

Dialysis

Evaluation and management services unrelated to the dialysis procedure that cannot be rendered during the dialysis session may be reported in addition to the dialysis procedure. All evaluation and management services related to the patient's end stage renal disease that are rendered on a day when dialysis is performed and all other patient care services that are rendered during the dialysis procedure are included in the dialysis procedure, 90935-90947.

END STAGE RENAL DISEASE SERVICES

• **90918** End stage renal disease (ESRD) related services per full month; for patients under 2 years of age to include monitoring for the adequacy of nutrition, assessment of growth and development, and counseling of parents

• **90919** between the second and twelfth birthdays to include monitoring for the adequacy of nutrition, assessment of growth and development, and counseling of parents

• **90920** through age nineteen to include monitoring for the adequacy of nutrition, assessment of growth and development, and counseling of parents

• **90921** for patients twenty years of age and over

• **90922** End stage renal disease (ESRD) related services (less than full month), per day

HEMODIALYSIS

(For cannula declotting, see 36860, 36861)

(For prolonged physician attendance, see 99150, 99151)

90935 Hemodialysis procedure with single physician evaluation

90937 Hemodialysis procedure requiring repeated evaluation(s) with or without substantial revision of dialysis prescription

(90941-90944 have been deleted. To report, see 90935-90937)

PERITONEAL DIALYSIS

(For insertion of cannula or catheter, see 49420, 49421)

(For prolonged physician attendance, see 99150, 99151)

90945 Dialysis procedure other than hemodialysis (eg, peritoneal, hemofiltration), with single physician evaluation

90947 Dialysis procedure other than hemodialysis (eg, peritoneal, hemofiltration) requiring repeated evaluations, with or without substantial revision of dialysis prescription

(90951-90958 have been deleted. To report, see 90935, 90937)

(90966-90985 have been deleted. To report, see 90945, 90947)

MISCELLANEOUS DIALYSIS PROCEDURES

(90988 has been deleted. To report, see 90918-90922)

90989 Dialysis training, patient, including helper where applicable, any mode, completed course

(90990, 90992 have been deleted. To report, see 90989 and 90993)

90993 Dialysis training, patient, including helper where applicable, any mode, course not completed, per training session

(90995 has been deleted. To report, see 90918-90921)

90997 Hemoperfusion (eg, with activated charcoal or resin)

(90998 has been deleted. To report, see 90922)

90999 Unlisted dialysis procedure, inpatient or outpatient

Gastroenterology

(For duodenal intubation and aspiration, see 89100-89105)

(For gastrointestinal radiologic procedures, see 74210-74363)

(For esophagoscopy procedures, see 43200-43228; upper GI endoscopy 43234-43258; endoscopy, small bowel and stomal 44360-44393; proctosigmoidoscopy 45300-45321; sigmoidoscopy 45330-45337; colonoscopy 45355-45385; anoscopy 46600-46614)

91000 Esophageal intubation and collection of washings for cytology, including preparation of specimens (separate procedure)

91010 Esophageal motility study;

91011 with mecholyl or similar stimulant

91012 with acid perfusion studies

91020 Esophagogastric manometric studies

91030 Esophagus, acid perfusion (Bernstein) test for esophagitis

91032 Esophagus, acid reflux test, with intraluminal pH electrode for detection of gastroesophageal reflux;

91033 prolonged recording

91052 Gastric analysis test with injection of stimulant of gastric secretion (eg, histamine, insulin, pentagastrin, calcium and secretin)

(For gastric biopsy by capsule, peroral, via tube, one or more specimens, see 43600)

(For gastric laboratory procedures, see also 89130-89141)

91055 Gastric intubation, washings, and preparing slides for cytology (separate procedure)

(For gastric lavage, therapeutic, see 91105)

91060 Gastric saline load test

(For biopsy by capsule, small intestine, per oral, via tube (one or more specimens), see 44100)

91065 Breath hydrogen test (eg, for detection of lactase deficiency)

(91090 has been deleted)

91100 Intestinal bleeding tube, passage, positioning and monitoring

91105 Gastric intubation, and aspiration or lavage for treatment (eg, for ingested poisons)

(For cholangiography, see 47500, 74320)

(For abdominal paracentesis, see 49080, 49081; with instillation of medication, see 96535)

(For peritoneoscopy, see 49300; with biopsy, see 49301)

(For peritoneoscopy and guided transhepatic cholangiography, see 49302; with biopsy, see 49303)

(For for splenoportography, see 38200, 75810)

91122 Anorectal manometry

91299 Unlisted diagnostic gastroenterology procedure

Ophthalmology

OPHTHALMOLOGICAL DIAGNOSTIC AND TREATMENT SERVICES

(For surgical procedures, see Surgery, Eye and Ocular Adnexa, 65091 et seq)

DEFINITIONS

INTERMEDIATE OPHTHALMOLOGICAL SERVICES: A level of service pertaining to the evaluation of a new or existing condition complicated with a new diagnostic or management problem not necessarily relating to the primary diagnosis, including history, general medical observation, external ocular and adnexal examination and other diagnostic procedures as indicated; may include the use of mydriasis.

For example:

a. Review of history, external examination, ophthalmoscopy, biomicroscopy for an acute complicated condition (eg, iritis) not requiring comprehensive ophthalmological services.

b. Review of interval history, external examination, ophthalmoscopy, biomicroscopy and tonometry in established patient with known cataract not requiring comprehensive ophthalmological services.

COMPREHENSIVE OPHTHALMOLOGICAL SERVICES: A level of service in which a general evaluation of the complete visual system is made. The comprehensive services constitute a single service entity but need not be performed at one session. The service includes history, general medical observation, external and ophthalmoscopic examination, gross visual fields and basic sensorimotor examination. It often includes, as indicated; biomicroscopy, examination with cycloplegia or mydriasis and tonometry. It always includes initiation of diagnostic and treatment programs as indicated.

For example:

The comprehensive services required for diagnosis and treatment of a patient with symptoms indicating possible disease of the visual system, such as glaucoma, cataract or retinal disease, or to rule out disease of the visual system, new or established patient.

"Initiation of diagnostic and treatment program" includes the prescription of medication, lenses and other therapy and arranging for special ophthalmological diagnostic or treatment services, consultations, laboratory procedures and radiological services as may be indicated.

Prescription of lenses may be deferred to a subsequent visit, but in any circumstance is not reported separately. ("Prescription of lenses" does not include anatomical facial measurements for or writing of laboratory specifications for spectacles. For Spectacle Services, see 92340 et seq).

SPECIAL OPHTHALMOLOGICAL SERVICES: Services in which a special evaluation of part of the visual system is made, which goes beyond the services usually included under general ophthalmological services, or in which special treatment is given.

For example:

Fluorescein angioscopy, quantitative visual field examination, or extended color vision examination (such as Nagel's anomaloscope) should be specifically reported as special ophthalmological services.

Medical diagnostic evaluation by the physician is an integral part of all ophthalmological services. Technical procedures (which may or may not be performed by the physician personally) are often part of the service, but should not be mistaken to constitute the service itself.

Intermediate and comprehensive ophthalmological services constitute integrated services in which medical diagnostic evaluation cannot be separated from the examining techniques used. Itemization of service components, such as slit lamp examination, keratometry, ophthalmoscopy, retinoscopy, tonometry, motor evaluation is not applicable.

GENERAL OPHTHALMOLOGICAL SERVICES

NEW PATIENT

A new patient is one who has not received any professional services from the physician or another physician of the same specialty who belongs to the same group practice within the past three years.

92002 Ophthalmological services: medical examination and evaluation with initiation of diagnostic and treatment program; intermediate, new patient

92004 comprehensive, new patient, one or more visits

ESTABLISHED PATIENT

An established patient is one who has received professional services from the physician or another physician of the same specialty who belongs to the same group practice within the past three years.

92012 Ophthalmological services: medical examination and evaluation, with initiation or continuation of diagnostic and treatment program; intermediate, established patient

92014 comprehensive, established patient, one or more visits

(For surgical procedures, see Surgery, Eye and Ocular Adnexa, 65091 et seq)

SPECIAL OPHTHALMOLOGICAL SERVICES

92015 Determination of refractive state

92018 Ophthalmological examination and evaluation, under general anesthesia, with or without manipulation of globe for passive range of motion or other manipulation to facilitate diagnostic examination; complete

92019 limited

92020 Gonioscopy with medical diagnostic evaluation (separate procedure)

(For gonioscopy under general anesthesia, see 92018)

92060 Sensorimotor examination with multiple measurements of ocular deviation and medical diagnostic evaluation (eg, restrictive or paretic muscle with diplopia) (separate procedure)

92065 Orthoptic and/or pleoptic training, with continuing medical direction and evaluation

92070 Fitting of contact lens for treatment of disease, including supply of lens

92081 Visual field examination, unilateral or bilateral, with medical diagnostic evaluation; limited examination (eg, tangent screen, Autoplot, arc perimeter, or single stimulus level automated test, such as Octopus 3 or 7 equivalent)

92082 intermediate examination (eg, at least 2 isopters on Goldmann perimeter, or semiquantitative, automated suprathreshold screening program, Humphrey suprathreshold automatic diagnostic test, Octopus program 33)

92083 extended examination (eg, Goldmann visual fields with at least 3 isopters plotted and static determination within the central 30°, or quantitative, automated threshold perimetry, Octopus program G-1, 32 or 42, Humphrey visual field analyzer full threshold programs 30-2, 24-2, or 30/60-2)

(Gross visual field testing (eg, confrontation testing) is a part of general ophthalmological services and is not reported separately)

92100 Serial tonometry (separate procedure) with multiple measurements of intraocular pressure over an extended time period with medical diagnostic evaluation, same day (eg, diurnal curve or medical treatment of acute elevation of intraocular pressure)

92120 Tonography with medical diagnostic evaluation, recording indentation tonometer method or perilimbal suction method

92130 Tonography with water provocation

92140 Provocative tests for glaucoma, with medical diagnostic evaluation, without tonography

OPHTHALMOSCOPY

Routine ophthalmoscopy is part of general and special ophthalmologic services whenever indicated. It is a non-itemized service and is not reported separately.

92225 Ophthalmoscopy, extended as for retinal detachment (may include use of contact lens, drawing or sketch, and/or fundus biomicroscopy), with medical diagnostic evaluation; initial

92226 subsequent

92230 Ophthalmoscopy, with medical diagnostic evaluation; with fluorescein angioscopy (observation only)

92235 with fluorescein angiography (includes multiframe photography)

92250 with fundus photography

92260 with ophthalmodynamometry

(For ophthalmoscopy under general anesthesia, see 92018)

OTHER SPECIALIZED SERVICES

92265 Oculoelectromyography, one or more extraocular muscles, one or both eyes, with medical diagnostic evaluation

92270 Electro-oculography, with medical diagnostic evaluation

92275 Electroretinography, with medical diagnostic evaluation

92280 Visually evoked potential (response) study, with medical diagnostic evaluation

(For electronystagmography for vestibular function studies, see 92541 et seq)

(For ophthalmic echography (diagnostic ultrasound), see 76511-76529)

92283 Color vision examination, extended, eg, anomaloscope or equivalent

(Color vision testing with pseudoisochromatic plates (such as HRR or Ishihara) is not reported separately. It is included in the appropriate general or ophthalmological service)

92284 Dark adaptation examination, with medical diagnostic evaluation

92285 External ocular photography with medical diagnostic evaluation for documentation of medical progress (eg, close-up photography, slit lamp photography, goniophotography, stereo-photography)

92286 Special anterior segment photography with medical diagnostic evaluation; with specular endothelial microscopy and cell count

92287 with fluorescein angiography

CONTACT LENS SERVICES

The prescription of contact lens includes specification of optical and physical characteristics (such as power, size, curvature, flexibility, gas-permeability). It is NOT a part of the general ophthalmological services.

The fitting of contact lens includes instruction and training of the wearer and incidental revision of the lens during the training period.

Follow-up of successfully fitted extended wear lenses is reported as part of a general ophthalmological service (92012 et seq).

The supply of contact lenses may be reported as part of the service of fitting. It may also be reported separately by using 92391 or 92396 and modifier '-26' or 09926 for the service of fitting without supply.

(For therapeutic or surgical use of contact lens, see 68340, 92070)

92310 Prescription of optical and physical characteristics of and fitting of contact lens, with medical supervision of adaptation; corneal lens, both eyes, except for aphakia

(For prescription and fitting of one eye, add modifier -52 or 09952)

92311 corneal lens for aphakia, one eye

92312 corneal lens for aphakia, both eyes

92313 corneoscleral lens

92314 Prescription of optical and physical characteristics of contact lens, with medical supervision of adaptation and direction of fitting by independent technician; corneal lens, both eyes, except for aphakia

(For prescription and fitting of one eye, add modifier -52 or 09952)

92315 corneal lens for aphakia, one eye

92316 corneal lens for aphakia, both eyes

92317 corneoscleral lens

92325 Modification of contact lens (separate procedure), with medical supervision of adaptation

92326 Replacement of contact lens

OCULAR PROSTHETICS, ARTIFICIAL EYE

92330 Prescription, fitting, and supply of ocular prosthesis (artificial eye), with medical supervision of adaptation

(If supply is not included, use modifier -26 or 09926; to report supply separately, see 92393)

92335 Prescription of ocular prosthesis (artificial eye) and direction of fitting and supply by independent technician, with medical supervision of adaptation

SPECTACLE SERVICES (INCLUDING PROSTHESIS FOR APHAKIA)

Prescription of spectacles, when required, is an integral part of general ophthalmological services and is not reported separately. It includes specification of lens type (monofocal, bifocal, other), lens power, axis, prism, absorptive factor, impact resistance, and other factors.

Fitting of spectacles is a separate service; when provided by the physician, it is reported as indicated by 92340-92371. Fitting includes measurement of anatomical facial characteristics, the writing of laboratory specifications, and the final adjustment of the spectacles to the visual axes and anatomical topography. Presence of physician is not required.

Supply of materials is a separate service component; it is not part of the service of fitting spectacles.

92340 Fitting of spectacles, except for aphakia; monofocal

92341 bifocal

92342 multifocal, other than bifocal

92352 Fitting of spectacle prosthesis for aphakia; monofocal

92353 multifocal

92354 Fitting of spectacle mounted low vision aid; single element system

92355 telescopic or other compound lens system

92358 Prosthesis service for aphakia, temporary (disposable or loan, including materials)

92370 Repair and refitting spectacles; except for aphakia

92371 spectacle prosthesis for aphakia

SUPPLY OF MATERIALS

92390 Supply of spectacles, except prosthesis for aphakia and low vision aids

92391 Supply of contact lenses, except prosthesis for aphakia

(For supply of contact lenses reported as part of the service of fitting, see 92310-92313)

(For replacement of contact lens, see 92326)

92392 Supply of low vision aids (A low vision aid is any lens or device used to aid or improve visual function in a person whose vision cannot be normalized by conventional spectacle correction. Includes reading additions up to 4D.)

92393 Supply of ocular prosthesis (artificial eye)

(For supply reported as part of the service of fitting, see 92330)

92395 Supply of permanent prosthesis for aphakia; spectacles

(For temporary spectacle correction, see 92358)

92396 contact lenses

(For supply reported as part of the service of fitting, see 92311, 92312)

(See 99070 for the supply of other materials, drugs, trays, etc.)

OTHER PROCEDURES

92499 Unlisted ophthalmological service or procedure

Special Otorhinolaryngologic Services

Diagnostic or treatment procedures usually included in a comprehensive otorhinolaryngologic evaluation or office visit, are reported as an integrated medical service, using appropriate descriptors from the 99201 series. Itemization of component procedures (eg, otoscopy, rhinoscopy, tuning fork test) does not apply.

Special otorhinolaryngologic services are those diagnostic and treatment services not usually included in a comprehensive otorhinolaryngologic evaluation or office visit. These services are reported separately, using descriptors from the 92500 series.

All services include medical diagnostic evaluation. Technical procedures (which may or may not be performed by the physician personally) are often part of the service, but should not be mistaken to constitute the service itself.

(For laryngoscopy with stroboscopy, use 31579)

92502 Otolaryngologic examination under general anesthesia

92504 Binocular microscopy (separate diagnostic procedure)

92506 Medical evaluation, speech, language and/or hearing problems

92507 Speech, language or hearing therapy, with continuing medical supervision; individual

92508 group

92511 Nasopharyngoscopy with endoscope (separate procedure)

92512 Nasal function studies (eg, rhinomanometry)

92516 Facial nerve function studies

92520 Laryngeal function studies

VESTIBULAR FUNCTION TESTS, WITH OBSERVATION AND EVALUATION BY PHYSICIAN, WITHOUT ELECTRICAL RECORDING

92531 Spontaneous nystagmus, including gaze

92532 Positional nystagmus

92533 Caloric vestibular test, each irrigation (binaural, bithermal stimulation constitutes four tests)

92534 Optokinetic nystagmus

VESTIBULAR FUNCTION TESTS, WITH RECORDING (eg, ENG, PENG), AND MEDICAL DIAGNOSTIC EVALUATION

92541 Spontaneous nystagmus test, including gaze and fixation nystagmus, with recording

92542 Positional nystagmus test, minimum of 4 positions, with recording

92543 Caloric vestibular test, each irrigation (binaural, bithermal stimulation constitutes four tests), with recording

92544 Optokinetic nystagmus test, bidirectional, foveal or peripheral stimulation, with recording

92545 Oscillating tracking test, with recording

92546 Torsion swing test, with recording

92547 Use of vertical electrodes in any or all of above tests counts as one additional test

(For unlisted vestibular tests, see 92599)

AUDIOLOGIC FUNCTION TESTS WITH MEDICAL DIAGNOSTIC EVALUATION

(For evaluation of speech, language and/or hearing problems through observation and assessment of performance, see 92506)

The audiometric tests listed below imply the use of calibrated electronic equipment. Other hearing tests (such as whispered voice, tuning fork) are considered part of the general otorhinolaryngologic services and are not reported separately. All descriptors refer to testing both ears. Use the modifier -52 or 09952, if a test is applied to one ear instead of to two ears. All descriptors (except 92559), apply to testing of individuals; for testing of groups, use 92559 and specify test(s) used.

92551 Screening test, pure tone, air only

92552 Pure tone audiometry (threshold); air only

92553 air and bone

92555 Speech audiometry; threshold only

92556 threshold and discrimination

92557 Basic comprehensive audiometry (92553 and 92556 combined), (pure tone, air and bone, and speech, threshold and discrimination)

(For hearing aid evaluation and selection, see 92590-92595)

92559 Audiometric testing of groups

92560 Bekesy audiometry; screening

92561 diagnostic

92562 Loudness balance test, alternate binaural or monaural

92563 Tone decay test

92564 Short increment sensitivity index (SISI)

92565 Stenger test, pure tone

(92566 has been deleted. To report, use 92567)

92567 Tympanometry (impedance testing)

92568 Acoustic reflex testing

92569 Acoustic reflex decay test

92571 Filtered speech test

92572 Staggered spondaic word test

92573 Lombard test

92574 Swinging story test

92575 Sensorineural acuity level test

92576 Synthetic sentence identification test

92577 Stenger test, speech

92578 Delayed auditory feedback test

92580 Electrodermal audiometry

(92581 has been deleted. To report, use 92585)

92582 Conditioning play audiometry

92583 Select picture audiometry

92584 Electrocochleography

92585 Brainstem evoked response recording (evoked response (EEG) audiometry)

92589 Central auditory function test(s) (specify)

92590 Hearing aid examination and selection; monaural

92591 binaural

92592 Hearing aid check; monaural

92593 binaural

92594 Electroacoustic evaluation for hearing aid; monaural

92595 binaural

92596 Ear protector attenuation measurements

OTHER PROCEDURES

92599 Unlisted otorhinolaryngological service or procedure

Cardiovascular

THERAPEUTIC SERVICES

92950 Cardiopulmonary resuscitation (eg, in cardiac arrest)

(See also critical care services, 99291, 99292)

92953 Temporary transcutaneous pacing

(For physician direction of ambulance or rescue personnel outside the hospital, see 99288)

92960 Cardioversion, elective, electrical conversion of arrhythmia, external

92970 Cardioassist-method of circulatory assist; internal

92971 external

(For balloon atrial-septostomy, see 33738)

(For placement of catheters for use in circulatory assist devices such as intra-aortic balloon pump, see 33970)

92975 Thrombolysis, coronary; by intracoronary infusion, including selective coronary angiography

92977 by intravenous infusion

(For thrombolysis of vessels other than coronary, see 37201, 75896)

▲92982 Percutaneous transluminal coronary balloon angioplasty; single vessel

92984 each additional vessel

92986 Percutaneous balloon valvuloplasty; aortic valve

92990 pulmonary valve

• 92995 Percutaneous transluminal coronary atherectomy, with or without balloon angioplasty; single vessel

• 92996 each additional vessel

CARDIOGRAPHY

(For echocardiography, see 93307-93350)

93000 Electrocardiogram, routine ECG with at least 12 leads; with interpretation and report

93005 tracing only, without interpretation and report

93010 interpretation and report only

(For ECG monitoring, see 99150, 99151)

93012 Telephonic or telemetric transmission of electrocardiogram rhythm strip;

93014 physician review with interpretation and report only

▲**93015** Cardiovascular stress test using maximal or submaximal treadmill or bicycle exercise; continuous electrocardiographic monitoring, and/or pharmacological stress, with physician supervision, with interpretation and report

93017 tracing only, without interpretation and report

93018 interpretation and report only

93024 Ergonovine provocation test

93040 Rhythm ECG, one to three leads; with interpretation and report

93041 tracing only without interpretation and report

93042 interpretation and report only

(93045 has been deleted. To report, use 93615)

93201 Phonocardiogram with or without ECG lead; with supervision during recording with interpretation and report (when equipment is supplied by the physician)

93202 tracing only, without interpretation and report (eg, when equipment is supplied by the hospital, clinic)

93204 interpretation and report

93205 Phonocardiogram with ECG lead, with indirect carotid artery and/or jugular vein tracing, and/or apex cardiogram; with interpretation and report

93208 tracing only, without interpretation and report

93209 interpretation and report only

93210 Phonocardiogram, intracardiac

93220 Vectorcardiogram (VCG), with or without ECG; with interpretation and report

93221 tracing only, without interpretation and report

93222 interpretation and report only

93224 Electrocardiographic monitoring for 24 hours by continuous original ECG waveform recording and storage, with visual superimposition scanning; includes recording, scanning analysis with report, physician review and interpretation

93225 recording (includes hook-up, recording, and disconnection)

93226 scanning analysis with report

93227 physician review and interpretation

93230 Electrocardiographic monitoring for 24 hours by continuous original ECG waveform recording and storage without superimposition scanning utilizing a device capable of producing a full miniaturized printout; includes recording, microprocessor-based analysis with report, physician review and interpretation

93231 recording (includes hook-up, recording, and disconnection)

93232 microprocessor-based analysis with report

93233 physician review and interpretation

93235 Electrocardiographic monitoring for 24 hours by continuous computerized monitoring and non-continuous recording, and real-time data analysis utilizing a device capable of producing intermittent full-sized waveform tracings, possibly patient activated; includes monitoring and real time data analysis with report, physician review and interpretation

93236 monitoring and real-time data analysis with report

93237 physician review and interpretation

(93240 has been deleted. To report, use 93799)

93255 Apexcardiography

(93258, 93259, 93262, 93263, 93266 have been deleted. To report, see 93224-93237)

93268 Patient demand single or multiple event recording with presymptom or postsymptom memory loop, transmission, physician review and interpretation

(93269 has been deleted. To report, see 93268)

(93270-93277 have been deleted. To report, see 93224-93237)

93278 Signal-averaged electrocardiography (SAECG), with or without ECG

(For interpretation and report only, use 93278 with modifier -26)

(For unlisted cardiographic procedure, see 93799)

CARDIAC FLUOROSCOPY

93280 Cardiac fluoroscopy

(For chest fluoroscopy, see 71034, 76000)

ECHOCARDIOGRAPHY

(Echocardiography includes obtaining ultrasonic signals from the heart and great arteries, with two-dimensional image and/or Doppler ultrasonic signal documentation, and interpretation and report. When interpretation is performed separately use modifier -26 or 09926.)

(93300, 93305 have been deleted)

93307 Echocardiography, real-time with image documentation (2D) with or without M-mode recording; complete

93308 follow-up or limited study

(93309 has been deleted. To report, see 93307, 93308)

▲**93312** Echocardiography, real time with image documentation (2D) (with or without M-Mode recording), transesophageal; including probe placement, image acquisition, interpretation and report

• **93313** placement of transesophageal probe only

• **93314** image acquisition, interpretation and report only

93320 Doppler echocardiography, pulsed wave and/or continuous wave with spectral display; complete

93321 follow-up or limited study

▲**93325** Doppler color flow velocity mapping (list separately in addition to code for echocardiography 76825, 76826, 76827, 76828, 93307, 93308, 93320, 93321)

93350 Echocardiography, real-time with image documentation (2D), with or without M-mode recording, during rest and cardiovascular stress test using maximal or submaximal treadmill or bicycle exercise, including electrocardiographic monitoring, with interpretation and report

CARDIAC CATHETERIZATION

Cardiac catheterization procedure includes introduction, positioning and repositioning of catheter(s), when necessary, recording of intracardiac and intravascular pressure, obtaining blood samples for measurement of blood gases and/or dye (or other) dilution curves and cardiac output measurements (dye dilution, Fick or other method, with or without rest and exercise and/or other studies) with or without electrode catheter placement, final evaluation and report.

(For radiological supervision and interpretation, see 75500-75766)

93501 Right heart catheterization

(For bundle of His recording, see 93600)

93503 Insertion and placement of flow directed catheter (eg, Swan-Ganz) for monitoring purposes

(For subsequent monitoring, see 99150, 99151)

93505 Endomyocardial biopsy

93510 Left heart catheterization, retrograde, from the brachial artery, axillary artery or femoral artery; percutaneous

93511 by cutdown

93514 Left heart catheterization by left ventricular puncture

(93515 has been deleted. To report, use 93524)

93524 Combined transseptal and retrograde left heart catheterization

93526 Combined right heart catheterization and retrograde left heart catheterization

93527 Combined right heart catheterization and transseptal left heart catheterization through intact septum (with or without retrograde left heart catheterization)

93528 Combined right heart catheterization with left ventricular puncture (with or without retrograde left heart catheterization)

93529 Combined right heart catheterization and left heart catheterization through existing septal opening (with or without retrograde left heart catheterization)

(93535 has been deleted. To report, see 33971, 93536)

93536 Percutaneous insertion of intra-aortic balloon catheter

(For removal of balloon catheter, see 33971)

When injection procedures are performed in conjunction with cardiac catheterization, these services do not include introduction of catheters but do include repositioning of catheters when necessary and use of automatic power injectors. The technical details of angiography, supervision of filming and processing, interpretation and report are not included. For radiological services, see appropriate section.

93541 Injection procedure during cardiac catheterization; for pulmonary angiography

(For radiological supervision and interpretation, see 75741-75746)

93542 for selective right ventricular or right atrial angiography

93543 for selective left ventricular or left atrial angiography

(For radiological supervision and interpretation, see 75500-75507)

93544 for aortography

(For radiological supervision and interpretation, see 75600-75625)

93545 for selective coronary angiography (injection of radiopaque material may be by hand)

(For radiological supervision and interpretation, see 75750-75754)

Codes 93546-93553 include the introduction of catheter (percutaneous or cutdown), placement or repositioning, and injection of the contrast media or dye.

93546 Combined left heart catheterization and left ventricular angiography

93547 Combined left heart catheterization, selective coronary angiography, one or more coronary arteries, and selective left ventricular angiography (this code number is to be used when procedure 93510 is combined with procedures 93543 and 93545)

93548 Combined left heart catheterization, selective coronary angiography, one or more coronary arteries, selective left ventriculography, with aortic root aortography

93549 Combined right and left heart catheterization, selective coronary angiography, one or more coronary arteries, and selective left ventricular angiography; (this code number is to be used when procedure 93547 is combined with right heart catheterization)

93550 with selective visualization of bypass graft (this code number is to be used when procedure 93549 is combined with procedure 93551)

93551 Selective opacification of aortocoronary bypass grafts, one or more coronary arteries (injection of radiopaque material may be made by hand)

93552 Combined left heart catheterization, selective coronary angiography, one or more coronary arteries, selective left ventricular cineangiography and visualization of bypass grafts; (this code number is to be used when procedure 93551 is combined with procedure 93547)

93553 with aortic root aortography (this code number is to be used when procedure 93548 is combined with procedure 93551)

(For radiological supervision and interpretation, see 75762-75766)

Codes 93561 and 93562 are not to be used with cardiac catheterization codes.

93561 Indicator dilution studies such as dye or thermal dilution, including arterial and/or venous catheterization; with cardiac output measurement (separate procedure)

93562 subsequent measurement of cardiac output

(For radioisotope method of cardiac output, see 78472, 78473, or 78481)

(93570 has been deleted. To report, use 92982)

(For unlisted cardiac catheterization procedure, see 93799)

INTRACARDIAC ELECTROPHYSIOLOGICAL PROCEDURES

93600 Bundle of His recording

93602 Intra-atrial recording

93603 Right ventricular recording

(93604, 93606 have been deleted. To report, see 93603, 93607, and 93609 as appropriate)

(93605 has been deleted. To report, use 93609)

93607 Left ventricular recording

(93608 has been deleted. To report, use 93609)

93609 Intraventricular and/or intra-atrial mapping of tachycardia site(s) with catheter manipulation to record from multiple sites to identify origin of tachycardia

93610 Intra-atrial pacing

93612 Intraventricular pacing

(93614 has been deleted)

93615 Esophageal recording of atrial electrogram with or without ventricular electrogram(s);

93616 with pacing

93618 Induction of arrhythmia by electrical pacing

(For intracardiac phonocardiogram, see 93210)

93620 Comprehensive electrophysiologic evaluation with right atrial pacing and recording, right ventricular pacing and recording, His bundle recording, and induction of arrhythmia (This code is to be used when 93600 is combined with 93602, 93603, 93610, 93612, and 93618);

93621 with left atrial recordings from coronary sinus or left atrium, with or without pacing

93622 with left ventricular recordings, with or without pacing

93623 Programmed stimulation and pacing after intravenous drug infusion (Use this code with 93620, 93621, 93622)

93624 Electrophysiologic follow-up study with pacing and recording to test effectiveness of therapy

(93630 has been deleted. To report, use 93631 and 33261)

93631 Intra-operative cardiac pacing and mapping

93640 Electrophysiologic evaluation of cardioverter-defibrillator lead and/or device

93650 Intracardiac catheter ablation of arrhythmogenic focus or tract(s), including intracardiac mapping, with or without temporary pacemaker placement

93660 Autonomic nervous system evaluation of cardiovascular function with tilt table evaluation, with or without pharmacological intervention

OTHER VASCULAR STUDIES

(For arterial cannulization and recording of direct arterial pressure, see 36620)

(For radiographic injection procedures, see 36000-36299)

(For vascular cannulization for hemodialysis, see 36800-36820)

(For chemotherapy for malignant disease, see 96500-96549)

(For penile plethysmography, see 54240)

(93700 has been deleted. To report, see 93850-93960)

(93710 has been deleted. To report, use 93860)

93720 Plethysmography, total body; with interpretation and report

93721 tracing only, without interpretation and report

93722 interpretation and report only

(For regional plethysmography, see 93850-93910)

(93725-93730 have been deleted. To report, see 93875-93971)

93731 Electronic analysis of dual-chamber internal pacemaker system (may include rate, pulse amplitude and duration, configuration of wave form, and/or testing of sensory function of pacemaker); without reprogramming

93732 with reprogramming

93733 telephonic analysis

93734 Electronic analysis of single-chamber internal pacemaker system (may include rate, pulse amplitude and duration, configuration of wave form, and/or testing of sensory function of pacemaker); without reprogramming

93735 with reprogramming

93736 telephonic analysis

93737 Electronic analysis of cardioverter/defibrillator; without reprogramming

93738 with reprogramming

93740 Temperature gradient studies

(93750 has been deleted. To report, see 93875-93971)

93760 Thermogram; cephalic

93762 peripheral

93770 Determination of venous pressure

(For central venous cannulization and pressure measurements, see 36488-36491, 36500)

(93780, 93781 have been deleted)

93784 Ambulatory blood pressure monitoring, utilizing a system such as magnetic tape and/or computer disk, for 24 hours or longer; including recording, scanning analysis, interpretation and report

93786 recording only

93788 scanning analysis with report

93790 physician review with interpretation and report

(93791-93796 have been deleted. To report, see 93731-93736)

OTHER PROCEDURES

93797 Physician services for outpatient cardiac rehabilitation; without continuous ECG monitoring (per session)

93798 with continuous ECG monitoring (per session)

93799 Unlisted cardiovascular service or procedure

Non-Invasive Vascular Diagnostic Studies

Vascular studies include patient care required to perform the studies, supervision of the studies and interpretation of study results with copies for patient records of hard copy output with analysis of all data, including bidirectional vascular flow or imaging when provided. The use of a simple hand-held or other Doppler device that does not produce hard copy output, or that produces a record that does not permit analysis of bidirectional vascular flow, is considered to be part of the physical examination of the vascular system and is not separately reported.

To report unilateral non-invasive diagnostic studies, use modifier -52 or 09952.

Duplex scan: An ultrasonic scanning procedure with display of both two-dimensional structure and motion with time and Doppler ultrasonic signal documentation with spectral analysis and/or color flow velocity mapping or imaging.

CEREBROVASCULAR ARTERIAL STUDIES

(93850, 93860 have been deleted. To report, see 93875-93882)

(93870 has been deleted. To report, see 93880 and 93882)

93875 Noninvasive physiologic studies of extracranial arteries, bilateral, (eg, periorbital flow direction with arterial compression, ocular plethysmography, analog velocity waveform spectral analysis, Doppler ultrasound evaluation)

93880 Duplex scan of extracranial arteries; complete bilateral study

93882 follow-up or limited study

93886 Transcranial Doppler study of the intracranial arteries; complete study

93888 follow-up or limited study

EXTREMITY ARTERIAL STUDIES (INCLUDING DIGITS)

(93890, 93910 have been deleted. To report, see 93920, 93931)

93920 Non-invasive physiologic studies of extremity arteries, bilateral, with or without exercise (eg, segmental blood pressure measurements, continuous wave Doppler analog wave form analysis, evocative pressure response to exercise or reactive hyperemia, photoplethysmographic or pulse volume digit wave form analysis, flow velocity signals); upper extremity arteries

93921 lower extremity arteries

93925 Duplex scan of lower extremity arteries or arterial bypass grafts; complete bilateral study

93926 follow-up or limited study

93930 Duplex scan of upper extremity arteries or arterial bypass grafts; complete bilateral study

93931 follow-up or limited study

EXTREMITY VENOUS STUDIES (INCLUDING DIGITS)

(93950, 93960 have been deleted. To report, see 93965-93971)

93965 Non-invasive physiologic studies of extremity veins, bilateral, (eg, continuous Doppler studies with evaluation of venous flow patterns and responses to compression and other maneuvers, phleborheography, impedance plethysmography, quantitative photoplethysmography)

93970 Duplex scan of extremity veins including responses to compression and other maneuvers; complete bilateral study

93971 follow-up or limited study

VISCERAL AND PENILE VASCULAR STUDIES

93975 Duplex scan of arterial inflow and venous outflow of abdominal, pelvic, and/or retroperitoneal organs; complete study

93976 follow-up or limited study

93978 Duplex scan of aorta, inferior vena cava, iliac vasculature, or bypass grafts; complete study

93979 follow-up or limited study

• **93980** Duplex scan of arterial inflow and venous outflow of penile vessels; complete study

• **93981** follow-up or limited study

Pulmonary

Items 94010-94799 include laboratory procedure(s), interpretation and physician's services (except surgical and anesthesia services as listed in the section on Surgery), unless otherwise stated. For laboratory procedures only, see section on Pathology and Laboratory.

94010 Spirometry, including graphic record, total and timed vital capacity, expiratory flow rate measurement(s), and/or maximal voluntary ventilation

94060 Bronchospasm evaluation: spirometry as in 94010, before and after bronchodilator (aerosol or parenteral) or exercise

94070 Prolonged postexposure evaluation of bronchospasm with multiple spirometric determinations after test dose of bronchodilator (aerosol only) antigen, exercise, cold air, methocholine or other chemical agent, with spirometry as in 94010

94150 Vital capacity, total (separate procedure)

94160 Vital capacity screening tests: total capacity, with timed forced expiratory volume (state duration), and peak flow rate

94200 Maximum breathing capacity, maximal voluntary ventilation

94240 Functional residual capacity or residual volume: helium method, nitrogen open circuit method, or other method

94250 Expired gas collection, quantitative, single procedure (separate procedure)

94260 Thoracic gas volume

(For plethysmography, see 93720-93722)

94350 Determination of maldistribution of inspired gas: multiple breath nitrogen washout curve including alveolar nitrogen or helium equilibration time

94360 Determination of resistance to airflow, oscillatory or plethysmographic methods

94370 Determination of airway closing volume, single breath tests

94375 Respiratory flow volume loop

94400 Breathing response to CO_2 (CO_2 response curve)

94450 Breathing response to hypoxia (hypoxia response curve)

94620 Pulmonary stress testing, simple or complex

94640 Nonpressurized inhalation treatment for acute airway obstruction

94642 Aerosol inhalation of pentamidine for pneumocystis carinii pneumonia treatment or prophylaxis

94650 Intermittent positive pressure breathing (IPPB) treatment, air or oxygen, with or without nebulized medication; initial demonstration and/or evaluation

94651 subsequent

94652 newborn infants

94656 Ventilation assist and management, initiation of pressure or volume preset ventilators for assisted or controlled breathing; first day

94657 subsequent days

94660 Continuous positive airway pressure ventilation (CPAP), initiation and management

94662 Continuous negative pressure ventilation (CNP), initiation and management

94664 Aerosol or vapor inhalations for sputum mobilization, bronchodilation, or sputum induction for diagnostic purposes; initial demonstration and/or evaluation

94665 subsequent

94667 Manipulation chest wall, such as cupping, percussing, and vibration to facilitate lung function; initial demonstration and/or evaluation

94668 subsequent

94680 Oxygen uptake, expired gas analysis; rest and exercise, direct, simple

94681 including CO_2 output, percentage oxygen extracted

94690 rest, indirect (separate procedure)

(94700, 94705, 94710 have been deleted. For blood gas determination, see 82800 et seq)

(For single arterial puncture, see 36600)

(94715 has been deleted. To report, use 82820)

94720 Carbon monoxide diffusing capacity, any method

94725 Membrane diffusion capacity

94750 Pulmonary compliance study, any method

94760 Noninvasive ear or pulse oximetry for oxygen saturation; single determination

94761 multiple determinations (eg, during exercise)

94762 by continuous overnight monitoring (separate procedure)

94770 Carbon dioxide, expired gas determination by infrared analyzer

(For bronchoscopy, see 31622-31659)

(For placement of flow directed catheter, see 93503)

(For venipuncture, see 36410)

(For central venous catheter placement, see 36488-36491)

(For arterial puncture, see 36600)

(For arterial catheterization, see 36620)

(For thoracentesis, see 32000)

(For phlebotomy, therapeutic, see 99195)

(For lung biopsy, needle, see 32405)

(For intubation, orotracheal or nasotracheal, see 31500)

94772 Circadian respiratory pattern recording (pediatric pneumogram), 12 to 24 hour continuous recording, infant

(Separate procedure codes for electromyograms, EEG, ECG, and recordings of respiration are excluded when 94772 is reported.)

94799 Unlisted pulmonary service or procedure

Allergy and Clinical Immunology

ALLERGY SENSITIVITY TESTS: the performance and evaluation of selective cutaneous and mucous membrane tests in correlation with the history, physical examination, and other observations of the patient. The number of tests performed should be judicious and dependent upon the history, physical findings, and clinical judgment. All patients should not necessarily receive the same tests nor the same number of sensitivity tests.

IMMUNOTHERAPY (DESENSITIZATION, HYPOSENSITIZATION): the parenteral administration of allergenic extracts as antigens at periodic intervals, usually on an increasing dosage scale to a dosage which is maintained as maintenance therapy. Indications for immunotherapy are determined by appropriate diagnostic procedures coordinated with clinical judgment and knowledge of the natural history of allergic diseases.

OTHER THERAPY: for medical conferences on the use of mechanical and electronic devices (precipitators, air conditioners, air filters, humidifiers, dehumidifiers), climatotherapy, physical therapy, occupational and recreational therapy, see 95105.

ALLERGY TESTING

(95000-95003 have been deleted. To report, use 95004)

• **95004** Percutaneous tests (scratch, puncture, prick) with allergenic extracts, immediate type reaction, specify number of tests

(95005, 95006, 95007 have been deleted. To report, use 95010)

• **95010** Percutaneous tests (scratch, puncture, prick) sequential and incremental, with drugs, biologicals or venoms, immediate type reaction, specify number of tests

(95011 has been deleted. To report, use 95010)

(95014 has been deleted. To report, use 95015)

• **95015** Intracutaneous (intradermal) tests, sequential and incremental, with drugs, biologicals, or venoms, immediate type reaction, specify number of tests

(95016-95018 have been deleted. To report, use 95015)

(95020-95023 have been deleted. To report, use 95024)

• **95024** Intracutaneous (intradermal) tests with allergenic extracts, immediate type reaction, specify number of tests

95027 Skin end point titration

• **95028** Intracutaneous (intradermal) tests with allergenic extracts, delayed type reaction, including reading, specify number of tests

(95030-95034 have been deleted. To report, use 95028)

95040 Patch or application tests; up to 10 tests

95041 11-20 tests

95042 21-30 tests

95043 more than 30 tests

95050 Photo patch tests; up to 10 tests

95051 more than 10 tests

95056 Photo tests

95060 Ophthalmic mucous membrane tests

95065 Direct nasal mucous membrane test

95070 Inhalation bronchial challenge testing (not including necessary pulmonary function tests); with histamine, methacholine, or similar compounds

95071 with antigens or gases, specify

(For pulmonary function tests, see 94060, 94070)

▲**95075** Ingestion challenge test (sequential and incremental ingestion of test items, eg, food, drug or other substance such as metabisulfite)

(95077 has been deleted)

95078 Provocative testing (eg, Rinkel test)

(95080-95082 have been deleted)

(For allergy laboratory tests, see 86000-86999)

(For intravenous therapy for severe or intractable allergic disease, see 90798)

OTHER MEDICAL SERVICES

95105 Medical conference services (eg, use of mechanical and electric devices, climatotherapy, breathing exercises and/or postural drainage)

ALLERGEN IMMUNOTHERAPY

Codes 95115-95199 include the professional services necessary for allergen immunotherapy. Office visit codes may be used in addition to allergen immunotherapy, if and only if, other identifiable services are provided at that time.

95115 Professional services for allergen immunotherapy not including provision of allergenic extracts; single injection

95117 multiple injections

95120 Professional services for allergen immunotherapy in prescribing physician's office or institution, including provision of allergenic extract; single antigen

95125 multiple antigens (specify number of injections)

95130 single stinging insect venom

95131 two stinging insect venoms

95132 three stinging insect venoms

95133 four stinging insect venoms

95134 five stinging insect venoms

95135 Professional services for the supervision and provision of antigens for allergen immunotherapy (specify number of vials); single antigen, single dose vials

95140 multiple antigens, single dose vials

95145 Professional services for the supervision and provision of antigens for allergen immunotherapy (specify number of treatments or total volume); single stinging insect venom, multiple dose vials

95146 two single stinging insect venoms, multiple dose vials

95147 three single stinging insect venoms, multiple dose vials

95148 four single stinging insect venoms, multiple dose vials

95149 five single stinging insect venoms, multiple dose vials

95150 Professional service for the supervision and provision of antigens for allergen immunotherapy (specify number of treatments or total volume); single or multiple antigens, one multiple dose vial

95155 single or multiple antigens, two or more multiple dose vials

(95160 has been deleted. To report, see 95145-95149)

95170 whole body extract of biting insect or other arthropod

95180 Rapid desensitization procedure, each hour (eg, insulin, penicillin, horse serum)

95199 Unlisted allergy/clinical immunologic service or procedure

(For skin testing of bacterial, viral, fungal extracts, see 95030-95034, 86485-86586)

(For special reports on allergy patients, see 99080)

(For testing procedures such as radioallergosorbent testing (RAST), rat mast cell technique (RMCT), mast cell degranulation test (MCDT), lymphocytic transformation test (LTT), leukocyte histamine release (LHR), migration inhibitory factor test (MIF), transfer factor test (TFT), nitroblue tetrazolium dye test (NTD), see Immunology section in Pathology or use 95199)

Neurology and Neuromuscular Procedures

Neurologic services are typically consultative, and any of the levels of consultation (99241-99263) may be appropriate.

In addition, services and skills outlined under Evaluation and Management levels of service appropriate to neurologic illnesses should be coded similarly.

All EEG services listed below (95805-95827) except 95817, 95821 include tracing, interpretation and report. For interpretation of EEG only, use modifier -26 or 09926.

95805 Multiple sleep latency testing (MSLT), recording, analysis and interpretation of physiological measurements of sleep during multiple nap opportunities

95816 Electroencephalogram (EEG) including recording awake and drowsy, with hyperventilation and/or photic stimulation; standard or portable, same facility

95817 portable, to an alternative facility

95819 Electroencephalogram (EEG) including recording awake and asleep, with hyperventilation and/or photic stimulation; standard or portable, same facility

95821 portable, to an alternate facility

95822 Electroencephalogram (EEG); sleep only

95823 physical or pharmacological activation only

95824 cerebral death evaluation only

95826 intracerebral (depth) EEG only

95827 all night sleep only

(For ambulatory 24 hour EEG monitoring, see 95950)

(For EEG during nonintracranial surgery, use 95955)

(For Wada activation test, use 95958)

95828 Polysomnography (recording, analysis and interpretation of the multiple simultaneous physiological measurements of sleep)

(For recording of circadian respiratory patterns of infants, see 94772)

95829 Electrocorticogram at surgery (separate procedure)

95830 Insertion by physician of sphenoidal electrodes for electroencephalographic (EEG) recording

95831 Muscle testing, manual (separate procedure); extremity (excluding hand) or trunk, with report

95832 hand (with or without comparison with normal side)

95833 total evaluation of body, excluding hands

95834 total evaluation of body, including hands

95842 Muscle testing, electrical: reaction of degeneration, chronaxie, galvanic/tetanus ratio, one or more extremities, one or more methods

(95845 has been deleted. To report, use 95999)

▲**95851** Range of motion measurements and report (separate procedure); each extremity (excluding hand) or each trunk section (spine)

95852 hand, with or without comparison with normal side

95857 Tensilon test for myasthenia gravis;

95858 with electromyographic recording

95860 Electromyography; one extremity and related paraspinal areas

95861 two extremities and related paraspinal areas

95863 three extremities and related paraspinal areas

95864 four extremities and related paraspinal areas

95867 Electromyography, cranial nerve supplied muscles; unilateral

95868 bilateral

95869 Electromyography, limited study of specific muscles (eg, thoracic spinal muscles)

(For anal or urethral sphincter, detrusor, urethra, perineum or abdominal musculature, see 51785-51792)

(For eye muscles, see 92265)

95872 Electromyography, single fiber, any technique

95875 Ischemic limb exercise with EMG, with lactic acid determination

95880 Assessment of higher cerebral function with medical interpretation; aphasia testing

95881 developmental testing

95882 cognitive testing and others

● **95883** Neuropsychological testing battery (eg, Halstead-Reitan, LURIA, WAIS-R) with report, per hour

95900 Nerve conduction, velocity and/or latency study; motor, each nerve

95904 sensory, each nerve

95920 Intraoperative neurophysiology testing, per hour

(Use code 95920 in addition to the evoked potential study performed, 92280, 92585, 95925)

95925 Somatosensory testing (eg, cerebral evoked potentials), one or more nerves

(For visual evoked potentials, see 92280)

(For brainstem evoked response recording, see 92585)

(For auditory evoked potentials, see 92585)

95933 Orbicularis oculi (blink) reflex, by electrodiagnostic testing

95935 "H" or "F" reflex study, by electrodiagnostic testing

95937 Neuromuscular junction testing (repetitive stimulation, paired stimuli), each nerve, any one method

▲95950 Monitoring for identification and lateralization of cerebral seizure focus by attached electrodes; electroencephalographic (8 channel EEG) recording and interpretation, each 24 hours

▲95951 combined electroencephalographic (EEG) and video recording and interpretation, each 24 hours

(95952 has been deleted. To report, see 95950)

● 95953 Monitoring for localization of cerebral seizure focus by computerized portable 16 or more channel EEG; electroencephalographic (EEG) recording and interpretation, each 24 hours

95954 Pharmacological activation during prolonged monitoring for localization of cerebral seizure focus

95955 Electroencephalogram (EEG) during nonintracranial surgery (eg, carotid surgery)

● 95956 Monitoring for localization of cerebral seizure focus by cable or radio, 16 or more channel telemetry; electroencephalographic (EEG) recording and interpretation, each 24 hours

95958 Wada activation test for hemispheric function, including electroencephalographic (EEG) monitoring

95961 Functional cortical mapping by stimulation of electrodes on brain surface, or of depth electrodes, to provoke seizures or identify vital cortex, other than in operating room; initial hour of physician attendance

95962 each additional hour of physician attendance

95999 Unlisted neurological or neuromuscular diagnostic procedure

Chemotherapy Administration

Procedures 96400-96549 are independent of the patient's visit. Either may occur independently on any date of service, or they may occur sequentially on the same day.

Preparation of chemotherapy agent(s) is included in the service for administration of the agent.

Regional (isolation) chemotherapy perfusion should be reported using the codes for arterial infusion. Placement of the intra-arterial catheter should be reported using the appropriate code from the Cardiovascular Surgery section.

(Report separate codes for each parenteral method of administration employed when chemotherapy is administered by different techniques.)

96400 Chemotherapy administration, subcutaneous or intramuscular, with or without local anesthesia

96408 Chemotherapy administration, intravenous; push technique

96410 infusion technique, up to one hour

96412 infusion technique, one to 8 hours, each additional hour

96414 infusion technique, initiation of prolonged infusion (more than 8 hours), requiring the use of a portable or implantable pump

(For pump or reservoir refilling, see 96520, 96530)

96420 Chemotherapy administration, intra-arterial; push technique

96422 infusion technique, up to one hour

96423 infusion technique, one to 8 hours, each additional hour

96425 infusion technique, initiation of prolonged infusion (more than 8 hours), requiring the use of a portable or implantable pump

(For pump or reservoir refilling, see 96520, 96530)

▲**96440** Chemotherapy administration into pleural cavity, requiring and including thoracentesis

▲**96445** Chemotherapy administration into peritoneal cavity, requiring and including peritoneocentesis

▲**96450** Chemotherapy administration, into CNS (eg, intrathecal), requiring and including lumbar puncture

(For intravesical (bladder) chemotherapy administration, see 51720)

(For insertion of subarachnoid catheter and reservoir for infusion of drug, see 63750, 63780; for insertion of intraventricular catheter and reservoir, see 61210, 61215)

(96500-96512 have been deleted. To report, see 96408-96414)

(96535-96540 have been deleted. To report, see 96440, 96450, 96530)

96520 Refilling and maintenance of portable pump

(96524, 96526 have been deleted. To report, see 96420-96425)

96530 Refilling and maintenance of implantable pump or reservoir

(Access of pump port is included in filling of implantable pump)

● **96542** Chemotherapy injection, subarachnoid or intraventricular via subcutaneous reservoir, single or multiple agents

96545 Provision of chemotherapy agent

(For radioactive isotope therapy, see 79000-79999)

96549 Unlisted chemotherapy procedure

Special Dermatological Procedures

Dermatologic services are typically consultative, and any of the five levels of consultation (99241-99263) may be appropriate.

In addition, services and skills outlined under Evaluation and Management levels of service appropriate to dermatologic illnesses should be coded similarly.

(For intralesional injections, see 11900, 11901)

(For Tzanck smear, use 87207)

96900 Actinotherapy (ultraviolet light)

96910 Photochemotherapy; tar and ultraviolet B (Goeckerman treatment) or petrolatum and ultraviolet B

96912 psoralens and ultraviolet A (PUVA)

96913 Photochemotherapy (Goeckerman and/or PUVA) for severe photoresponsive dermatoses requiring at least four to eight hours of care under direct supervision of the physician (includes application of medication and dressings)

96999 Unlisted special dermatological service or procedure

Physical Medicine

(Performed or supervised by physician)

(For muscle testing, range of joint motion, electromyography, see 95831 et seq)

(For biofeedback training by EMG, see 90900)

(For transcutaneous nerve stimulation (TNS), see 64550)

MODALITIES

(Physician or therapist is required to be in constant attendance)

(97000 has been deleted. To report, use 97010-97039)

97010 Physical medicine treatment to one area; hot or cold packs

97012 traction, mechanical

97014 electrical stimulation (unattended)

97016 vasopneumatic devices

97018 paraffin bath

97020 microwave

97022 whirlpool

97024 diathermy

97026 infrared

97028 ultraviolet

97039 unlisted modality (specify)

PROCEDURES

(Physician or therapist is required to be in constant attendance)

(97100 has been deleted. To report, use 97110-97139)

(97101 has been deleted. To report, use 97145)

97110 Physical medicine treatment to one area, initial 30 minutes, each visit; therapeutic exercises

97112 neuromuscular reeducation

97114 functional activities

97116 gait training

97118 electrical stimulation (manual)

97120 iontophoresis

97122 traction, manual

97124 massage

97126 contrast baths

97128 ultrasound

97139 unlisted procedure (specify)

97145 Physical medicine treatment to one area, each additional 15 minutes

(97200, 97201 have been deleted. To report, see 97010-97039, 97110-97145)

97220 Hubbard tank; initial 30 minutes, each visit

97221 each additional 15 minutes, up to one hour

97240 Pool therapy or Hubbard tank with therapeutic exercises; initial 30 minutes, each visit

97241 each additional 15 minutes, up to one hour

97260 Manipulation (cervical, thoracic, lumbosacral, sacroiliac, hand, wrist) (separate procedure), performed by physician; one area

97261 each additional area

(For manipulation under general anesthesia, see appropriate anatomic section in Musculoskeletal System)

▲**97500** Orthotics training (dynamic bracing, splinting), upper and/or lower extremities; initial 30 minutes, each visit

97501 each additional 15 minutes

(Codes 97500, 97501 should not be reported with 97116)

97520 Prosthetic training; initial 30 minutes, each visit

97521 each additional 15 minutes

97530 Kinetic activities to increase coordination, strength and/or range of motion, one area (any two extremities or trunk); initial 30 minutes, each visit

97531 each additional 15 minutes

97540 Training in activities of daily living (self care skills and/or daily life management skills); initial 30 minutes, each visit

97541 each additional 15 minutes

• **97545** Work hardening/conditioning; initial 2 hours

• **97546** each additional hour

TESTS AND MEASUREMENTS

(For muscle testing, manual or electrical, joint range of motion, electromyography or nerve velocity determination, see 95831-95904)

97700 Office visit, including one of the following tests or measurements, with report

a. Orthotic "check-out"
b. Prosthetic "check-out"
c. Activities of daily living "check-out"; initial 30 minutes, each visit

97701 each additional 15 minutes

97720 Extremity testing for strength, dexterity, or stamina; initial 30 minutes, each visit

97721 each additional 15 minutes

(97740, 97741 have been deleted. To report, see 97530, 97531)

97752 Muscle testing with torque curves during isometric and isokinetic exercise, mechanized or computerized evaluations with printout

OTHER PROCEDURES

97799 Unlisted physical medicine service or procedure

(98900-98902 have been deleted. To report, use appropriate category and level of Evaluation and Management codes)

(98910-98912 have been deleted. To report, see 99361-99362)

(98920-98922 have been deleted. To report, see 99371-99373)

Special Services and Reports

The procedures with code numbers 99000 through 99090 provide the reporting physician with the means of identifying the completion of special reports and services that are an adjunct to the basic services rendered. The specific number assigned indicates the special circumstances under which a basic procedure is performed.

MISCELLANEOUS SERVICES

99000 Handling and/or conveyance of specimen for transfer from the physician's office to a laboratory

99001 Handling and/or conveyance of specimen for transfer from the patient in other than a physician's office to a laboratory (distance may be indicated)

99002 Handling, conveyance, and/or any other service in connection with the implementation of an order involving devices (eg, designing, fitting, packaging, handling, delivery or mailing) when devices such as orthotics, protectives, prosthetics are fabricated by an outside laboratory or shop but which items have been designed, and are to be fitted and adjusted by the attending physician

(For routine collection of venous blood, use 36415)

(99012, 99013, 99014, 99015 have been deleted. To report, see 99371-99373)

99024 Postoperative follow-up visit, included in global service

(As a component of a surgical "package", see Guideline 2, SURGERY)

99025 Initial (new patient) visit when starred (*) surgical procedure constitutes major service at that visit

99050 Services requested after office hours in addition to basic service

99052 Services requested between 10:00 PM and 8:00 AM in addition to basic service

99054 Services requested on Sundays and holidays in addition to basic service

99056 Services provided at request of patient in a location other than physician's office which are normally provided in the office

99058 Office services provided on an emergency basis

(99062, 99064, 99065 have been deleted. To report, see 99281-99285)

99070 Supplies and materials (except spectacles), provided by the physician over and above those usually included with the office visit or other services rendered (list drugs, trays, supplies, or materials provided)

(For spectacles, see 92390-92395)

99071 Educational supplies, such as books, tapes, and pamphlets, provided by the physician for the patient's education at cost to physician

99075 Medical testimony

99078 Physician educational services rendered to patients in a group setting (eg, prenatal, obesity, or diabetic instructions)

99080 Special reports such as insurance forms, or the review of medical data to clarify a patient's status—more than the information conveyed in the usual medical communications or standard reporting form

99082 Unusual travel (eg, transportation and escort of patient)

99090 Analysis of information data stored in computers (eg, ECGs, blood pressures, hematologic data)

QUALIFYING CIRCUMSTANCES FOR ANESTHESIA

(For explanation of these services, see Guideline 7, ANESTHESIA)

99100 Anesthesia for patient of extreme age, under one year and over seventy

99116 Anesthesia complicated by utilization of total body hypothermia

99135 Anesthesia complicated by utilization of controlled hypotension

99140 Anesthesia complicated by emergency conditions (specify)

(An emergency is defined as existing when delay in treatment of the patient would lead to a significant increase in the threat to life or body part.)

PROLONGED SERVICES

99150 Prolonged physician attendance requiring physician detention beyond usual service (eg, operative standby, monitoring ECG, EEG, intrathoracic pressures, intravascular pressures, blood gases during surgery, standby for newborn care following cesarean section, or maternal-fetal monitoring); 30 minutes to one hour

99151 more than one hour

(For long-term recorded ECG monitoring, see 93224-93237)

(99152 has been deleted. To report, use 99440)

(99154 has been deleted. To report, use 01996)

(99155, 99156 have been deleted. To report, use appropriate category and level of Evaluation and Management codes)

(99160, 99162 have been deleted. To report, see 99291, 99292)

(99165, 99166 have been deleted. To report, use 99199)

(For monitoring cardiac output, see 78470, 93561, 93562)

(For monitoring intra-aortic balloon counterpulsation, see 33972)

(99170 has been deleted. To report, use 91105)

(99171-99174 have been deleted. To report, see 99291, 99292 or 99231-99233)

OTHER SERVICES

99175 Ipecac or similar administration for individual emesis and continued observation until stomach adequately emptied of poison

(For diagnostic intubation, see 82926-82932, 89130-89141)

(For gastric lavage for diagnostic purposes, see 91055)

99178 Administration and medical interpretation of developmental tests

99180 Hyperbaric oxygen therapy; initial

99182 subsequent

99185 Hypothermia; regional

99186 total body

99190 Assembly and operation of pump with oxygenator or heat exchanger (with or without ECG and/or pressure monitoring); each hour

99191 3/4 hour

99192 1/2 hour

99195 Phlebotomy, therapeutic (separate procedure)

99199 Unlisted special service or report

Appendix A

Modifiers

-20 Microsurgery: When the surgical services are performed using the techniques of microsurgery, requiring the use of an operating microscope, modifier '-20' may be added to the surgical procedure or the separate five digit modifier code 09920 may be used. Modifier '-20' is not to be used when a magnifying surgical loupe is used, whether attached to the eyeglasses or on a headband. A special report may be appropriate to document the necessity of the microsurgical approach.

-21 Prolonged Evaluation and Management Services: When the service(s) provided is prolonged or otherwise greater than that usually required for the highest level of evaluation and management service within a given category, it may be identified by adding modifier '-21' to the evaluation and management code number or by use of the separate five digit modifier code 09921. A report may also be appropriate.

-22 Unusual Procedural Services: When the service(s) provided is greater than that usually required for the listed procedure, it may be identified by adding modifier '-22' to the usual procedure number or by use of the separate five digit modifier code 09922. A report may also be appropriate.

-23 Unusual Anesthesia: Occasionally, a procedure, which usually requires either no anesthesia or local anesthesia, because of unusual circumstances must be done under general anesthesia. This circumstance may be reported by adding the modifier '-23' to the procedure code of the basic service or by use of the separate five digit modifier code 09923.

-24 Unrelated Evaluation and Management Service by the Same Physician During a Postoperative Period: The physician may need to indicate that an evaluation and management service was performed during a postoperative period for a reason(s) unrelated to the original procedure. This circumstance may be reported by adding the modifier '-24' to the appropriate level of E/M service, or the separate five digit modifier 09924 may be used.

-25 Significant, Separately Identifiable Evaluation and Management Service by the Same Physician on the Day of a Procedure: The physician may need to indicate that on the day a procedure or service identified by a CPT code was performed, the patient's condition required a significant, separately identifiable E/M service above and beyond the usual preoperative and postoperative care associated with the procedure that was performed. This circumstance may be reported by adding the modifier '-25' to the appropriate level of E/M service, or the separate five digit modifier 09925 may be used.

-26 Professional Component: Certain procedures are a combination of a physician component and a technical component. When the physician component is reported separately, the service may be identified by adding the modifier '-26' to the usual procedure number or the service may be reported by use of the five digit modifier code 09926.

-32 Mandated Services: Services related to *mandated* consultation and/or related services (eg, PRO, 3rd party payor) may be identified by adding the modifier '-32' to the basic procedure or the service may be reported by use of the five digit modifier 09932.

-47 Anesthesia by Surgeon: Regional or general anesthesia provided by the surgeon may be reported by adding the modifier '-47' to the basic service or by use of the separate five digit modifier code 09947. (This does not include local anesthesia.)
Note: Modifier '-47' or 09947 would not be used as a modifier for the anesthesia procedures 00100-01999.

-50 Bilateral Procedure: Unless otherwise identified in the listings, bilateral procedures that are performed at the same operative session, should be identified by the appropriate five digit code describing the first procedure. The second (bilateral) procedure is identified either by adding modifier '-50' to the procedure number or by use of the separate five digit modifier code 09950.

-51 Multiple Procedures: When multiple procedures are performed on the same day or at the same session, the major procedure or service may be reported as listed. The secondary additional, or lesser procedure(s) or service(s) may be identified by adding the modifier '-51' to the secondary procedure or service code(s) or by use of the separate five digit modifier code 09951. This modifier may be used to report multiple medical procedures performed at the same session, as well as a combination of medical and surgical procedures, or several surgical procedures performed at the same operative session.

-52 Reduced Services: Under certain circumstances a service or procedure is partially reduced or eliminated at the physician's election. Under these circumstances the service provided can be identified by its usual procedure number and the addition of the modifier '-52', signifying that the service is reduced. This provides a means of reporting reduced services without disturbing the identification of the basic service. Modifier code 09952 may be used as an alternative to modifier '-52'.

-54 Surgical Care Only: When one physician performs a surgical procedure and another provides preoperative and/or postoperative management, surgical services may be identified by adding the modifier '-54' to the usual procedure number or by use of the separate five digit modifier code 09954.

-55 Postoperative Management Only: When one physician performs the postoperative management and another physician has performed the surgical procedure, the postoperative component may be identified by adding the modifier '-55' to the usual procedure number or by use of the separate five digit modifier code 09955.

-56 Preoperative Management Only: When one physician performs the preoperative care and evaluation and another physician performs the surgical procedure, the preoperative component may be identified by adding the modifier '-56' to the usual procedure number or by use of the separate five digit modifier code 09956.

-62 Two Surgeons: Under certain circumstances the skills of two surgeons (usually with different skills) may be required in the management of a specific surgical procedure. Under such circumstances the separate services may be identified by adding the modifier '-62' to the procedure number used by each surgeon for reporting his services. Modifier code 09962 may be used as an alternative to modifier '-62'.

-66 Surgical Team: Under some circumstances, highly complex procedures (requiring the concomitant services of several physicians, often of different specialties, plus other highly skilled, specially trained personnel, various types of complex equipment) are carried out under the "surgical team" concept. Such circumstances may be identified by each participating physician with the addition of the modifier '-66' to the basic procedure number used for reporting services. Modifier code 09966 may be used as an alternative to modifier '-66'.

-76 Repeat Procedure by Same Physician: The physician may need to indicate that a procedure or service was repeated subsequent to the original service. This circumstance may be reported by adding the modifier '-76' to the repeated service or the separate five digit modifier code 09976 may be used.

-77 Repeat Procedure by Another Physician: The physician may need to indicate that a basic procedure performed by another physician had to be repeated. This situation may be reported by adding modifier '-77' to the repeated service or the separate five digit modifier code 09977 may be used.

-78 Return to the Operating Room for a Related Procedure During the Postoperative Period: The physician may need to indicate that another procedure was performed during the postoperative period of the initial procedure. When this subsequent procedure is related to the first, and requires the use of the operating room, it may be reported by adding the modifier '-78' to the related procedure, or by using the separate five digit modifier 09978. (For repeat procedures on the same day, see -76).

-79 Unrelated Procedure or Service by the Same Physician During the Postoperative Period: The physician may need to indicate that the performance of a procedure or service during the postoperative period was unrelated to the original procedure. This circumstance may be reported by using the modifier '-79' or by using the separate five digit modifier 09979. (For repeat procedures on the same day, see -76).

-80 Assistant Surgeon: Surgical assistant services may be identified by adding the modifier '-80' to the usual procedure number(s) or by use of the separate five digit modifier code 09980.

-81 Minimum Assistant Surgeon: Minimum surgical assistant services are identified by adding the modifier '-81' to the usual procedure number or by use of the separate five digit modifier code 09981.

-82 Assistant Surgeon (when qualified resident surgeon not available): The unavailability of a qualified resident surgeon is a prerequisite for use of modifier '-82' appended to the usual procedure code number(s) or by use of the separate five digit modifier code 09982.

-90 Reference (Outside) Laboratory: When laboratory procedures are performed by a party other than the treating or reporting physician, the procedure may be identified by adding the modifier '-90' to the usual procedure number or by use of the separate five digit modifier code 09990.

-99 Multiple Modifiers: Under certain circumstances two or more modifiers may be necessary to completely delineate a service. In such situations modifier '-99' should be added to the basic procedure, and other applicable modifiers may be listed as part of the description of the service. Modifier code 09999 may be used as an alternative to modifier '-99'.

-53- modifer used to show the computer that you were unable to complete the service & that you may come back at another time to try the service.

-57- modifier that is added to the E/M code to show that it was during that particular visit that the physician decided that the surgery should be performed.

-58- modifier used when the coder is trying to show that another procedure may need to be done during the post-op time of the first procedure - and that the second procedure is related to the first.

-59- modifier- used to report that 2 or more procedures were done by the same MD at the same time -or- at different sessions, but that they are related to each other.

-91 modifer- used to repeat lab work on the same day

Appendix B

Summary of Additions, Deletions and Revisions

Code

00534 Anesthesia code added

10140 Terminology revised

10141 Code deleted. To report, see 10140

11060 Code deleted. To report, see 11300-11313

11061 Code deleted. To report, see 11300-11313

11062 Code deleted. To report, see 11300-11313

11100 Terminology revised

11101 Terminology revised

11200 Terminology revised

11300 Shaving of lesion code added

11301 Shaving of lesion code added

11302 Shaving of lesion code added

11303 Shaving of lesion code added

11305 Shaving of lesion code added

11306 Shaving of lesion code added

11307 Shaving of lesion code added

11308 Shaving of lesion code added

11310 Shaving of lesion code added

11311 Shaving of lesion code added

11312 Shaving of lesion code added

11313 Shaving of lesion code added

11450 Terminology revised

11451 Terminology revised

11462 Terminology revised

11463 Terminology revised

11470 Terminology revised

11471 Terminology revised

11975 Terminology revised

11976 Terminology revised

11977 Reinsertion of contraceptive capsules code added

16040 Excision of burn wound code added

16041 Excision of burn wound code added

16042 Excision of burn wound code added

Appendices

17105 Terminology revised

17250 Terminology revised

19240 Terminology revised

19290 Placement of breast needle/wire code added

19291 Placement of breast needle/wire code added

20693 Terminology revised

21300 Terminology revised

21310 Terminology revised

21315 Terminology revised

21336 Treatment of fracture code added

21337 Terminology revised

21340 Terminology revised

21343 Terminology revised

21344 Treatment of fracture code added

21345 Terminology revised

21347 Terminology revised

21348 Treatment of fracture code added

21355 Terminology revised

21356 Treatment of fracture code added

21360 Terminology revised

21365 Terminology revised

21366 Treatment of fracture code added

21400 Terminology revised

21408 Treatment of fracture code added

21421 Terminology revised

21422 Terminology revised

21423 Treatment of fracture code added

21431 Terminology revised

21432 Terminology revised

21433 Terminology revised

21435 Terminology revised

21436 Treatment of fracture code added

21440 Terminology revised

21445 Terminology revised

21450 Terminology revised

21451 Terminology revised

21452 Terminology revised

21453 Terminology revised

21454 Terminology revised

21455 Code deleted. To report, see 21453

21461 Terminology revised

21470 Terminology revised

21480 Terminology revised

21485 Terminology revised

21493 Terminology revised

21495 Terminology revised

21800 Terminology revised

21805 Terminology revised

21810 Terminology revised

21820 Terminology revised

21825 Terminology revised

23500 Terminology revised

23510 Code deleted. To report, see 23500, 23505, 23515

23515 Terminology revised

23520 Terminology revised

23530 Terminology revised

23540 Terminology revised

23550 Terminology revised

23570 Terminology revised

23575 Terminology revised

23580 Code deleted. To report, see 23570, 23575, 23585

23585 Terminology revised

23600 Terminology revised

23605 Terminology revised

23610 Code deleted. To report, see 23600, 23605, 23615

23615 Terminology revised

23616 Treatment of fracture code added

23620 Terminology revised

23630 Terminology revised

23650 Terminology revised

23658 Code deleted. To report, see 23650, 23655, 23660, 23665, 23670

23660 Terminology revised

23665 Terminology revised

23670 Terminology revised

23675 Terminology revised

23680 Terminology revised

24006 Arthrotomy code added

24500 Terminology revised

24505 Terminology revised

24506 Code deleted. To report, see 24516

24510 Code deleted. To report, see 24500, 24505, 24515, 24516

24515 Terminology revised

24516 Treatment of fracture code added

24530 Terminology revised

24531 Code deleted. To report, see 24535

24535 Terminology revised

24536 Code deleted. To report, see 24535

24538 Terminology revised

24540 Code deleted. To report, see 24530, 24535, 24538, 24545, 24546

24542 Code deleted. To report, see 24530, 24535, 24538, 24545, 24546

24545 Terminology revised

24546 Treatment of fracture code added

24560 Terminology revised

24570 Code deleted. To report, see 24560, 24565, 24575

24575 Terminology revised

24576 Terminology revised

24578 Code deleted. To report, see 24576, 24577, 24579

24579 Terminology revised

24580 Code deleted. To report, see 24530, 24560, 24576, 24650, 24670

24581 Code deleted. To report, see 24535, 24565, 24577, 24675

24583 Code deleted. To report, see 24535, 24538, 24545, 24560, 24565, 24577

24585 Code deleted. To report, see 24538, 24545, 24575, 24579, 24665, 24666, 24685

24586 Terminology revised

24587 Terminology revised

24588 Code deleted. To report, see 24586, 24587

24610 Code deleted. To report, see 24586, 24600, 24605, 24615

24615 Terminology revised

24620 Terminology revised

24625 Code deleted. To report, see 24620, 24635

24635 Terminology revised

24640 Terminology revised

24650 Terminology revised

24660 Code deleted. To report, see 24650, 24655, 24665, 24666

24665 Terminology revised

24666 Terminology revised

24670 Terminology revised

24680 Code deleted. To report, see 24670, 24675, 24685

24685 Terminology revised

25020 Terminology revised

25500 Terminology revised

25510 Code deleted. To report, see 25500, 25505, 25515

25515 Terminology revised

25520 Treatment of fracture code added

25525 Treatment of fracture code added

25526 Treatment of fracture code added

25530 Terminology revised

25540 Code deleted. To report, see 25530, 25535, 25545

25545 Terminology revised

25560 Terminology revised

25570 Code deleted. To report, see 25560, 25565, 25574, 25575

25574 Treatment of fracture code added

25575 Terminology revised

25600 Terminology revised

25610 Code deleted. To report, see 25605

25611 Terminology revised

25615 Code deleted. To report, see 25600, 25605, 25611, 25620

25620 Terminology revised

25622 Terminology revised

25626 Code deleted. To report, see 25622, 25624, 25628

25628 Terminology revised

25630 Terminology revised

25640 Code deleted. To report, see 25630, 25635, 25645

25645 Terminology revised

25650 Terminology revised

25660 Terminology revised

25665 Code deleted. To report, see 25650, 25660, 25670

25670 Terminology revised

25675 Terminology revised

25676 Terminology revised

25680 Terminology revised

25685 Terminology revised

25690 Terminology revised

26600 Terminology revised

26607 Terminology revised

26608 Percutaneous skeletal fixation code added

26610 Code deleted. To report, see 26605, 26607, 26608

26615 Terminology revised

26641 Terminology revised

26645 Terminology revised

26650 Terminology revised

26655 Code deleted. To report, see 26645, 26650, 26665

26660 Code deleted. To report, see 26650, 26665

26665 Terminology revised

26670 Terminology revised

26676 Terminology revised

26680 Code deleted. To report, see 26670, 26675, 26676, 26685

26685 Terminology revised

26700 Terminology revised

26706 Terminology revised

26710 Code deleted. To report, see 26700, 26705, 26706, 26715

26715 Terminology revised

26720 Terminology revised

26725 Terminology revised

26727 Terminology revised

26730 Code deleted. To report, see 26720, 26725, 26727, 26735

26735 Terminology revised

26740 Terminology revised

26744 Code deleted. To report, see 26740, 26742, 26746

26746 Terminology revised

26750 Terminology revised

26756 Terminology revised

26760 Code deleted. To report, see 26750, 26755, 26756, 26765

26765 Terminology revised

26770 Terminology revised

26776 Terminology revised

26780 Code deleted. To report, see 26770, 26775, 26776, 26785

26785 Terminology revised

27190 Code deleted. To report, see 27193, 27194

27191 Code deleted. To report, see 27193, 27194

27192 Code deleted. To report, see 27215, 27216

27193 Treatment of fracture code added

27194 Treatment of fracture code added

27195 Code deleted. To report, see 27193

27196 Code deleted. To report, see 27194

27200 Terminology revised

27201 Code deleted. To report, see 27200, 27202

27202 Terminology revised

27210 Code deleted. To report, see 27193, 27194, 27215, 27216, 27217, 27218

27212 Code deleted. To report, see 27193, 27194, 27215, 27216, 27217, 27218

27214 Code deleted. To report, see 27215, 27216, 27217, 27218

27215 Treatment of fracture code added

27216 Percutaneous skeletal fixation code added

27217 Treatment of fracture/ dislocation code added

27218 Treatment of fracture/ dislocation code added

27220 Terminology revised

27224 Code deleted. To report, see 27226, 27227

27225 Code deleted. To report, see 27227, 27228

27226 Treatment of fracture code added

27227 Treatment of fracture code added

27228 Treatment of fracture code added

27230 Terminology revised

27232 Terminology revised

27234 Code deleted. To report, see 27230, 27232, 27235, 27236

27235 Terminology revised

27236 Terminology revised

27238 Terminology revised

27240 Terminology revised

27242 Code deleted. To report, see 27238, 27240, 27244, 27245

27244 Terminology revised

27245 Treatment of fracture code added

27246 Terminology revised

27248 Terminology revised

27250 Terminology revised

27253 Terminology revised

27254 Terminology revised

27255 Code deleted. To report, see 27226, 27227, 27253, 27254

27256 Terminology revised

27258 Terminology revised

27265 Terminology revised

27266 Terminology revised

27496 Decompression fasciotomy code added

27497 Decompression fasciotomy code added

27498 Decompression fasciotomy code added

27499 Decompression fasciotomy code added

27500 Terminology revised

27501 Treatment of fracture code added

27502 Terminology revised

27503 Treatment of fracture code added

27504 Code deleted. To report, see 27500, 27501, 27502, 27503, 27506, 27507, 27509, 27511, 27513

27506 Terminology revised

27507 Treatment of fracture code added

27508 Terminology revised

27509 Percutaneous skeletal fixation code added

27510 Terminology revised

27511 Treatment of fracture code added

27512 Code deleted. To report, see 27508, 27510, 27514

27513 Treatment of fracture code added

27514 Terminology revised

27516 Terminology revised

27517 Terminology revised

27518 Code deleted. To report, see 27516, 27517, 27519

27519 Terminology revised

27520 Terminology revised

27522 Code deleted. To report, see 27520, 27524

27524 Terminology revised

27530 Terminology revised

27532 Terminology revised

27534 Code deleted. To report, see 27530, 27532, 27535, 27536

27535 Treatment of fracture code added

27536 Terminology revised

27537 Code deleted. To report, see 27535, 27536

27538 Terminology revised

27540 Terminology revised

27550 Terminology revised

27554 Code deleted. To report, see 27550, 27552, 27556, 27557, 27558

27556 Terminology revised

27558 Treatment of dislocation code added

27560 Terminology revised

27564 Code deleted. To report, see 27560, 27562, 27566

27566 Terminology revised

27600 Terminology revised

27601 Terminology revised

27602 Terminology revised

27750 Terminology revised

27752 Terminology revised

27754 Code deleted. To report, see 27750, 27752, 27756, 27758

27756 Terminology revised

27758 Terminology revised

27759 Treatment of fracture code added

27760 Terminology revised

27762 Terminology revised

27764 Code deleted. To report, see 27760, 27762, 27766

27766 Terminology revised

27780 Terminology revised

27782 Code deleted. To report, see 27780, 27781, 27784

27784 Terminology revised

27786 Terminology revised

27790 Code deleted. To report, see 27786, 27788, 27792

27792 Terminology revised

27800 Code deleted. To report, see 27750

27802 Code deleted. To report, see 27752

27804 Code deleted. To report, see 27750, 27752, 27756, 27758, 27759

27806 Code deleted. To report, see 27756, 27758, 27759

27808 Terminology revised

27812 Code deleted. To report, see 27808, 27810, 27814

27814 Terminology revised

27816 Terminology revised

27820 Code deleted. To report, see 27816, 27818, 27822, 27823

27822 Terminology revised

27823 Terminology revised

27824 Treatment of fracture code added

27825 Treatment of fracture code added

27826 Treatment of fracture code added

27827 Treatment of fracture code added

27828 Treatment of fracture code added

27829 Treatment of joint code added

27830 Terminology revised

27832 Terminology revised

27840 Terminology revised

27842 Terminology revised

27844 Code deleted. To report, see 27840, 27842, 27846, 27848

27846 Terminology revised

27848 Terminology revised

27892 Decompression fasciotomy code added

27893 Decompression fasciotomy code added

27894 Decompression fasciotomy code added

28400 Terminology revised

28405 Terminology revised

28406 Terminology revised

28410 Code deleted. To report, see 28400, 28405, 28406, 28415, 28420

28415 Terminology revised

28430 Terminology revised

28436 Terminology revised

28440 Code deleted. To report, see 28430, 28435, 28436, 28445

28445 Terminology revised

28450 Terminology revised

28456 Terminology revised

28460 Code deleted. To report, see 28450, 28455, 28456, 28465

28465 Terminology revised

28470 Terminology revised

28476 Terminology revised

28480 Code deleted. To report, see 28470, 28475, 28476, 28485

28485 Terminology revised

28490 Terminology revised

28496 Terminology revised

28500 Code deleted. To report, see 28490, 28495, 28496, 28505

28505 Terminology revised

28510 Terminology revised

28520 Code deleted. To report, see 28510, 28515, 28525

28525 Terminology revised

28530 Terminology revised

28531 Treatment of fracture code added

28540 Terminology revised

28546 Terminology revised

28550 Code deleted. To report, see 28540, 28545, 28546, 28555

28555 Terminology revised

28570 Terminology revised

28576 Percutaneous skeletal fixation code added

28580 Code deleted. To report, see 28570, 28575, 28576, 28585

28585 Terminology revised

28600 Terminology revised

28606 Terminology revised

28610 Code deleted. To report, see 28600, 28605, 28606, 28615

28615 Terminology revised

28630 Terminology revised

28636 Percutaneous skeletal fixation code added

28640 Code deleted. To report, see 28630, 28635, 28636, 28645

28645 Terminology revised

28660 Terminology revised

28666 Percutaneous skeletal fixation code added

28670 Code deleted. To report, see 28660, 28665, 28666, 28675

28675 Terminology revised

29850 Arthroscopic fracture treatment code added

29851 Arthroscopic fracture treatment code added

29855 Arthroscopic fracture treatment code added

29856 Arthroscopic fracture treatment code added

30460 Rhinoplasty code added

30462 Rhinoplasty code added

30620 Terminology revised

31719 Code deleted. To report, see 31730

31730 Introduction of stent/tube code added

33500 Terminology revised

33501 Repair of coronary fistula code added

33510 Terminology revised

33511 Terminology revised

33512 Terminology revised

33513 Terminology revised

33514 Terminology revised

33516 Terminology revised

33517 Coronary artery bypass graft code added

33518 Coronary artery bypass graft code added

33519 Coronary artery bypass graft code added

33521 Coronary artery bypass graft code added

33522 Coronary artery bypass graft code added

33523 Coronary artery bypass graft code added

33530 Terminology revised

33533 Coronary artery bypass graft code added

33534 Coronary artery bypass graft code added

33535 Coronary artery bypass graft code added

33536 Coronary artery bypass graft code added

33800 Aortopexy code added

35450 Terminology revised

35470 Terminology revised

35480 Transluminal atherectomy code added

35481 Transluminal atherectomy code added

35482 Transluminal atherectomy code added

35483 Transluminal atherectomy code added

35484 Transluminal atherectomy code added

35485 Transluminal atherectomy code added

35490 Transluminal atherectomy code added

35491 Transluminal atherectomy code added

35492 Transluminal atherectomy code added

35493 Transluminal atherectomy code added

35494 Transluminal atherectomy code added

35495 Transluminal atherectomy code added

36005 Injection for contrast venography code added

36415 Terminology revised

37205 Transcatheter placement of stent code added

37206 Transcatheter placement of stent code added

37207 Transcatheter placement of stent code added

37208 Transcatheter placement of stent code added

43842 Gastroplasty code added

43843 Gastroplasty code added

43844 Terminology revised

43845 Code deleted. To report, see 43842, 43843

47505 Injection for cholangiography code added

49315 Laparoscopic appendectomy code added

49427 Injection to evaluate shunt code added

49905 Omental flap code added

50727 Revision of urostomy code added

50728 Revision of urostomy code added

50780 Terminology revised

50782 Ureteroneocystostomy code added

50783 Ureteroneocystostomy code added

50785 Terminology revised

52335 Terminology revised

52339 Cystourethroscopy code added

55740 Code deleted. To report, use 55899

56000 Code deleted. To report, see 56405

56100 Code deleted. To report, see 56605

56200 Code deleted. To report, see 56810

56300 Laparoscopy code added

56301 Laparoscopy code added

56302 Laparoscopy code added

56303 Laparoscopy code added

56304 Laparoscopy code added

56305 Laparoscopy code added

56306 Laparoscopy code added

56307 Laparoscopy code added

56308 Laparoscopy code added

56309 Laparoscopy code added

56350 Hysteroscopy code added

56351 Hysteroscopy code added

56352 Hysteroscopy code added

56353 Hysteroscopy code added

56354 Hysteroscopy code added

56355 Hysteroscopy code added

56356 Hysteroscopy code added

56400 Code deleted. To report, see 56405

56405 Incision and drainage code added

56600 Code deleted. To report, see 56605

56605 Biopsy code added

56606 Biopsy code added

56620 Terminology revised

56625 Terminology revised

56630 Terminology revised

56631 Vulvectomy code added

56633 Vulvectomy code added

56634 Vulvectomy code added

56635 Code deleted. To report, see 56634, 56637

56637 Vulvectomy code added

56640 Terminology revised

56810 Perineoplasty code added

57282 Terminology revised

57415 Removal of foreign body code added

57450 Code deleted

57451 Code deleted

57460 Colposcopy code added

58100 Terminology revised

58102 Code deleted

58200 Terminology revised

58210 Terminology revised

58240 Terminology revised

58260 Terminology revised

58262 Vaginal hysterectomy code added

58263 Vaginal hysterectomy code added

58345 Transcervical fallopian tube catheterization code added

58980 Code deleted. To report, see 56300

58982 Code deleted. To report, see 56301

58983 Code deleted. To report, see 56302

58984 Code deleted. To report, see 56303

58985 Code deleted. To report, see 56304

58986 Code deleted. To report, see 56305

58987 Code deleted. To report, see 56306

58988 Code deleted. To report, see 56307

58990 Code deleted. To report, see 56350

58992 Code deleted. To report, see 56352

58994 Code deleted. To report, see 56354

58995 Code deleted. To report, see 56352, 56354, 56356

58996 Code deleted. To report, see 56356

59420 Code deleted. To report, see evaluation and management codes

59812 Terminology revised

61531 Electrode implant for seizure monitoring code added

61533 Terminology revised

61760 Electrode implant for seizure monitoring code added

61780 Code deleted. To report, see 61760

62278 Terminology revised

62279 Terminology revised

62282 Terminology revised

62291 Terminology revised

65860 Laser eye surgery code added

66761 Terminology revised

66825 Repositioning of lens prosthesis code added

68760 Terminology revised

68761 Closure of lacrimal punctum code added

74400 Terminology revised

74742 Radiological supervision and interpretation code added

75809 Radiological supervision and interpretation code added

75960 Radiological supervision and interpretation code added

75962 Terminology revised

75964 Terminology revised

75966 Terminology revised

75968 Terminology revised

75978 Terminology revised

75992 Radiological supervision and interpretation code added

75993 Radiological supervision and interpretation code added

75994 Radiological supervision and interpretation code added

75995 Radiological supervision and interpretation code added

75996 Radiological supervision and interpretation code added

76096 Terminology revised

76097 Code deleted. To report, see 19291, 76096

76825 Terminology revised

76826 Fetal echocardiography code added

76827 Fetal echocardiography code added

76828 Fetal echocardiography code added

76872 Terminology revised

80019 Terminology revised

80031 Code deleted. To report, see Therapeutic Drug Assay section

80040 Code deleted. To report, see 83520

80042 Code deleted. To report, see 87197

80050 Terminology revised

80052 Code deleted. To report, see codes for specific tests

80053 Code deleted. To report, see 80050 and codes for specific tests

80055 Terminology revised

80056 Code deleted. To report, see codes for specific tests

80057 Code deleted. To report, see codes for specific tests

80058 Terminology revised

80059 Terminology revised

80060 Code deleted. To report, see codes for specific tests

80061 Terminology revised

80062 Code deleted. To report, see 80061 and/or codes for specific tests

80063 Code deleted. To report, see codes for specific tests

80064 Code deleted. To report, see codes for specific tests

80065 Code deleted. To report, see codes for specific tests

80066 Code deleted. To report, see codes for specific tests

80067 Code deleted. To report, see codes for specific tests

80068 Code deleted. To report, see codes for specific tests

80070 Code deleted. To report, see 80091

80071 Code deleted. To report, see codes for specific tests

80072 Terminology revised

80073 Code deleted. To report, see 80002-80019

80075 Code deleted. To report, see codes for specific tests

80080 Code deleted. To report, see 84153

80082 Code deleted. To report, see codes for specific tests

80084 Code deleted. To report, see codes for specific tests

80085 Code deleted. To report, see codes for specific tests

80086 Code deleted. To report, see codes for specific tests

80088 Code deleted. To report, see codes for specific tests

80089 Code deleted. To report, see codes for specific tests

80090 Terminology revised

80091 Thyroid panel code added

80092 Thyroid panel code added

80099 Code deleted. To report, see codes for specific tests

80100 Drug testing code added

80101 Drug testing code added

80102 Drug testing code added

80103 Drug testing code added

80150 Therapeutic drug assay code added

80152 Therapeutic drug assay code added

80154 Therapeutic drug assay code added

80156 Therapeutic drug assay code added

80158 Therapeutic drug assay code added

80160 Therapeutic drug assay code added

80162 Therapeutic drug assay code added

80164 Therapeutic drug assay code added

80166 Therapeutic drug assay code added

80168 Therapeutic drug assay code added

80170 Therapeutic drug assay code added

80172 Therapeutic drug assay code added

80174 Therapeutic drug assay code added

80176 Therapeutic drug assay code added

80178 Therapeutic drug assay code added

80182 Therapeutic drug assay code added

80184 Therapeutic drug assay code added

80185 Therapeutic drug assay code added

80186 Therapeutic drug assay code added

80188 Therapeutic drug assay code added

80190 Therapeutic drug assay code added

80192 Therapeutic drug assay code added

80194 Therapeutic drug assay code added

80196 Therapeutic drug assay code added

80198 Therapeutic drug assay code added

80200 Therapeutic drug assay code added

80202 Therapeutic drug assay code added

80299 Therapeutic drug assay code added

81000 Terminology revised

81002 Terminology revised

81003 Urinalysis code added

81005 Terminology revised

81025 Urinalysis code added

81050 Urinalysis code added

82003 Terminology revised

82005 Code deleted

82009 Terminology revised

82011 Code deleted. To report, see 80196

82012 Code deleted

82015 Code deleted

82024 Terminology revised

82030 Terminology revised

82035 Code deleted

82042 Terminology revised

82043 Chemistry code added

82044 Chemistry code added

82055 Terminology revised

82060 Code deleted. To report, use 82055

82065 Code deleted. To report, use 82055

82070 Code deleted. To report, use 82055

82072 Code deleted

82075 Terminology revised

82076 Code deleted. To report, see 82055, 84600

82078 Code deleted. To report, see 82055, 84600

82085 Terminology revised

82086 Code deleted. To report, use 82085

82087 Code deleted. To report, use 82088

82088 Terminology revised

82089 Code deleted. To report, use 82088

82095 Code deleted. To report, use 80100, 80101, 80103

82096 Code deleted. To report, use code for specific drug and 80103

82100 Code deleted. To report, use 80100 and 80101

82101 Terminology revised

82103 Chemistry code added

82104 Chemistry code added

82105 Chemistry code added

82106 Chemistry code added

82108 Terminology revised

82112 Code deleted. To report, see 80150

82126 Code deleted

82131 Chemistry code added

82134 Code deleted

82137 Code deleted. To report, use 84420

82138 Code deleted. To report, use 80152

82140 Terminology revised

82141 Code deleted. To report, use 82140

82142 Code deleted

82145 Terminology revised

82150 Terminology revised

82156 Code deleted. To report, use 82150

82157 Terminology revised

82159 Code deleted. To report, use 82160

82160 Terminology revised

82163 Terminology revised

82164 Terminology revised

82165 Code deleted

82168 Code deleted. To report, see code for specific method

82170 Code deleted. To report, use 83015, 83018

82172 Terminology revised

82175 Terminology revised

82190 Chemistry code added

82205 Terminology revised

82210 Code deleted. To report, see 80100-80103, 82205

82225 Code deleted. To report, see 83015, 83018

82230 Code deleted. To report, see 83015, 83018

82231 Code deleted. To report, use 82232

82232 Terminology revised

82235 Code deleted

82236 Code deleted

82239 Chemistry code added

82240 Terminology revised

82245 Code deleted. To report, see 81000, 81002, 81005

82250 Terminology revised

82251 Terminology revised

82260 Code deleted. To report, use 82250

82265 Code deleted. To report, see 82143

82268 Code deleted. To report, see 83015, 83018

82273 Terminology revised

82280 Code deleted. To report, see code for specific method

82285 Code deleted. To report, see code for specific method

82290 Code deleted. To report, use 84311

82291 Code deleted. To report, use 84311

82300 Terminology revised

82305 Code deleted. To report, see 82486, 82491

82306 Terminology revised

82307 Terminology revised

82308 Terminology revised

82310 Terminology revised

82315 Code deleted. To report, use 82310

82320 Code deleted. To report, use 82310

82325 Code deleted. To report, use 82310

82330 Terminology revised

82335 Code deleted

82340 Terminology revised

82355 Terminology revised

82360 Terminology revised

82372 Code deleted. To report, see 80156

82374 Terminology revised

82378 Chemistry code added

82380 Terminology revised

82382 Terminology revised

82387 Chemistry code added

82390 Terminology revised

82397 Chemistry code added

82400 Code deleted. To report, use code for specific method

82405 Code deleted

82415 Terminology revised

82418 Code deleted. To report, use code for specific method

82420 Code deleted. To report, use code for specific method

82425 Code deleted. To report, use code for specific method

82435 Terminology revised

82436 Terminology revised

82437 Code deleted

82443 Code deleted. To report, use code for specific method

82470 Code deleted

82484 Code deleted. To report, use 82480 and 82482

82486 Terminology revised

82487 Terminology revised

82488 Terminology revised

82489 Terminology revised

82491 Chemistry code added

82495 Terminology revised

82512 Code deleted. To report, use 80154

82520 Terminology revised

82525 Terminology revised

82526 Code deleted. To report, use 82525

82528 Terminology revised

82529 Code deleted. To report, use 82533

82530 Chemistry code added

82531 Code deleted

82532 Code deleted

82533 Terminology revised

82534 Code deleted. To report, use 82533

82540 Terminology revised

82545 Code deleted. To report, use 82540

82546 Code deleted. To report, use 82540 and 82565

82550 Terminology revised

82553 Chemistry code added

82554 Chemistry code added

82555 Code deleted

82565 Terminology revised

82585 Terminology revised

82595 Terminology revised

82600 Terminology revised

82601 Code deleted. To report, use 80103 and 82600

82606 Code deleted

82607 Terminology revised

82614 Code deleted

82620 Code deleted. To report, see 82130

82624 Code deleted

82626 Terminology revised

82627 Chemistry code added

82628 Code deleted. To report, see 80100-80103, 80299

82633 Terminology revised

82634 Terminology revised

82635 Code deleted

82636 Code deleted. To report, see 80100-80103, 80154

82639 Code deleted. To report, use code for specific method

82640 Code deleted

82641 Code deleted

82643 Code deleted. To report, see 80162

82649 Terminology revised

82656 Code deleted. To report, see 80166

82660 Code deleted. To report, see 80100, 80101

82668 Terminology revised

82670 Terminology revised

82673 Code deleted. To report, use 82677

82674 Code deleted. To report, use 82677

82676 Code deleted. To report, use 82677

82677 Terminology revised

82678 Code deleted. To report, use 82679

82679 Terminology revised

82690 Terminology revised

82691 Code deleted. To report, see 82690

82692 Code deleted. To report, use 80168

82693 Chemistry code added

82694 Code deleted. To report, use 82696

82696 Terminology revised

82705 Terminology revised

82710 Terminology revised

82720 Code deleted

82725 Terminology revised

82727 Code deleted. To report, use 81005

82728 Terminology revised

82730 Code deleted. To report, see 85384, 85385

82735 Terminology revised

82740 Code deleted. To report, use 82735

82741 Code deleted. To report, see code for specific method

82745 Code deleted

82746 Terminology revised

82747 Chemistry code added

82750 Code deleted. To report, use code for specific method

82755 Code deleted

82756 Code deleted

82760 Terminology revised

82763 Code deleted. To report, use 82760 and administration codes

82765 Code deleted. To report, use 82760

82780 Code deleted. To report, use code for specific method

82784 Terminology revised

82785 Terminology revised

82786 Code deleted

82787 Chemistry code added

82790 Code deleted

82791 Code deleted

82792 Terminology revised

82793 Code deleted

82795 Code deleted

82820 Chemistry code added

82926 Terminology revised

82927 Code deleted. To report, use 82926

82928 Terminology revised

82929 Code deleted. To report, use 82928

82931 Code deleted. To report, use 82928

82932 Code deleted. To report, use 82928

82938 Terminology revised

82941 Terminology revised

82942 Code deleted

82943 Terminology revised

82944 Code deleted

82947 Terminology revised

82948 Terminology revised

82949 Code deleted

82954 Code deleted. To report, use 82947

82962 Chemistry code added

82965 Terminology revised

82975 Terminology revised

82977 Terminology revised

82985 Terminology revised

82995 Code deleted. To report, use 80172

83000 Code deleted

83001 Terminology revised

83002 Terminology revised

83003 Terminology revised

83008 Terminology revised

83010 Terminology revised

83011 Code deleted. To report, use 83010

83012 Terminology revised

83015 Terminology revised

83018 Terminology revised

83020 Terminology revised

83026 Chemistry code added

83036 Terminology revised

83040 Code deleted. To report, see 83050

83052 Code deleted. To report, use 85660

83053 Code deleted. To report, use 85660

83070 Terminology revised

83071 Terminology revised

83086 Code deleted. To report, see 82128

83087 Code deleted. To report, see 82128

83093 Code deleted. To report, use code for specific method for quantitative, and for qualitative, see 81005

83094 Code deleted. To report, use code for specific method for quantitative, and for qualitative, see 81005

83095 Code deleted. To report, use code for specific method for quantitative, and for qualitative, see 81005

83150 Terminology revised

83485 Code deleted

83486 Code deleted

83491 Terminology revised

83492 Code deleted. To report, use 83491

83493 Code deleted

83494 Code deleted. To report, use 83491

83495 Code deleted. To report, use 83491

83496 Code deleted. To report, use 83491

83497 Terminology revised

83498 Terminology revised

83500 Terminology revised

83505 Terminology revised

83510 Code deleted. To report, use 83500 and 83505

83518 Chemistry code added

83519 Chemistry code added

83520 Chemistry code added

83523 Code deleted. To report, use 80174

83524 Code deleted.

83525 Terminology revised

83528 Terminology revised

83530 Code deleted

83540 Terminology revised

83545 Code deleted. To report, use 83540

83546 Code deleted. To report, use 83540

83550 Terminology revised

83555 Code deleted. To report, use 83550

83565 Code deleted. To report, use 83550

83570 Terminology revised

83571 Code deleted. To report, use 83570

83576 Code deleted. To report, see code for specific method

83578 Code deleted

83582 Terminology revised

83583 Code deleted

83584 Code deleted

83586 Terminology revised

83587 Code deleted. To report, use 83593

83588 Code deleted. To report, use 83586

83589 Code deleted. To report, use 83586

83590 Code deleted

83593 Terminology revised

83597 Code deleted

83599 Code deleted. To report, use 83586

83600 Code deleted. To report, use code for specific method

83610 Code deleted. To report, use 83615

83615 Terminology revised

83620 Code deleted. To report, use 83615

83624 Code deleted

83625 Terminology revised

83626 Code deleted

83628 Code deleted. To report, use 83625

83629 Code deleted. To report, use 83615

83631 Code deleted. To report, use 83615

83632 Terminology revised

83645 Code deleted. To report, see quantitative code or screening for toxicity

83650 Code deleted. To report, use 83645

83655 Terminology revised

83660 Code deleted. To report, use 83655

83661 Terminology revised

83662 Chemistry code added

83670 Terminology revised

83675 Code deleted. To report, see 83670

83680 Code deleted. To report, see 83670

83685 Code deleted. To report, use 80176

83690 Terminology revised

83700 Code deleted. To report, see 82465, 83718-83721, 84478

83705 Code deleted. To report, see 82465, 83718-83721, 84478

83715 Terminology revised

83717 Terminology revised

83718 Terminology revised

83719 Terminology revised

83720 Code deleted

83721 Chemistry code added

83725 Code deleted. To report, see 80178

83727 Terminology revised

83728 Code deleted. To report, see 80100-80103, 80299

83730 Code deleted

83735 Terminology revised

83740 Code deleted. To report, use 83735

83750 Code deleted. To report, use 83735

83755 Code deleted. To report, use 83735

83760 Code deleted. To report, use 83735

83765 Code deleted. To report, use 83735

83775 Terminology revised

83785 Terminology revised

83795 Code deleted

83799 Code deleted. To report, use 83925

83805 Terminology revised

83825 Terminology revised

83830 Code deleted. To report, use 83825

83835 Terminology revised

83842 Code deleted. To report, see code for specific method

83845 Code deleted. To report, see 80100-80103

83858 Terminology revised

83859 Code deleted

83860 Code deleted. To report, see 80100-80103, 83925

83861 Code deleted. To report, see 80100-80103, 83925

83862 Code deleted. To report, see 80100-80103, 83925

83864 Terminology revised

83865 Code deleted. To report, use 83864

83873 Terminology revised

83874 Terminology revised

83875 Code deleted

83880 Code deleted. To report, see 83925

83883 Chemistry code added

83885 Terminology revised

83890 Molecular diagnostic code added

83892 Molecular diagnostic code added

83894 Molecular diagnostic code added

83895 Code deleted

83896 Molecular diagnostic code added

83898 Molecular diagnostic code added

83900 Code deleted

83910 Code deleted

83912 Terminology revised

83913 Code deleted. To report, see 83898

83916 Terminology revised

83917 Code deleted

83920 Code deleted. To report, use code for specific method

83925 Chemistry code added

83938 Code deleted

83945 Terminology revised

83946 Code deleted. To report, use 80154

83947 Code deleted. To report, see 82009, 82010

83948 Code deleted. To report, see 80100-80103, 83925

83949 Code deleted

83965 Code deleted. To report, use code for specific method

83970 Terminology revised

83971 Code deleted. To report, use code for specific method

83972 Code deleted. To report, use code for specific method

83973 Code deleted. To report, use 84375

83975 Code deleted. To report, use code for specific method

83985 Code deleted. To report, use code for specific method

83995 Code deleted. To report, use code for specific method

84005 Code deleted

84021 Code deleted. To report, see 80100, 80101, 84022

84022 Terminology revised

84030 Terminology revised

84031 Code deleted

84033 Code deleted. To report, use code for specific method

84035 Terminology revised

84037 Code deleted. To report, use 84035

84038 Code deleted. To report, use code for specific method

84039 Code deleted

84040 Code deleted

84045 Code deleted. To report, see 80185

84060 Terminology revised

84061 Chemistry code added

84065 Code deleted. To report, use 84066

84066 Terminology revised

84075 Terminology revised

84080 Terminology revised

84081 Terminology revised

84082 Code deleted

84083 Code deleted

84090 Code deleted

84100 Terminology revised

84118 Code deleted. To report, use 84120

84119 Terminology revised

84120 Terminology revised

84121 Code deleted. To report, use 84120

84126 Terminology revised

84127 Chemistry code added

84128 Code deleted

84132 Terminology revised

84134 Chemistry code added

84135 Terminology revised

84136 Code deleted. To report, use 84135

84138 Terminology revised

84139 Code deleted. To report, use 84138

84141 Code deleted. To report, see 80188

84142 Code deleted. To report, see 80190, 80192

84144 Terminology revised

84146 Terminology revised

84147 Code deleted. To report, see 80100-80103

84149 Code deleted

84150 Terminology revised

84153 Chemistry code added

84155 Terminology revised

84170 Code deleted

84175 Terminology revised

84176 Code deleted

84180 Code deleted

84181 Chemistry code added

84182 Chemistry code added

84185 Code deleted

84190 Code deleted. To report, use 84175

84195 Code deleted

84200 Code deleted. To report, use 84175

84205 Code deleted. To report, use code for specific method

84206 Terminology revised

84207 Terminology revised

84208 Code deleted. To report, use 89060

84210 Terminology revised

84220 Terminology revised

84230 Code deleted. To report, use 80194

84231 Code deleted. To report, see 83520

84232 Code deleted

84233 Terminology revised

84236 Code deleted. To report, use 84233 and 84234

84244 Terminology revised

84255 Terminology revised

84260 Terminology revised

84270 Chemistry code added

84275 Terminology revised

84285 Terminology revised

84295 Terminology revised

84305 Chemistry code added

84307 Chemistry code added

84310 Code deleted

84311 Chemistry code added

84318 Code deleted

84324 Code deleted. To report, see code for specific method

84395 Code deleted

84402 Chemistry code added

84403 Terminology revised

84405 Code deleted. To report, use 84403

84406 Code deleted. To report, see 84270

84407 Code deleted. To report, use code for specific method

84408 Code deleted. To report, see 80100-80103, 80299

84409 Code deleted. To report, use code for specific method

84410 Code deleted. To report, use code for specific method

84420 Code deleted. To report, use 80198

84430 Terminology revised

84432 Chemistry code added

84434 Code deleted. To report, use 84022

84435 Code deleted

84436 Terminology revised

84437 Terminology revised

84439 Terminology revised

84443 Terminology revised

84444 Terminology revised

84445 Terminology revised

84447 Code deleted. To report, see 80100-80103

84448 Code deleted. To report, see 80100-80103

84450 Terminology revised

84455 Code deleted. To report, use 84450

84460 Terminology revised

84465 Code deleted. To report, use 84460

84466 Chemistry code added

84472 Code deleted. To report, use code for specific method

84474 Code deleted. To report, use code for specific method

84476 Code deleted. To report, see 84022

84478 Terminology revised

84479 Terminology revised

84480 Terminology revised

84481 Terminology revised

84482 Chemistry code added

84483 Code deleted. To report, see 80100-80103, 80299

84488 Terminology revised

84490 Terminology revised

84510 Terminology revised

84520 Terminology revised

84525 Terminology revised

84565 Code deleted

84570 Code deleted

84575 Code deleted

84584 Code deleted

84588 Terminology revised

84589 Terminology revised

84590 Terminology revised

84595 Code deleted. To report, use 82380 and 84590

84600 Terminology revised

84605 Code deleted

84610 Code deleted

84613 Code deleted

84615 Code deleted. To report, use code for specific method

84630 Terminology revised

84635 Code deleted. To report, use 84630

84681 Terminology revised

84695 Code deleted. To report, see 80170

84702 Terminology revised

84800 Code deleted. To report, see 84437

84810 Code deleted. To report, use 80200

84830 Chemistry code added

84999 Terminology revised

85000 Code deleted. To report, use 85002

85002 Terminology revised

85005 Code deleted

85007 Terminology revised

85008 Hematology and coagulation code added

85012 Code deleted

85013 Hematology and coagulation code added

85014 Terminology revised

85018 Terminology revised

85095 Terminology revised

85100 Code deleted. To report, use 85095 and 85097

85101 Code deleted. To report, see 85095

85103 Code deleted. To report, see 88305

85105 Code deleted. To report, see 88305

85109 Code deleted

85130 Hematology and coagulation code added

85170 Terminology revised

85171 Code deleted

85172 Code deleted

85242 Code deleted

85244 Terminology revised

85245 Hematology and coagulation code added

85246 Hematology and coagulation code added

85247 Hematology and coagulation code added

85300 Terminology revised

85302 Terminology revised

85303 Hematology and coagulation code added

85305 Terminology revised

85306 Hematology and coagulation code added

85310 Code deleted

85311 Code deleted

85320 Code deleted

85330 Code deleted. To report, see 85335

85335 Hematology and coagulation code added

85337 Hematology and coagulation code added

85340 Code deleted

85341 Code deleted

85362 Terminology revised

85363 Code deleted

85364 Code deleted

85365 Code deleted. To report, use 86320

85366 Hematology and coagulation code added

85367 Code deleted

85368 Code deleted. To report, use 85366

85369 Code deleted

85370 Hematology and coagulation code added

85371 Code deleted. To report, see 85384, 85385

85372 Code deleted

85376 Code deleted. To report, use 85384, 85385

85377 Code deleted. To report, use 85384, 85385

85378 Hematology and coagulation code added

85379 Hematology and coagulation code added

85384 Hematology and coagulation code added

85385 Hematology and coagulation code added

85390 Terminology revised

85392 Code deleted

85395 Code deleted

85398 Code deleted

85400 Terminology revised

85415 Hematology and coagulation code added

85426 Code deleted. To report, see 85245-85247

85475 Hematology and coagulation code added

85525 Hematology and coagulation code added

85538 Code deleted. To report, see 88319

85544 Code deleted

85548 Code deleted. To report, see 85008

85549 Terminology revised

85555 Terminology revised

85556 Code deleted

85557 Terminology revised

85560 Code deleted. To report, see 88319

85575 Terminology revised

85576 Code deleted

85577 Code deleted

85580 Code deleted. To report, use 85590

85590 Terminology revised

85595 Terminology revised

85597 Hematology and coagulation code added

85611 Hematology and coagulation code added

85612 Terminology revised

85613 Hematology and coagulation code added

85615 Code deleted

85618 Code deleted

85630 Code deleted. To report, use 85029, 85030

85632 Code deleted

85650 Code deleted

85651 Terminology revised

85665 Code deleted

85667 Code deleted

85700 Code deleted

85705 Hematology and coagulation code added

85710 Code deleted

85711 Code deleted

86000 Terminology revised

86002 Code deleted

86004 Code deleted. To report, see 86940, 86941

86006 Code deleted. To report, see 83519, 86336 and code for specific method

86007 Code deleted

86008 Code deleted

86009 Code deleted

86011 Code deleted. To report, see 86021

86012 Code deleted. To report, see 86978

86013 Code deleted

86014 Code deleted. To report, see 86022

86016 Code deleted. To report, see 86850

86019 Code deleted. To report, see 86860

86024 Code deleted. To report, see 86885, 86886

86031 Code deleted. To report, see 86880

86032 Code deleted. To report, see 86885

86033 Code deleted. To report, see 86886

86034 Code deleted. To report, see 86880-86886 and 86971

86038 Terminology revised

86039 Immunology code added

86064 Code deleted. To report, see 82103, 82104

86066 Code deleted. To report, see 82104

86067 Code deleted. To report, see 82104

86068 Code deleted. To report, see 86920-86922

86070 Code deleted. To report, see 86920

86080 Code deleted. To report, see 86900-86910

86082 Code deleted. To report, see 86900, 86901

86083 Code deleted. To report, see 86850, 86901

86084 Code deleted. To report, see 86156, 86157

86085 Code deleted. To report, see 86904

86095 Code deleted. To report, see 86905

86100 Code deleted

86105 Code deleted

86115 Code deleted

86128 Code deleted

86130 Code deleted. To report, see 86891

86147 Immunology code added

86149 Code deleted

86151 Code deleted. To report, see 82378

86156 Immunology code added

86157 Immunology code added

86158 Code deleted

86159 Code deleted. To report, see 86160 and 86161

86160 Immunology code added

86161 Immunology code added

86162 Terminology revised

86163 Code deleted. To report, see 86160 and 86161

86164 Code deleted. To report, see 86160 and 86161

86185 Terminology revised

86225 Terminology revised

86226 Immunology code added

86235 Terminology revised

86243 Terminology revised

86244 Code deleted. To report, see 82105, 82106

86255 Terminology revised

86256 Terminology revised

86265 Code deleted. To report, see 86930

86266 Code deleted. To report, see 86931

86267 Code deleted. To report, see 86932

86277 Terminology revised

86280 Terminology revised

86281 Code deleted. To report, see 85475

86282 Code deleted. To report, see 86940

86283 Code deleted. To report, see 86941

86287 Terminology revised

86288 Code deleted

86289 Terminology revised

86290 Terminology revised

86291 Terminology revised

86293 Terminology revised

86295 Terminology revised

86296 Terminology revised

86298 Code deleted

86300 Code deleted. To report, see 86308

86302 Immunology code added

86305 Code deleted. To report, use 86309

86306 Immunology code added

86308 Immunology code added

86309 Immunology code added

86310 Terminology revised

86311 Terminology revised

86312 Code deleted. To report, see 86687-86689

86314 Code deleted. To report, use 86689

86316 Terminology revised

86317 Terminology revised

86318 Terminology revised

86319 Code deleted. To report, see 80100-80103

86320 Terminology revised

86325 Terminology revised

86329 Terminology revised

86332 Terminology revised

86333 Code deleted. To report, see 86332

86335 Code deleted

86337 Terminology revised

86338 Code deleted. To report, see 86337

86340 Terminology revised

86342 Code deleted. To report, see 86945

86349 Code deleted. To report, see 86950

86353 Terminology revised

86357 Code deleted

86358 Code deleted. To report, see 86180, 88342, 88346

86376 Terminology revised

86377 Code deleted. To report, see 86376

86385 Code deleted. To report, see 86910

86386 Code deleted. To report, see 86910

86403 Terminology revised

86404 Code deleted. To report, see 86965

86405 Code deleted

86410 Code deleted. To report, see 86970

86411 Code deleted. To report, see 86971

86412 Code deleted. To report, see 86972

86417 Code deleted. To report, see 86975

86418 Code deleted. To report, see 86976

86419 Code deleted. To report, see 86977

86420 Code deleted. To report, see 86978

86421 Terminology revised

86423 Code deleted. To report, see 86421

86430 Terminology revised

86431 Immunology code added

86455 Code deleted. To report, use 86586

86485 Immunology code added

86540 Code deleted. To report, see 86735

86586 Immunology code added

86587 Code deleted. To report, see 86985

86588 Immunology code added

86594 Code deleted. To report, see 86376 and 86800

86595 Code deleted

86600 Code deleted

86602 Antibody code added

86603 Antibody code added

86606 Antibody code added

86609 Antibody code added

86612 Antibody code added

86615 Antibody code added

86618 Antibody code added

86619 Antibody code added

86622 Antibody code added

86625 Antibody code added

86628 Antibody code added

86630 Code deleted

86631 Antibody code added

86632 Antibody code added

86635 Antibody code added

86638 Antibody code added

86641 Antibody code added

86644 Antibody code added

86645 Antibody code added

86648 Antibody code added

86650 Code deleted. To report, use 86781

86651 Antibody code added

86652 Antibody code added

86653 Antibody code added

86654 Antibody code added

86658 Antibody code added

86662 Code deleted. To report, use 86650

86663 Antibody code added

86664 Antibody code added

86665 Antibody code added

86668 Antibody code added

86671 Antibody code added

86674 Antibody code added

86677 Antibody code added

86681 Code deleted. To report, see 86255, 86256

86682 Antibody code added

86684 Antibody code added

86685 Code deleted. To report, see 86255, 86256

86687 Terminology revised

86688 Antibody code added

86689 Terminology revised

86692 Antibody code added

86694 Antibody code added

86695 Antibody code added

86698 Antibody code added

86701 Antibody code added

86702 Antibody code added

86703 Antibody code added

86710 Antibody code added

86713 Antibody code added

86717 Antibody code added

86720 Antibody code added

86723 Antibody code added

86727 Antibody code added

86729 Antibody code added

86732 Antibody code added

86735 Antibody code added

86738 Antibody code added

86741 Antibody code added

86744 Antibody code added

86747 Antibody code added

86750 Antibody code added

86753 Antibody code added

86756 Antibody code added

86759 Antibody code added

86762 Antibody code added

86765 Antibody code added

86768 Antibody code added

86771 Antibody code added

86774 Antibody code added

86777 Antibody code added

86778 Antibody code added

86781 Antibody code added

86784 Antibody code added

86787 Antibody code added

86790 Antibody code added

86793 Antibody code added

86800 Terminology revised

86812 Terminology revised

86813 Terminology revised

86816 Terminology revised

86817 Terminology revised

86849 Immunology code added

86850 Transfusion medicine code added

86860 Transfusion medicine code added

86870 Transfusion medicine code added

86880 Transfusion medicine code added

86886 Transfusion medicine code added

86890 Transfusion medicine code added

86891 Transfusion medicine code added

86900 Transfusion medicine code added

86901 Transfusion medicine code added

86903 Transfusion medicine code added

86904 Transfusion medicine code added

86905 Transfusion medicine code added

86906 Transfusion medicine code added

86910 Transfusion medicine code added

86915 Transfusion medicine code added

86920 Transfusion medicine code added

86921 Transfusion medicine code added

86922 Transfusion medicine code added

86927 Transfusion medicine code added

86930 Transfusion medicine code added

86931 Transfusion medicine code added

86932 Transfusion medicine code added

86940 Transfusion medicine code added

86941 Transfusion medicine code added

86945 Transfusion medicine code added

86950 Transfusion medicine code added

86965 Transfusion medicine code added

86970 Transfusion medicine code added

86971 Transfusion medicine code added

86972 Transfusion medicine code added

86975 Transfusion medicine code added

86976 Transfusion medicine code added

86977 Transfusion medicine code added

86978 Transfusion medicine code added

86985 Transfusion medicine code added

86999 Terminology revised

88150 Terminology revised

88156 Cytopathology code added

88157 Cytopathology code added

88371 Protein analysis of tissue code added

88372 Protein analysis of tissue code added

90918 End stage renal disease service code added

90919 End stage renal disease service code added

90920 End stage renal disease service code added

90921 End stage renal disease service code added

90922 End stage renal disease service code added

90995 Code deleted. To report, see 90918-90921

90998 Code deleted. To report, see 90922

92982 Terminology revised

92995 Percutaneous coronary atherectomy code added

92996 Percutaneous coronary atherectomy code added

93015 Terminology revised

93312 Terminology revised

93313 Echocardiography code added

93314 Echocardiography code added

93325 Terminology revised

93980 Penile vascular study code added

93981 Penile vascular study code added

94700 Code deleted. To report, see 82800 et seq

94705 Code deleted. To report, see 82800 et seq

94710 Code deleted. To report, see 82800 et seq

94715 Code deleted. To report, use 82820

95000 Code deleted. To report, use 95004

95001 Code deleted. To report, use 95004

95002 Code deleted. To report, use 95004

95003 Code deleted. To report, use 95004

95004 Allergy skin test code added

95005 Code deleted. To report, use 95010

95006 Code deleted. To report, use 95010

95007 Code deleted. To report, use 95010

95010 Allergy skin test code added

95011 Code deleted. To report, use 95010

95014 Code deleted. To report, use 95015

95015 Allergy skin test code added

95016 Code deleted. To report, use 95015

95017 Code deleted. To report, use 95015

95018 Code deleted. To report, use 95015

95020 Code deleted. To report, use 95024

95021 Code deleted. To report, use 95024

95022 Code deleted. To report, use 95024

95023 Code deleted. To report, use 95024

95024 Allergy skin test code added

95028 Allergy skin test code added

95030 Code deleted. To report, use 95028

95031 Code deleted. To report, use 95028

95032 Code deleted. To report, use 95028

95033 Code deleted. To report, use 95028

95034 Code deleted. To report, use 95028

95075 Terminology revised

95851 Terminology revised

95883 Neuropsychological testing code added

95950 Terminology revised

95951 Terminology revised

95952 Code deleted. To report, see 95950

95953 Monitoring for seizure code added

95956 Monitoring for seizure code added

96440 Terminology revised

96445 Terminology revised

96450 Terminology revised

96542 Chemotherapy administration code added

97500 Terminology revised

97545 Work hardening/ conditioning code added

97546 Work hardening/ conditioning code added

99218 Hospital observation service code added

99219 Hospital observation service code added

99220 Hospital observation service code added

99221 Terminology revised

99283 Terminology revised

99291 Terminology revised

99295 Neonatal intensive care code added

99296 Neonatal intensive care code added

99297 Neonatal intensive care code added

99303 Terminology revised

99438 Code deleted

Appendix C

Short Procedure Tape Revision

Code

Code	Action	Description
00534	Add:	Anesth, Cardioverter/defib
10140	Revise:	Drainage of hematoma/fluid
10141	Delete	
11060	Delete	
11061	Delete	
11062	Delete	
11300	Add:	Shave skin lesion
11301	Add:	Shave skin lesion
11302	Add:	Shave skin lesion
11303	Add:	Shave skin lesion
11305	Add:	Shave skin lesion
11306	Add:	Shave skin lesion
11307	Add:	Shave skin lesion
11308	Add:	Shave skin lesion
11310	Add:	Shave skin lesion
11311	Add:	Shave skin lesion
11312	Add:	Shave skin lesion
11313	Add:	Shave skin lesion
11975	Revise:	Insert contraceptive cap
11977	New:	Remove/reinsert contra cap
16040	Add:	Burn wound excision
16041	Add:	Burn wound excision
16042	Add:	Burn wound excision
19290	Add:	Place needle wire, breast
19291	Add:	Place needle wire, breast
21336	Add:	Repair nasal septal fracture
21344	Add:	Repair of sinus fracture
21348	Add:	Repair of nose/jaw fracture
21356	Add:	Repair cheek bone fracture
21366	Add:	Repair cheek bone fracture
21408	Add:	Repair eye socket fracture
21423	Add:	Repair mouth roof fracture
21436	Add:	Repair craniofacial fracture
21455	Delete	

23510 Delete

23580 Delete

23610 Delete

23616 Add: Repair humerus fracture

23658 Delete

24006 Add: Release elbow joint

24506 Delete

24510 Delete

24516 Add: Repair humerus fracture

24531 Delete

24536 Delete

24540 Delete

24542 Delete

24546 Add: Repair humerus fracture

24570 Delete

24578 Delete

24580 Delete

24581 Delete

24583 Delete

24585 Delete

24588 Delete

24610 Delete

24625 Delete

24660 Delete

24680 Delete

25510 Delete

25520 Add: Repair fracture of radius

25525 Add: Repair fracture of radius

25526 Add: Repair fracture of radius

25540 Delete

25570 Delete

25574 Add: Treat fracture radius & ulna

25575 Revise: Treat fracture radius & ulna

25610 Delete

25615 Delete

25626 Delete

25640 Delete

25665 Delete

26608 Add: Treat metacarpal fracture

26610 Delete

26655 Delete

26660 Delete

26680 Delete

26710 Delete

26730 Delete

26744 Delete

26760 Delete

26780 Delete

27190 Delete

27191 Delete

27192 Delete

27193 Add: Treat pelvic ring fracture

27194 Add: Treat pelvic ring fracture

27195 Delete

27196 Delete

27201 Delete

27210 Delete

27212 Delete

27214 Delete

27215 Add: Treat pelvic fracture(s)

27216 Add: Treat pelvic ring fracture

27217 Add: Treat pelvic ring fracture

27218 Add: Treat pelvic ring fracture

27224 Delete

27225 Delete

27226 Add: Treat hip fracture

27227 Add: Treat hip fracture(s)

27228 Add: Treat hip fracture(s)

27234 Delete

27242 Delete

27245 Add: Repair of thigh fracture

27255 Delete

27496 Add: Decompression of thigh/knee

27497 Add: Decompression of thigh/knee

27498 Add: Decompression of thigh/knee

27499 Add: Decompression of thigh/knee

27501 Add: Treatment of thigh fracture

27503 Add: Treatment of thigh fracture

27504 Delete

27507 Add: Treatment of thigh fracture

27509 Add: Treatment of thigh fracture

27511 Add: Treatment of thigh fracture

27512 Delete

27513 Add: Treatment of thigh fracture

27518 Delete

27522 Delete

27534 Delete

27535 Add: Repair of knee fracture

27537 Delete

27554 Delete

27558 Add: Repair of knee dislocation

Code	Action	Description
27564	Delete	
27754	Delete	
27759	Add:	Repair of tibia fracture
27764	Delete	
27782	Delete	
27790	Delete	
27800	Delete	
27802	Delete	
27804	Delete	
27806	Delete	
27812	Delete	
27820	Delete	
27824	Add:	Treat lower leg fracture
27825	Add:	Repair lower leg fracture
27826	Add:	Repair lower leg fracture
27827	Add:	Repair lower leg fracture
27828	Add:	Repair lower leg fracture
27829	Add:	Repair lower leg joint
27844	Delete	
27892	Add:	Decompression of leg
27893	Add:	Decompression of leg
27894	Add:	Decompression of leg
28406	Revise:	Repair heel fracture
28410	Delete	
28436	Revise:	Repair ankle fracture
28440	Delete	
28460	Delete	
28480	Delete	
28500	Delete	
28520	Delete	
28531	Add:	Repair sesamoid bone fracture
28546	Revise:	Repair foot dislocation
28550	Delete	
28576	Add:	Repair foot dislocation
28580	Delete	
28606	Revise:	Repair foot dislocation
28610	Delete	
28636	Add:	Repair toe dislocation
28640	Delete	
28666	Add:	Repair toe dislocation
28670	Delete	
29850	Add:	Knee arthroscopy/ surgery
29851	Add:	Knee arthroscopy/ surgery

29855 Add: Tibial arthroscopy/surgery

29856 Add: Tibial arthroscopy/surgery

30460 Add: Revision of nose

30462 Add: Revision of nose

31719 Delete

31730 Add: Intro windpipe wire/tube

33501 Add: Repair heart vessel fistula

33517 Add: Coronary arteries bypass

33518 Add: Coronary arteries bypass

33519 Add: Coronary arteries bypass

33521 Add: Coronary arteries bypass

33522 Add: Coronary arteries bypass

33523 Add: Coronary arteries bypass

33533 Add: Coronary arteries bypass

33534 Add: Coronary arteries bypass

33535 Add: Coronary arteries bypass

33536 Add: Coronary arteries bypass

33800 Add: Aortic suspension

35480 Add: Atherectomy, open

35481 Add: Atherectomy, open

35482 Add: Atherectomy, open

35483 Add: Atherectomy, open

35484 Add: Atherectomy, open

35485 Add: Atherectomy, open

35490 Add: Atherectomy, percutaneous

35491 Add: Atherectomy, percutaneous

35492 Add: Atherectomy, percutaneous

35493 Add: Atherectomy, percutaneous

35494 Add: Atherectomy, percutaneous

35495 Add: Atherectomy, percutaneous

36005 Add: Injection, venography

37205 Add: Transcatheter stent

37206 Add: Transcatheter stent

37207 Add: Transcatheter stent

37208 Add: Transcatheter stent

Code	Action	Description
43842	Add:	Gastroplasty for obesity
43843	Add:	Gastroplasty for obesity
43845	Delete	
47505	Add:	Injection for liver x-rays
49315	Add:	Laparoscopic appendectomy
49427	Add:	Inject, abdomen-venous shunt
49905	Add:	Omental flap
50727	Add:	Revision of ureter
50728	Add:	Revision of ureter
50782	Add:	Reimplant ureter in bladder
50783	Add:	Reimplant ureter in bladder
52339	Add:	Cystoscopy, tumor resection
55740	Delete	
56000	Delete	
56100	Delete	
56200	Delete	
56300	Add:	Laparoscopy; pelvis dx
56301	Add:	Laparoscopy; tubal cautery
56302	Add:	Laparoscopy; tubal block
56303	Add:	Laparoscopy; excise lesions
56304	Add:	Laparoscopy; lysis
56305	Add:	Laparoscopy; biopsy
56306	Add:	Laparoscopy; aspiration
56307	Add:	Laparoscopy; remove adnexa
56308	Add:	Laparoscopy; hysterectomy
56309	Add:	Laparoscopy; remove myoma
56350	Add:	Hysteroscopy; diagnostic
56351	Add:	Hysteroscopy; biopsy
56352	Add:	Hysteroscopy; lysis
56353	Add:	Hysteroscopy; resect septum
56354	Add:	Hysteroscopy; remove myoma
56355	Add:	Hysteroscopy; remove body
56356	Add:	Hysteroscopy; ablation
56400	Delete	
56405	Add:	I & D of vulva/perineum
56600	Delete	
56605	Add:	Biopsy of vulva/perineum
56606	Add:	Biopsy of vulva/perineum

56625 Revise: Complete removal of vulva

56631 Add: Remove vulva/ lymph node

56633 Add: Remove vulva/ lymph node

56634 Add: Remove vulva/ lymph node

56635 Delete

56637 Add: Remove vulva/ lymph nodes

56810 Add: Repair of perineum

57415 Add: Removal vaginal foreign body

57450 Delete

57451 Delete

57460 Add: Vagina exam/ cervix excision

58102 Delete

58262 Add: Vaginal hysterectomy

58263 Add: Vaginal hysterectomy

58345 Add: Place catheter tube

58980 Delete

58982 Delete

58983 Delete

58984 Delete

58985 Delete

58986 Delete

58987 Delete

58988 Delete

58990 Delete

58992 Delete

58994 Delete

58995 Delete

58996 Delete

59420 Delete

61531 Add: Implant brain electrodes

61760 Add: Implant brain electrodes

61780 Delete

65860 Add: Incise inner eye adhesions

66825 Add: Reposition intraocular lens

68761 Add: Close tear duct opening

74742 Add: X-ray fallopian tube

75809 Add: Nonvascular shunt, x-ray

75960 Add: Transcatheter intro, stent

75992 Add: Atherectomy, x-ray exam

75993 Add: Atherectomy, x-ray exam

75994 Add: Atherectomy, x-ray exam

75995 Add: Atherectomy, x-ray exam

75996 Add: Atherectomy, x-ray exam

76096 Revise: X-ray of needle wire, breast

76097 Delete

76826 Add: Echo exam of fetal heart

76827 Add: Echo exam of fetal heart

76828 Add: Echo exam of fetal heart

76872 Revise: Echo exam, transrectal

80031 Delete

80040 Delete

80042 Delete

80052 Delete

80053 Delete

80056 Delete

80057 Delete

80060 Delete

80061 Revise: Lipid panel

80062 Delete

80063 Delete

80064 Delete

80065 Delete

80066 Delete

80067 Delete

80068 Delete

80070 Delete

80071 Delete

80073 Delete

80075 Delete

80080 Delete

80082 Delete

80084 Delete

80085 Delete

80086 Delete

80088 Delete

80089 Delete

80090 Revise: TORCH antibody panel

80091 Add: Thyroid panel

80092 Add: Thyroid panel w/ TSH

80099 Delete

80100 Add: Drug testing

80101 Add: Drug testing

80102 Add: Drug testing

80103 Add: Drug analysis, tissue prep

80150 Add: Assay, amikacin

80152 Add: Assay, amitryptyline

80154 Add: Assay, benzodiazepines

80156 Add: Assay, carbamazepine

80158 Add: Assay, cyclosporine

80160	Add:	Assay, desipramine
80162	Add:	Assay, digoxin
80164	Add:	Assay, dipropylacetic acid
80166	Add:	Assay, doxepin
80168	Add:	Assay, ethosuximide
80170	Add:	Assay, gentamicin
80172	Add:	Assay, gold
80174	Add:	Assay, imipramine
80176	Add:	Assay, lidocaine
80178	Add:	Assay, lithium
80182	Add:	Assay, nortryptyline
80184	Add:	Assay, phenobarbital
80185	Add:	Assay, phenytoin, total
80186	Add:	Assay, phenytoin, free
80188	Add:	Assay, primidone
80190	Add:	Assay, procainamide
80192	Add:	Assay, procainamide metabol
80194	Add:	Assay, quinidine
80196	Add:	Assay, salicylate
80198	Add:	Assay, theophylline
80200	Add:	Assay, tobramycin
80202	Add:	Assay, vancomycin
80299	Add:	Quantitative assay, drug
81002	Revise:	Urinalysis nonauto w/o scope
81003	Add:	Urinalysis, auto, w/o scope
81025	Add:	Urine pregnancy test
81050	Add:	Urinalysis, volume measure
82003	Revise:	Assay, acetaminophen
82005	Delete	
82009	Revise:	Test for acetone/ ketones
82011	Delete	
82012	Delete	
82015	Delete	
82024	Revise:	Assay, ACTH
82035	Delete	
82043	Add:	Microalbumin, quantitative
82044	Add:	Microalbumin, semiquant
82055	Revise:	Assay, ethanol
82060	Delete	
82065	Delete	
82070	Delete	

82072 Delete

82076 Delete

82078 Delete

82085 Revise: Assay, aldolase

82086 Delete

82087 Delete

82088 Revise: Assay, aldosterone

82089 Delete

82095 Delete

82096 Delete

82100 Delete

82103 Add: Alpha-1-antitrypsin, total

82104 Add: Alpha-1-antitrypsin, pheno

82105 Add: Alpha-fetoprotein, serum

82106 Add: Alpha-fetoprotein; amniotic

82108 Revise: Assay, aluminum

82112 Delete

82126 Delete

82131 Add: Amino acids analysis

82134 Delete

82137 Delete

82138 Delete

82140 Revise: Assay, ammonia

82141 Delete

82142 Delete

82150 Revise: Assay, amylase

82156 Delete

82157 Revise: Assay, androstenedione

82159 Delete

82160 Revise: Assay, androsterone

82163 Revise: Assay, angiotensin II

82164 Revise: Angiotensin I enzyme test

82165 Delete

82168 Delete

82170 Delete

82172 Revise: Assay, apolipoprotein

82190 Add: Atomic absorption test

82210 Delete

82225 Delete

82230 Delete

82231 Delete

82232 Revise: Assay, Beta-2 protein

82235 Delete

82236 Delete

82239 Add: Assay, bile acids, total

82240 Revise: Bile acids, choleglycine

82245 Delete

82250 Revise: Assay, bilirubin

82251 Revise: Assay, bilirubin

82260 Delete

82265 Delete

82268 Delete

82273 Revise: Test for blood, other source

82280 Delete

82285 Delete

82290 Delete

82291 Delete

82300 Revise: Assay, cadmium

82305 Delete

82307 Revise: Assay, vitamin D

82308 Revise: Assay, calcitonin

82310 Revise: Assay, calcium

82315 Delete

82320 Delete

82325 Delete

82330 Revise: Assay, calcium

82335 Delete

82372 Delete

82378 Add: Carcinoembryonic antigen

82380 Revise: Assay, carotene

82387 Add: Assay, cathepsin-D

82390 Revise: Assay, ceruloplasmin

82397 Add: Chemiluminescent assay

82400 Delete

82405 Delete

82415 Revise: Assay, chloramphenicol

82418 Delete

82420 Delete

82425 Delete

82435 Revise: Assay, blood chlorides

82436 Revise: Assay, urine chlorides

82437 Delete

82443 Delete

82470 Delete

82484 Delete

82491 Add: Gas/liquid chromotography

82495 Revise: Assay, chromium

82512 Delete

82525 Revise: Assay, copper

82526 Delete

82528 Revise: Assay, corticosterone

82529 Delete

82530 Add: Assay, free cortisol

82531 Delete

82532 Delete

82533 Revise: Assay, total cortisol

82534 Delete

82540 Revise: Assay, creatine

82545 Delete

82546 Delete

82550 Revise: Assay, CK (CPK)

82553 Add: Creatine, MB fraction

82554 Add: Creatine, isoforms

82555 Delete

82565 Revise: Assay, creatinine

82585 Revise: Assay, cryofibrinogen

82595 Revise: Assay, cryoglobulin

82600 Revise: Assay, cyanide

82601 Delete

82606 Delete

82607 Revise: Assay, vitamin B-12

82614 Delete

82620 Delete

82624 Delete

82626 Revise: Dehydroepiandrosterone

82627 Add: Dehydroepiandrosterone

82628 Delete

82633 Revise: Desoxycorticosterone

82634 Revise: Deoxycortisol

82635 Delete

82636 Delete

82639 Delete

82640 Delete

82641 Delete

82643 Delete

82656 Delete

82660 Delete

82668 Revise: Assay, erythropoietin

82670 Revise: Assay, estradiol

82673 Delete

82674 Delete

82676 Delete

82677 Revise: Assay, estriol

82678 Delete

82679 Revise: Assay, estrone

82690 Revise: Assay, ethchlorvynol

82691 Delete

82692 Delete

82693 Add: Assay, ethylene glycol

82694 Delete

82696 Revise: Assay, etiocholanolone

82705 Revise: Fats/lipids, feces, qual

82710 Revise: Fats/lipids, feces, quant

82720 Delete

82727 Delete

82730 Delete

82735 Revise: Assay, fluoride

82740 Delete

82741 Delete

82745 Delete

82746 Revise: Folic acid, serum

82747 Add: Folic acid, RBC

82750 Delete

82755 Delete

82756 Delete

82760 Revise: Assay, galactose

82763 Delete

82765 Delete

82780 Delete

82784 Revise: Assay, gammaglobulin IgM

82785 Revise: Assay, gammaglobulin IgE

82786 Delete

82787 Add: Immunoglobulin subclasses

82790 Delete

82791 Delete

82793 Delete

82795 Delete

82820 Add: Hemoglobin-oxygen affinity

82927 Delete

82929 Delete

82931 Delete

82932 Delete

82938 Revise: Gastrin test

82941 Revise: Assay, gastrin

82942 Delete

82943 Revise: Assay, glucagon

82944 Delete

82947 Revise: Assay quantitative, glucose

82948 Revise: Reagent strip/blood glucose

82949 Delete

82954 Delete

82962 Add: Glucose blood test

82965 Revise: Assay, GDH enzyme

82975 Revise: Assay, glutamine

82977 Revise: Assay, GGT

82985 Revise: Assay, glycated protein

82995 Delete

83000 Delete

83001 Revise: Assay, gonadotropin (FSH)

83002 Revise: Assay, gonadotropin (LH)

83003 Revise: Assay, growth hormone (HGH)

83008 Revise: Assay, guanosine

83010 Revise: Quant assay, haptoglobin

83011 Delete

83012 Revise: Pheno assay, haptoglobins

83015 Revise: Heavy metal screen

83018 Revise: Quantitative screen, metals

83026 Add: Hemoglobin, copper sulfate

83036 Revise: Glycated hemoglobin test

83040 Delete

83052 Delete

83053 Delete

83070 Revise: Qualt assay hemosiderin

83071 Revise: Quant assay hemosiderin

83086 Delete

83087 Delete

83093 Delete

83094 Delete

83095 Delete

83150 Revise: Assay, HVA

83485 Delete

83486 Delete

83491 Revise: Assay, corticosteroids

83492 Delete

83493 Delete

83494 Delete

83495 Delete

83496 Delete

83497 Revise: Assay, 5-HIAA

83498 Revise: Assay, progesterone

83500 Revise: Assay, free hydroxyproline

83505 Revise: Assay, total hydroxyproline

83510 Delete

83518 Add: Immunoassay, dipstick

83519 Add: Immunoassay, analyte

83520 Add: Immunoassay

83523 Delete

83524 Delete

83525 Revise: Assay, insulin

83528 Revise: Assay, intrinsic factor

83530 Delete

83540 Revise: Assay, iron

83545 Delete

83546 Delete

83550 Revise: Iron binding test

83555 Delete

83565 Delete

83570 Revise: Assay, IDH enzyme

83571 Delete

83576 Delete

83578 Delete

83582 Revise: Assay, ketogenic steroids

83583 Delete

83584 Delete

83586 Revise: Assay, 17-ketosteroids

83587 Delete

83588 Delete

83589 Delete

83590 Delete

83593 Revise: Fractionation ketosteroids

83597 Delete

83599 Delete

83600 Delete

83610 Delete

83615 Revise: LDH enzyme test

83620 Delete

83624 Delete

83625 Revise: Assay, LDH enzymes

83626 Delete

83628 Delete

83629 Delete

83631 Delete

83632 Revise: Assay, placental lactogen

83645 Delete

83650 Delete

83655 Revise: Assay, lead

83660 Delete

83661 Revise: Assay, L/S ratio

83662 Add: L/S ratio, foam stability

83670 Revise: Assay, LAP enzyme

83675 Delete

83680 Delete

83685 Delete

83690 Revise: Assay, lipase

83700 Delete

83705 Delete

83720 Delete

83721 Add: Assay, blood lipoprotein

83725 Delete

83727 Revise: Assay, LRH hormone

83728 Delete

83730 Delete

83735 Revise: Assay, magnesium

83740 Delete

83750 Delete

83755 Delete

83760 Delete

83765 Delete

83775 Revise: Assay, MD enzyme

83795 Delete

83799 Delete

83825 Revise: Assay, mercury

83830 Delete

83835 Revise: Assay, metanephrines

83842 Delete

83845 Delete

83858 Revise: Assay, methsuximide

83859 Delete

83860 Delete

83861 Delete

83862 Delete

83864 Revise: Mucopoly-saccharides

83865 Delete

83873 Revise: Assay, CSF protein

83874 Revise: Assay, myoglobin

83875 Delete

83880 Delete

83883 Add: Nephelometry, not specified

83885 Revise: Assay, nickel

83890 Add: Molecular diagnostics

83892 Add: Molecular diagnostics

83894 Add: Molecular diagnostics

83895 Delete

83896 Add: Molecular diagnostics

83898 Add: Molecular diagnostics

83900 Delete

83910 Delete

83912 Revise: Molecular diagnostics

83913 Delete

83916 Revise: Oligoclonal bands

83917 Delete

83920 Delete

83925 Add: Assay, opiates

83938 Delete

83945 Revise: Assay, oxalate

83946 Delete

83947 Delete

83948 Delete

83949 Delete

83965 Delete

83970 Revise: Assay, parathormone

83971 Delete

83972 Delete

83973 Delete

83975 Delete

83985 Delete

83995 Delete

84005 Delete

84021 Delete

84022 Revise: Assay, phenothiazine

84031 Delete

84033 Delete

84035 Revise: Assay, phenylketones

84037 Delete

84038 Delete

84039 Delete

84040 Delete

84045 Delete

84060 Revise: Assay, acid phosphatase

84061 Add: Phosphatase, forensic exam

84065 Delete

84082 Delete

84083 Delete

84090 Delete

84100 Revise: Assay, phosphorus

84118 Delete

84121 Delete

84127 Add: Assay, feces porphyrins

84128 Delete

84132 Revise: Assay, serum potassium

84134 Add: Assay, prealbumin

84135 Revise: Assay, pregnanediol

84136 Delete

84138 Revise: Assay, pregnanetriol

84139 Delete

84141 Delete

84142 Delete

84146 Revise: Assay, prolactin

84147 Delete

84149 Delete

84150 Revise: Assay, prostaglandin

84153 Add: Assay, PSA

84155 Revise: Assay, total protein

84170 Delete

84176 Delete

84180 Delete

84181 Add: Western blot test

84182 Add: Western blot test

84185 Delete

84190 Delete

84195 Delete

84200 Delete

84205 Delete

84206 Revise: Assay, proinsulin

84208 Delete

84210 Revise: Assay, pyruvate

84220 Revise: Assay, pyruvate kinase

84230 Delete

84231 Delete

84232 Delete

84236 Delete

84244 Revise: Assay, renin

84260 Revise: Assay, serotonin

84270 Add: Sex hormone globulin (SHBG)

84275 Revise: Assay, sialic acid

84295 Revise: Assay, serum sodium

84305 Add: Assay, somatomedin

84307 Add: Assay, somatostatin

84310 Delete

84311 Add: Spectrophotometry

84318 Delete

84324 Delete

84395 Delete

84402 Add: Assay, free testosterone

84403 Revise: Assay, total testosterone

84405 Delete

84406 Delete

84407 Delete

84408 Delete

84409 Delete

84410 Delete

84420 Delete

84430 Revise: Assay, thiocyanate

84432 Add: Assay, thyroglobulin

84434 Delete

84435 Delete

84436 Revise: Assay, total thyroxine

84439 Revise: Assay, free thyroxine

84444 Revise: Thyrotropin factor

84445 Revise: Thyroid immunoglobulins TSI

84447 Delete

84448 Delete

84455 Delete

84465 Delete

84466 Add: Assay, transferrin

84472 Delete

84474 Delete

84476 Delete

84478 Revise: Assay, triglycerides

84480 Revise: Total assay, TT-3

84481 Revise: Free assay (FT-3)

84482 Add: T3 reverse assay

84483 Delete

84510 Revise: Assay, tyrosine

84520 Revise: Assay, urea nitrogen

84525 Revise: Reagent strip BUN

84565 Delete

84570 Delete

84575 Delete

84584 Delete

84588 Revise: Assay, vasopressin

84589 Revise: Assay, viscosity

84590 Revise: Assay, vitamin-A

84595 Delete

84605 Delete

84610 Delete

84613 Delete

84615 Delete

84630 Revise: Assay, zinc

84635 Delete

84695 Delete

84800 Delete

84810 Delete

84830 Add: Ovulation tests

85000 Delete

85005 Delete

85008 Add: Nondifferential WBC count

85012 Delete

85013 Add: Spun, microhematocrit

85018 Revise: Hemoglobin

85100 Delete

85101 Delete

85103 Delete

85105 Delete

85109 Delete

85130 Add: Chromogenic substrate assay

85170 Revise: Blood clot retraction

85171 Delete

85172 Delete

85242 Delete

85245 Add: Blood clot factor VIII test

85246 Add: Blood clot factor VIII test

85247 Add: Blood clot factor VIII test

85302 Revise: Blood clot inhibitor antigen

85303 Add: Blood clot inhibitor test

Code	Action	Description
85306	Add:	Blood clot inhibitor test
85310	Delete	
85311	Delete	
85320	Delete	
85330	Delete	
85335	Add:	Factor inhibitor test
85337	Add:	Thrombomodulin
85340	Delete	
85341	Delete	
85363	Delete	
85364	Delete	
85365	Delete	
85366	Add:	Fibrinogen test
85367	Delete	
85368	Delete	
85369	Delete	
85370	Add:	Fibrinogen test
85371	Delete	
85372	Delete	
85376	Delete	
85377	Delete	
85378	Add:	Fibrin degradation
85379	Add:	Fibrin degradation
85384	Add:	Fibrinogen
85385	Add:	Fibrinogen
85392	Delete	
85395	Delete	
85398	Delete	
85415	Add:	Fibrinolytic plasminogen
85426	Delete	
85475	Add:	Hemolysin, acid
85525	Add:	Neutralize heparin
85538	Delete	
85544	Delete	
85548	Delete	
85549	Revise:	Muramidase
85556	Delete	
85560	Delete	
85576	Delete	
85577	Delete	
85580	Delete	
85590	Revise:	Platelet count, manual
85595	Revise:	Platelet count, automated
85597	Add:	Platelet neutralization
85611	Add:	Prothrombin test
85613	Add:	Russell viper venom, diluted
85615	Delete	
85618	Delete	
85630	Delete	
85632	Delete	
85650	Delete	

85665 Delete

85667 Delete

85700 Delete

85705 Add: Thromboplastin inhibition

85710 Delete

85711 Delete

86002 Delete

86004 Delete

86006 Delete

86007 Delete

86008 Delete

86009 Delete

86011 Delete

86012 Delete

86013 Delete

86014 Delete

86016 Delete

86019 Delete

86024 Delete

86031 Delete

86032 Delete

86033 Delete

86034 Delete

86038 Revise: Antinuclear antibodies (ANA)

86039 Add: Antinuclear antibodies titer

86064 Delete

86066 Delete

86067 Delete

86068 Delete

86070 Delete

86080 Delete

86082 Delete

86083 Delete

86084 Delete

86085 Delete

86095 Delete

86100 Delete

86105 Delete

86115 Delete

86128 Delete

86130 Delete

86147 Add: Cardiolipin antibody

86149 Delete

86151 Delete

86156 Add: Cold agglutinin screen

86157 Add: Cold agglutinin, titer

86158 Delete

86159 Delete

86160 Add: Complement, antigen

86161 Add: Complement/ function activity

86163 Delete

86164 Delete

86185 Revise: Counterimmuno-electrophoresis

86226 Add: DNA antibody

86243 Revise: FC receptor

86244 Delete

86265 Delete

86266 Delete

86267 Delete

86277 Revise: Growth hormone antibody/HGH

86281 Delete

86282 Delete

86283 Delete

86287 Revise: Hepatitis B (HBsAG)

86288 Delete

86298 Delete

86300 Delete

86302 Add: Hepatitis C antibody

86305 Delete

86306 Add: Hepatitis, delta agent

86308 Add: Heterophile antibodies screen

86309 Add: Heterophile antibodies titer

86312 Delete

86314 Delete

86318 Revise: Immunoassay, infectious agent

86319 Delete

86329 Revise: Immunodiffusion

86332 Revise: Immune complex assay

86333 Delete

86335 Delete

86337 Revise: Insulin antibodies

86338 Delete

86342 Delete

86349 Delete

86357 Delete

86358 Delete

86376 Revise: Microsomal antibody

86377 Delete

86385 Delete

86386 Delete

86403 Revise: Particle agglutination test

86404 Delete

86405 Delete

86410 Delete

86411 Delete

86412 Delete

86417 Delete

86418 Delete

86419 Delete

86420 Delete

86423 Delete

86431 Add: Rheumatoid factor, quant

86455 Delete

86485 Add: Skin test, candida

86540 Delete

86586 Add: Skin test, unlisted

86587 Delete

86588 Add: Streptococcus, direct screen

86594 Delete

86595 Delete

86600 Delete

86602 Add: Antibody, actinomyces

86603 Add: Antibody, adenovirus

86606 Add: Antibody, Aspirgillus

86609 Add: Antibody, bacterium

86612 Add: Antibody, Blastomyces

86615 Add: Antibody, Bordetella

86618 Add: Antibody, Lyme disease

86619 Add: Antibody, Borrelia

86622 Add: Antibody, Brucella

86625 Add: Antibody, Campylobacter

86628 Add: Antibody, Candida

86630 Delete

86631 Add: Antibody, Chlamydia

86632 Add: Antibody, Chlamydia, IgM

86635 Add: Antibody, Coccidioides

86638 Add: Antibody, Q Fever

86641 Add: Antibody, Cryptococcus

86644 Add: Antibody, CMV

86645 Add: Antibody, CMV, IgM

86648 Add: Antibody, Diptheria

86650 Delete

86651 Add: Antibody, encephalitis

86652 Add: Antibody, encephalitis

86653 Add: Antibody, encephalitis

86654 Add: Antibody, encephalitis

86658 Add: Antibody, enterovirus

86662 Delete

86663 Add: Antibody, Epstein-Barr

86664 Add: Antibody, Epstein-Barr

86665 Add: Antibody, Epstein-Barr

86668 Add: Francisella Tularensis

86671 Add: Antibody, fungus

86674 Add: Antibody, Giardia Lamblia

86677 Add: Antibody, Helicobacter Pylori

86681 Delete

86682 Add: Antibody, helminth

86684 Add: Antibody, Hemophilus influenza

86685 Delete

86687 Revise: Antibody, HTLV I

86688 Add: Antibody, HTLV-II

86689 Revise: HTLV/HIV confirmatory test

86692 Add: Hepatitis, delta agent

86694 Add: Antibody, herpes simplex

86695 Add: Antibody, herpes simplex

86698 Add: Antibody, histoplasma

86701 Add: Antibody, HIV-1

86702 Add: Antibody, HIV-2

86703 Add: HIV-1/HIV-2, single assay

86710 Add: Antibody, influenza virus

86713 Add: Antibody, Legionella

86717 Add: Antibody, Leishmania

86720 Add: Antibody, Leptospira

86723 Add: Listeria Monocytogenes

86727 Add: Lymphocytic choriomeningitis

86729 Add: Lymphogranaloma Venereum

86732 Add: Antibody, mucormycosis

86735 Add: Antibody, mumps

86738 Add: Antibody, Mycoplasma

86741 Add: Neisseria Meningitidis

86744 Add: Antibody, Nocardia

86747 Add: Antibody, parvovirus

86750 Add: Antibody, malaria

86753 Add: Antibody, protozoa

86756 Add: Antibody, respiratory virus

86759 Add: Antibody, rotavirus

86762 Add: Antibody, rubella

86765 Add: Antibody, rubeola

86768 Add: Antibody, Salmonella

86771 Add: Antibody, Shigella

86774 Add: Antibody, tetanus

86777 Add: Antibody, Toxoplasma

86778 Add: Antibody, Toxoplasma, IgM

86781 Add: Confirm Treponema Pallidum

86784 Add: Antibody, trichinella

86787 Add: Antibody, varicella-zoster

86790 Add: Antibody, virus

86793 Add: Antibody, Yersinia

86800 Revise: Antibody, thyroglobulin

86813 Revise: HLA typing, A, B, or C

86816 Revise: HLA typing, DR/DQ

86817 Revise: HLA typing, DR/DQ

86849 Add: Immunology procedure

86850 Add: RBC antibody screen

86860 Add: RBC antibody elution

86870 Add: RBC antibody identification

86880 Add: Coombs test

86886 Add: Coombs test

86890 Add: Autologous blood process

86891 Add: Autologous blood, op salvage

86900 Add: Blood typing, ABO only

86901 Add: Blood typing, Rh (D)

86903 Add: Blood typing, antigen screen

86904 Add: Blood typing, antigen screen

86905 Add: Blood typing, RBC antigens

86906 Add: Blood typing, Rh phenotype

86910 Add: Blood typing, paternity test

86915 Add: Bone marrow

86920 Add: Compatibility test

86921 Add: Compatibility test

86922 Add: Compatibility test

86927 Add: Plasma, fresh frozen

86930 Add: Blood unit service

86931 Add: Blood unit service

86932 Add: Blood unit service

86940 Add: Hemolysins and agglutinins

86941 Add: Hemolysins and agglutinins

86945 Add: Blood product/ irradiation

Code	Action	Description
86950	Add:	Leukocyte transfusion
86965	Add:	Pooling of blood products
86970	Add:	Pretreatment RBC, drugs
86971	Add:	Pretreatment RBC, dilution
86972	Add:	Pretreatment RBC, separation
86975	Add:	Pretreatment serum, drugs
86976	Add:	RBC pretreatment, serum
86977	Add:	RBC pretreatment, serum
86978	Add:	RBC pretreatment, serum
86985	Add:	Split blood or products
86999	Revise:	Transfusion procedure
88156	Add:	TBS smear (Bethesda System)
88157	Add:	TBS smear (Bethesda System)
88371	Add:	Protein analysis/ Western
88372	Add:	Protein analysis w/probe
90918	Add:	Hemodialysis services
90919	Add:	Hemodialysis services
90920	Add:	Hemodialysis services
90921	Add:	Hemodialysis services
90922	Add:	Hemodialysis services
90995	Delete	
90998	Delete	
92995	Add:	Coronary atherectomy
92996	Add:	Coronary atherectomy
93313	Add:	Echo exam of heart
93314	Add:	Echo exam of heart
93980	Add:	Penile vascular study
93981	Add:	Penile vascular study
94700	Delete	
94705	Delete	
94710	Delete	
94715	Delete	
95000	Delete	
95001	Delete	
95002	Delete	
95003	Delete	
95004	Add:	Allergy skin tests
95005	Delete	
95006	Delete	

95007 Delete

95010 Add: Sensitivity skin tests

95011 Delete

95014 Delete

95015 Add: Sensitivity skin tests

95016 Delete

95017 Delete

95018 Delete

95020 Delete

95021 Delete

95022 Delete

95023 Delete

95024 Add: Allergy skin tests

95028 Add: Allergy skin tests

95030 Delete

95031 Delete

95032 Delete

95033 Delete

95034 Delete

95883 Add: Neuropsychological testing

95952 Delete

95953 Add: EEG monitoring/ computer

95956 Add: EEG monitoring/ cable/radio

96542 Add: Chemotherapy injection

97545 Add: Work hardening

97546 Add: Work hardening

99218 Add: Observation care

99219 Add: Observation care

99220 Add: Observation care

99295 Add: Neonatal critical care

99296 Add: Neonatal critical care

99297 Add: Neonatal critical care

99438 Delete

Instructions for the use of the CPT Index

MAIN TERMS

The index is organized by main terms. Each main term can stand alone, or be followed by up to 3 modifying terms. There are 4 primary classes of main entries:

1) Procedure or service. For example:
   Endoscopy; Anastomosis; Splint

2) Organ or other anatomic site. For example:
   Tibia; Colon; Salivary Gland

3) Condition. For example:
   Abscess; Entropion; Tetralogy of Fallot

4) Synonyms, Eponyms and Abbreviations. For example:
   EEG; Bricker Operation; Clagett Procedure

MODIFYING TERMS

A main term may be followed by a series of up to 3 indented terms that modify the main term. When modifying terms appear, one should review the list, as these subterms do have an effect on the selection of the appropriate code for the procedure.

CODE RANGES

Whenever more than one code applies to a given index entry, a code range is listed. If two sequential codes or several non-sequential codes apply, they will be separated by a comma. For example:

Debridement
   Mastoid Cavity 69220, 69222

If more than two sequential codes apply, they will be separated by a hyphen. For example:

Antibody
   Antitrypsin, Alpha-1 86064-86067

CROSS REFERENCES

Cross references provide instructions to the user. There are 2 types of cross references.

1) "SEE"—This directs the user to refer to the term listed after the word "SEE." This type of reference is used primarily for synonyms, eponyms and abbreviations.

2) "SEE ALSO"—This directs the user to look under another main term if the procedure is not listed under the first main index entry.

OTHER CONVENTIONS

As a space saving convention, certain words infer some meaning. This convention is primarily used when a procedure or service is listed as a subterm. For example:

Knee
   Incision (of)

In this example, the word in parentheses (of) does not appear in the index, but it is inferred. As another example:

Pancreas
   Anesthesia (for procedures on)

In this example, as there is no such entity as pancreas anesthesia, the words in parentheses are inferred. That is, anesthesia for procedures on the pancreas.

The alphabetic index is NOT a substitute for the main text of CPT. Even if only one code appears, the user must refer to the main text to ensure that the code selection is accurate.

A

B

E

F

G

H

L

M

N

O

Q

S

T

U

V

W

X

Y

Z

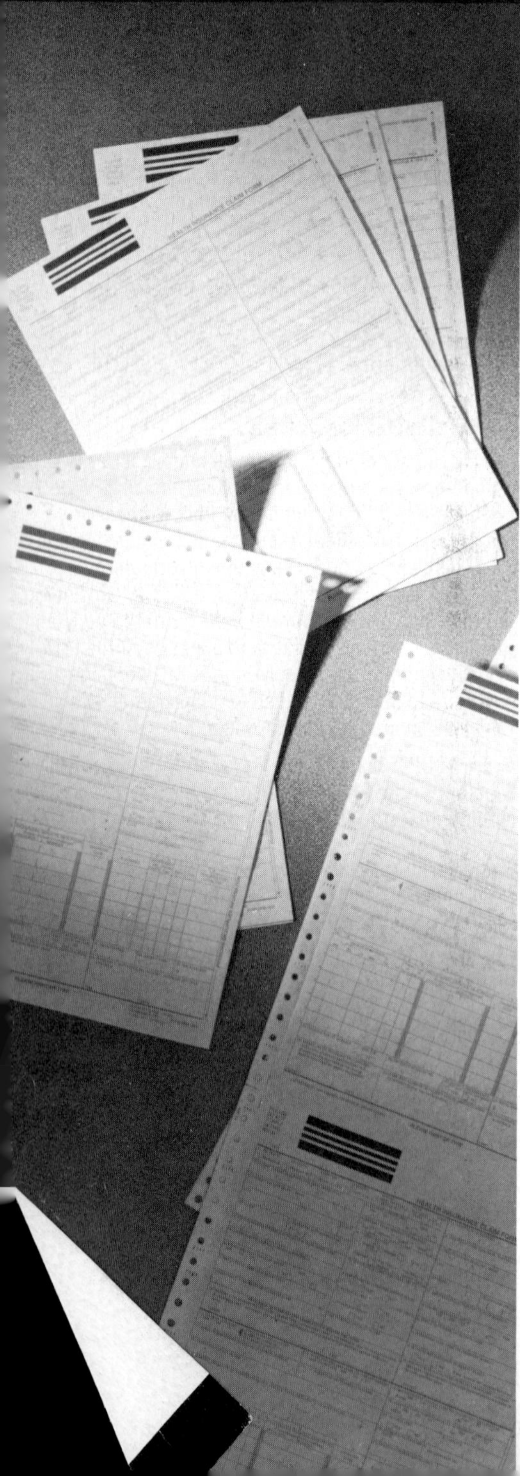